Sexual and Reproductive Health

Joseph Truglio • Rita S. Lee
Barbara E. Warren • Rainier Patrick Soriano
Editors

Sexual and Reproductive Health

A Practical Guide for Primary Care

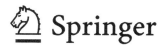 Springer

Editors
Joseph Truglio
Departments of Internal Medicine, Pediatrics
and Medical Education
Icahn School of Medicine Mount Sinai
New York, NY, USA

Barbara E. Warren
Department of Medical Education
Icahn School of Medicine Mount Sinai
New York, NY, USA

Rita S. Lee
Department of Medicine
University of Colorado School of Medicine
Aurora, CO, USA

Rainier Patrick Soriano
Brookdale Department of Geriatrics
and Palliative Medicine and Department
of Medical Education
Icahn School of Medicine at Mount Sinai
New York, NY, USA

ISBN 978-3-030-94631-9   ISBN 978-3-030-94632-6   (eBook)
https://doi.org/10.1007/978-3-030-94632-6

This Springer imprint is published by the registered company Springer Nature Switzerland AG
The registered company address is: Gewerbestrasse 11, 6330 Cham, Switzerland

Preface

Sexual and reproductive health (SRH) is a critical aspect of the overall health and wellness of patients. Primary care clinicians are in a unique position to partner with patients to improve SRH. This book is designed to serve as a point-of-care resource for primary care clinicians at all levels of training and practice. It aims to present an approach to SRH that is inclusive of all ages, genders, sexual orientations, and physical abilities. At all times, our editors and authors strive to use inclusive, patient-centered language, even when available data and current guidelines may operate within gender-binary frameworks, exclude certain groups, or conflate sexual practices with sexual orientation and gender identity. We hope that the frameworks we present will help you apply the best available evidence and guidelines in an equitable, just, and patient-centered way to each and every patient you see.

This book is divided into three parts. Part I presents an approach to SRH across the lifespan, including pediatrics, adolescents and young adults, adults, and older adults. Part II presents more in-depth content on specific domains of SRH, and specific populations that may require additional knowledge. While Parts I and II are inclusive of all genders, we recognize that many resources, studies, and guidelines exclude transgender and gender non-binary (TGNB) patients, and many social and political structures marginalize individuals who do not identify within cis-gender male-female binary identities. For these reasons, Part III of this book is dedicated to SRH for TGNB patients, including physical health, mental health, and legal considerations regarding SRH.

As with all aspects of medicine, evidence and best practices evolve over time. While the screening, diagnostic, and treatment recommendations described in this book are current and up to date at the time of publication, we recommend clinicians directly reference the primary literature professional guidelines when making clinical decisions.

Resources for further reading and updated guidelines include:

- The Centers for Disease Control and Prevention: Centers for Disease Control and Prevention (cdc.gov)

- The United States Preventive Services Task Force: Home page|United States Preventive Services Taskforce (uspreventiveservicestaskforce.org)
- The Fenway Institute: 05 – The Fenway Institute|Fenway Health: Health Care Is A Right, Not A Privilege.
- The World Professional Association for Transgender Health: WPATH World Professional Association for Transgender Health
- Thank you for your interest in this book, and your dedication to the care of your patients.

New York, NY, USA   Joseph Truglio, MD
Aurora, CO, USA   Rita S. Lee, MD
New York, NY, USA   Barbara E. Warren, PsyD
New York, NY, USA   Rainier Patrick Soriano, MD

Contents

Contributors

Joan Bosco Icahn School of Medicine at Mount Sinai, New York, NY, USA

Division of General Internal Medicine, Department of Medicine at Mount Sinai Beth Israel, New York, NY, USA

Jose Cortes Icahn School of Medicine at Mount Sinai, New York, NY, USA

David E. DeLaet Departments of Internal Medicine and Pediatrics, Icahn School of Medicine at Mount Sinai, New York, NY, USA

Alexandra Dembar Gustave L Levy, Mount Sinai School of Medicine, New York, NY, USA

A. C. Demidont Principal Medical Scientist, HIV Prevention Medical Affairs, New England, (CT, RI, MA, VT, NH, ME, Upstate NY), USA

Anne Franklin University of Colorado, Children's Hospital Colorado, Center for Cancer and Blood Disorders, Aurora, CO, USA

Robyn Gisbert Physical Therapy Program, Department of Physical Medicine and Rehabilitation, University of Colorado Anschutz Medical Campus, Aurora, CO, USA

Zil Goldstein Associate Medical Director, Callen-Lorde Community Health Center, New York City, NY, USA

Aaron Grotas Department of Urology, Mount Sinai, New York, NY, USA

Jo Hirschmann Center for Spirituality and Health, Icahn School of Medicine at Mount Sinai, New York, NY, USA

Mollie Jacobs Department of Family Medicine, University of Colorado, Aurora, CO, USA

Noelle Marie Javier Brookdale Department of Geriatrics and Palliative Medicine, Mount Sinai Hospital, New York, NY, USA

Scott K. Jelinek Department of Pediatrics, Icahn School of Medicine at Mount Sinai, New York, NY, USA

Dana Judd Physical Therapy Program, Department of Physical Medicine and Rehabilitation, University of Colorado Anschutz Medical Campus, Aurora, CO, USA

Marissa Kent Department of Urology, Mount Sinai, New York, NY, USA

John Koeppe Department of General Internal Medicine, University of Colorado at Denver and Health Sciences Center, Denver, CO, USA

Jennifer M. LeComte RISN/GIM, Rowan University School of Osteopathic Medicine, Sewell, NJ, USA

Barry Love Department of Pediatrics and Medicine, Icahn School of Medicine at Mount Sinai, New York, NY, USA

Srilakshmi Mitta Department of Obstetric Medicine, Brown University Medical School, Women & Infants' Hospital, Providence, RI, USA

Linda Overholser University of Colorado Denver Anschutz Medical Campus, Division of General Internal Medicine, Aurora, CO, USA

Mariecel Pilapil Department of Pediatrics, Department of Medicine, Zucker School of Medicine at Hofstra/Northwell, New Hyde Park, NY, USA

Asa Radix Callen-Lorde Community Health Center, New York, NY, USA

Zoe I. Rodriguez Department of Obstetrics, Gynecology and Reproductive Science, Icahn School of Medicine at Mount Sinai, New York, NY, USA

Jelinek Scott Pediatric Resident Physician, Department of Pediatrics, Icahn School of Medicine at Mount Sinai, New York, NY, USA

Sangyoon Jason Shin Icahn School of Medicine at Mount Sinai, New York, NY, USA

Mount Sinai Downtown – Union Square, New York, NY, USA

Rainier Patrick Soriano Brookdale Department of Geriatrics and Palliative Medicine and Department of Medical Education, Icahn School of Medicine at Mount Sinai, New York, NY, USA

Brookdale Department of Geriatrics and Palliative Medicine, The Mount Sinai Hospital, New York, NY, USA

Alexis Tchaconas Internal Medicine/Pediatrics, The Mount Sinai Hospital, New York, NY, USA

Joseph Truglio Departments of Internal Medicine, Pediatrics and Medical Education, Icahn School of Medicine Mount Sinai, New York, NY, USA

Jill Weiss Law Office of Jillian T. Weiss, Brooklyn, NY, USA

Linda Wesp Clinical Assistant Professor University of Wisconsin Milwaukee – College of Nursing, Milwaukee, WI, USA

Kevin Yan Icahn School of Medicine at Mount Sinai, New York, NY, USA

Division of General Internal Medicine, Department of Medicine at Mount Sinai West and Mount Sinai Morningside), New York, NY, USA

Eric Yarbrough Department of Psychiatry, NYU School of Medicine, New York, NY, USA

Part I
Sexual and Reproductive Health
Using a Lifespan Approach

Chapter 1
Sexual and Reproductive Health in the Pediatric Population

Mariecel Pilapil

Contents

Clinicians that care for the pediatric population are key players in the sexual and reproductive health of children. Healthy sexual development is a multifaceted process that involves the interplay of physical and anatomical changes, emotional development, and cultural beliefs. Although clinicians often think about sexuality and sexual development during adolescence, it is essential that healthcare professionals address sexual development and gender identity in a culturally effective and developmentally appropriate manner with children and their caregivers. In addition, pediatric clinicians have the opportunity to provide longitudinal sexual education in the larger context of preventative care [1]. In this chapter, we will discuss a general

M. Pilapil (✉)
Department of Pediatrics, Department of Medicine, Zucker School of Medicine at Hofstra/
Northwell, New Hyde Park, NY, USA
e-mail: mpilapil@northwell.edu

© Springer Nature Switzerland AG 2022
J. Truglio et al. (eds.), *Sexual and Reproductive Health*,
https://doi.org/10.1007/978-3-030-94632-6_1

approach to sexual and reproductive health in the pediatric population from birth to 11 years old as a guide for primary care clinicians.

Promoting Healthy Sexual Development and Sexuality in the Pediatric Population

The American Academy of Pediatrics (AAP) has published guidelines for the promotion of healthy sexual development and sexuality spanning birth to adolescence in *Bright Futures: Guidelines for Health Supervision of Infants, Children, and Adolescents* (4th Edition). Although these guidelines exist, it is also important for clinicians to individualize their approach according to the cultural attitudes of the families they care for.

Infancy (Birth to 11 Months)

The development of healthy intimacy begins as early as infancy and can affect the child's sexual development later on in life. The foundation of intimacy begins with the close physical and emotional relationship between the parent and child. The child needs to feel valued, loved, and important [2]. This healthy intimacy is dependent on the caregiver to establish a feeling of trust in the parent-child relationship. This can occur by meeting the infant's basic needs and through comforting, nonthreatening physical contact [3].

Knowledge of typical childhood sexual development is essential to enable clinicians to guide caregivers appropriately regarding sexual behaviors they may observe in children. During infancy, parents may notice sexual behaviors such as hand-to-genital contact. This is often distressing to parents and may cause concern regarding whether these are normative behaviors. The AAP recommends that clinicians address these behaviors as a normal aspect of the infant's awareness of his/her own body. As children progress through the stages of sexual development, they can engage in behaviors that may be sexual, and not necessarily abnormal. In fact, sexual behaviors have occurred in up to 73 percent of children by the time they are 13 years old [4]. Reassuring caregivers about normative behaviors and monitoring for concerning behaviors is dependent on the pediatric clinician (see Table 1.1). Clinicians should incorporate anticipatory guidance on sexual development into routine preventive care in much the same way as motor, verbal, and social development. Caregivers may be hesitant to discuss their concerns about their child's sexual development, so it is dependent on the clinician to destigmatize and normalize such conversations as part of routine health education.

Table 1.1 Common sexual behaviors in childhood

Age	Behavior
Preschool children (less than 4 years)	Exploring and touching genitalia Showing genitalia to others Trying to touch mother's or other women's breasts (crossing boundaries) Interested in being naked or seeing others naked (exhibitionism) Talking about bodily functions ("pee" or "poop")
Young children (4–6 years old)	Touching genitalia (masturbation) Attempting to see others naked Mimicking behavior of physical intimacy (kissing, holding hands) Talking about genitalia and using "naughty" words, often without understanding their meaning Interest in seeing genitalia of other children their own age
School-aged children (7–12 years old)	Touching genitalia (masturbation) Playing games with other children that involve sexual behavior ("truth or dare", "boyfriend/girlfriend", etc.) Looking at pictures of naked or partially naked people Viewing sexual content in media Desire for privacy Beginning sexual attraction to peers

Adapted from Sexual Development and Behavior in Children; The National Child Traumatic Stress Network

During infancy and throughout childhood, clinicians should counsel parents on how to effectively communicate with their children on issues related to sexual development. For example, parents should be encouraged to engage in proper naming of the genitalia (e.g., penis and vulva), which may promote discussion about sexuality between parents and children as they get older [2]. The foundation of healthy parent-child communication and intimacy begins during infancy.

Early Childhood (1 Through 4 Years)

During early childhood, sexual exploration is a normal, healthy part of development. At this age, children start to show interest in their own and others' genitalia [2]. Children at this age will often make references to elimination of urine or stool as well as regarding genitalia without inhibition or conformation with social etiquette [2].

Furthermore, children begin to become aware of gender and sex-based differences. They begin to learn that boys and girls are physically different and that they may have different gender roles and expression (i.e., hair styles, fashion, etc.). It is common for children to be interested in and identify with the clothing or roles of the other gender [2]. Caregivers may ask their pediatric clinicians about these behaviors, but they should be reassured that this form of sexual exploration is a normal part of development. While exploration of different forms of gender expression is expected during childhood, it is important to note that in studies of transgender and gender nonbinary adolescents and adults, evidence of discordance between biologic sex and gender identity and/or expression may begin at this age [5]. Some children may also display gender dysphoria – emotional distress due to a difference between gender identity and outward manifestation of gender. The persistence of gender dysphoria into adolescence and adulthood is variable and may depend on the intensity of gender dysphoria [6]. Thus, the overall trajectory of gender dysphoria at this age is difficult to predict, but pediatric clinicians can offer support and information regarding the stages of sexual development. Parental acceptance of their child regardless of how the child may identify or express their gender is crucial to the child's mental health and adjustment.

Sexual play and masturbation are normal and common at this age, though they may be concerning to parents. Clinicians should take the opportunity during regular preventative visits to provide anticipatory guidance about these behaviors. Masturbation may take several forms in children of this age including posturing, tightening of thighs, and handling of genitals [2]. These behaviors often occur as a soothing mechanism and may occur more commonly when the child is tired, for example.

Lastly, as children become increasingly verbal at this age, it is also important for clinicians to encourage parent-child communication about sexuality. Discussions at this age may include similarities and differences between boys' and girls' bodies and appropriate and inappropriate touching [7].

Middle Childhood (5 Through 11 Years)

During middle childhood, children begin to have more varied exposures to elements of sexuality including their parents, peers, and media. It is important for clinicians to address these various influences and provide accurate information regarding sexual and reproductive health.

The nature of parent-child communication about sexuality evolves during middle childhood, and caregivers should be encouraged to provide accurate sexual information and promote an open dialogue with children regarding sexuality. Parents and children may feel more embarrassed at this age to discuss these matters, but children should be given the opportunity to ask questions. At this age, peers become an increasing source of information, including those related to sexual and reproductive health, and parents and clinicians must be available to correct inaccuracies and misperceptions [2]. The anticipated physical changes during puberty should also be discussed with both patients and their caregivers (see below for physical sexual development).

The concept of intimacy continues to evolve as children enter middle childhood. Appropriate expressions of love and intimacy such as hugging, kissing, and holding hands begin to be explored. During this period, curiosity regarding adult sexual behavior increases, and children start to become interested in sexual content in media and other sources. Traditional media such as television, movies, music, and magazines contain a great deal of sexual content. In 2005, more than two-thirds of television programs contained sexual content [8]. Most studies on the influence of sexual media on engagement in sexual behaviors focus on adolescents, but the lessons may be extrapolated to school-age prepubertal children. Three longitudinal surveys of adolescents found that youth whose media exposure contained a large amount of sexual content were more likely to begin engaging in sexual intercourse earlier compared to adolescents whose media exposure contained less or no sexual content [9]. Young children, particularly those less than 8 years old, have difficulty distinguishing what is happening on screen versus real life, and caregivers should be aware of the content of their children's media exposure [9]. Additionally, although data is limited on its long-term effects, social media is emerging as a source of sexual content and should also be monitored by caregivers.

Transitioning to Adolescence

As the child approaches adolescence, it is also important for clinicians to begin to introduce an "adolescent-style" of care. Namely, this may include speaking to the child directly to obtain a history, seeing them alone, and setting expectations for an increasing responsibility for his/her own care with some shared decision-making.

In order to foster independence, it may be helpful to begin by asking the parent or caregiver to leave the room during a portion of the visit beginning at 10 or 11 years old [10]. This is often the first step to introduce pediatric patients into their increasing role in their own health care during adolescence. It is helpful for clinicians to allow parents time both in the beginning and at the end of the visit to voice concerns. In order to reduce potential resistance from parents, the pediatric clinician should explain the purpose of seeing patients alone during a portion of the visit and focus on the child's developmental level. Some useful phrases to address this topic with parents include [11]:

- "As children grow up, it is developmentally appropriate for them to gradually separate from their parents…and begin taking responsibility for their own health. This helps prepare them for adulthood."
- "Nothing replaces a parent/guardian and I hope to serve as another adult resource for your child in reinforcing healthy habits and decisions."

Discussions regarding patient confidentiality should also be introduced at this stage. It is important to explain to children that confidentiality is not unlimited – for example, a clinician may say, "I will not tell your parents what we talk about unless you give me permission or I am concerned about your safety" [10]. The focus should be on how confidentiality improves health care.

The AAP recommends that all pediatric providers have an office policy that clearly describes confidential services [12]. *Bright Futures* recommends that clinicians introduce the topic of confidentiality during the 11- to 14-year-old age range. Consent and confidentiality laws vary from state to state, and pediatric clinicians should familiarize themselves with state-specific laws. Specifically, the AAP recommends the Guttmacher Institute (https://www.guttmacher.org/) and the Center for Adolescent Health and the Law (https://www.cahl.org/) as resources for clinicians. For both parents and children, knowing how the patient-provider relationship will evolve may ease anxieties as patients transition into adolescence.

Assessing Physical Sexual Development

As part of the routine assessment of children, physical sexual development should be assessed at routine preventative visits. This begins with the initial exam after birth and continues through full sexual maturity into adolescence. Full assessment requires routine examination of breasts in females and genitalia in both males and females. The most commonly used system for assessment of physical sexual development is that of sexual maturity ratings (SMR), also known as "Tanner stages". This assessment involves descriptions of secondary sexual characteristics including breast changes (females), testicular changes (males), and pubic hair in both males and females [13, 14]. See Figs. 1.1 and 1.2. Most children who are 11 years old or younger generally fall into Tanner stage 1 or 2 prior to adolescence. Any signs of early puberty should be further assessed.

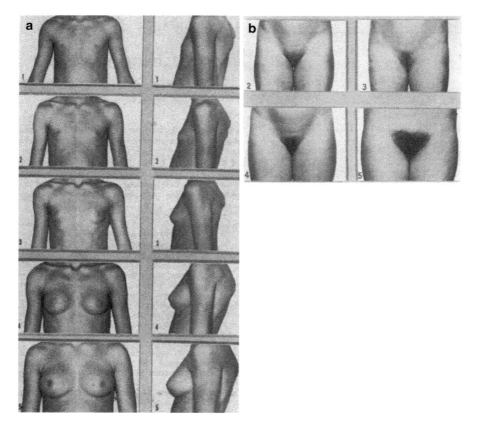

Fig. 1.1 Pubertal Changes in Girls. (**a**) Standards for breast ratings (**b**) Standards for pubic hair ratings (Reprinted with permission from Marshall and Tanner [13])

Fig. 1.2 Pubertal Changes in Boys. (Reprinted with permission from Marshall and, Tanner [13])

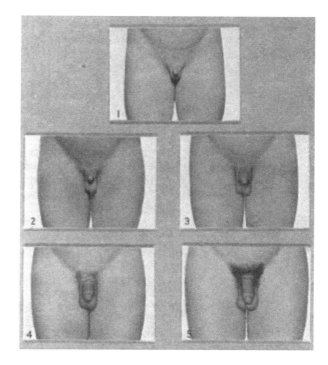

Ambiguous Genitalia

Ambiguous genitalia is a disorder of sexual development (DSD) in which the external genitalia do not have the typical appearance of either sex [15]. A 2006 consensus conference replaced the use of terms such as "pseudohermaphrodite," "hermaphrodite," and "intersex" with the broad term "disorders of sexual development (DSD)" [16]. The presence of ambiguous external genitalia is present in up to 1 in 1000 live births [15]. Although this diagnosis is rare, pediatric clinicians must be prepared to diagnose ambiguous genitalia and must be cognizant of the long-term consequences of this diagnosis.

Patients born with ambiguous genitalia should ideally be cared for by a specialized, multidisciplinary team incorporating expertise from urology, genetics, gynecology, and mental health professionals. The Accord Alliance (www.accordalliance.org) is a resource for both parents and clinicians that has published clinical guidelines on the management of disorders of sex development in childhood [15]. Upon assessment in the newborn nursery, it is important for all staff to be cognizant of the terminology they use and refer to the infant as "your baby" rather than "he," "she," or "it" [17]. A detailed history and physical examination are essential for evaluation.

Mothers should be asked about prenatal exposure to androgens, family history of androgen insensitivity or congenital adrenal hyperplasia, and consanguinity. Physical examination should include penile length, gonads, urethral opening, and clitoral size. Features which should alert the pediatric clinician to a possible DSD include bilateral undescended testes, microphallus, clitoromegaly, posterior labial fusion, and hypospadias with one other abnormal finding [16, 17].

If a DSD is suspected, initial studies should include a karyotype using fluorescence in situ hybridization (FISH), pelvic/abdominal ultrasonography, and assessment of adrenal and gonadal function. The results of these studies along with physical examination can help categorize the patient into one of three categories [16]:

1. Virilized XX
2. Undervirilized XY
3. Mixed sex chromosome pattern

Throughout the evaluation of a newborn with suspected DSD, it is of the utmost importance to provide psychological and social support to parents as well as accurate medical information regarding their child's condition. Sex of rearing decisions must be made jointly by the medical team and the family given what is known about the patient's DSD. The current approach is to assign a social sex, though some advocate delaying this decision until the child's gender identity is established [16].

Precocious Puberty

Precocious puberty is defined as the onset of pubertal changes in girls younger than 8 years and boys younger than 9 years, which are 2–2.5 standard deviations (SD) earlier than the population norm [18]. Precocious puberty has an estimated incidence of 1 in 5000 and 1 in 10,000 children, with a female predominance [19]. During routine assessment at well-child visits, signs of early puberty should be assessed through history and physical examination. Isolated pubertal changes such as premature thelarche (breast development) or premature adrenarche (pubic or axillary hair) in conjunction with prepubertal linear growth without neurologic features likely do not have true precocious puberty and can be monitored every 3–6 months for progression [18].

Precocious puberty can be categorized based on its cause as central vs. peripheral. In central precocious puberty, the hypothalamic-pituitary-gonadal (HPG) axis is activated and leads to early, but normal pubertal, development. In contrast, peripheral precocious puberty is the result of hormonal sources outside of the HPG axis such as an androgen- or estrogen-secreting tumor. Peripheral causes of precocious puberty lead to atypical sexual development that is often rapidly progressive [18].

Assessment of a child with suspected precocious puberty should include a physical exam with attention to secondary sexual characteristics including breast development (in females), scrotal and penile development (in males), and pubic and axillary hair. Growth charts should be reviewed to assess for a marked increase in linear growth [19]. Additional assessment should include bone age X-rays and pelvic ultrasound to assess uterine size and morphology. Referral to consultation with endocrinology in cases of suspected precocious puberty is essential. Based on neurologic exam findings and initial lab workup, imaging of the central nervous system (CNS) with CT or MRI to rule out CNS tumors or other lesions may be necessary [19]. Pediatric clinicians – particularly those who provide primary care – should be familiar with the workup of precocious puberty as they are often the first to detect the initial signs.

Addressing Gender and Sexuality in Prepubertal Children: Common Parental Concerns

Identifying Abnormal Sexual Behavior

Parents frequently present to their children's primary care providers with concerns regarding a sexual behavior they may have observed in their child. Although sexual behaviors are common in children, it is important for clinicians to be aware of concerning features of sexual behavior. Some red flags include behaviors that are threatening or forceful, developmentally inappropriate, and accompanied by negative emotions in children including anger or anxiety and involve children of very different ages [20]. If there is a concern that one of these red flags may be present, the first step is for caregivers (and the clinician) to elicit from the child what exactly happened. It is important that this is done in a nonthreatening way to encourage children to be open and honest. Factors such as developmental level, type/frequency of sexual behavior, parent response to behavior, situational factors (new siblings or caregivers), access to sexualized material, and abuse/neglect must be examined [21]. The Child Sexual Behavior Inventory (CSBI) is a parental report measure that may aid clinicians in further investigating sexual behaviors and is validated for children ages 2 through 12 years old [22]. This tool is completed by the mother (or other primary female caregiver), and the total score can be used as an indicator of sexual behavior. Though it was originally developed to assess children who had previously been sexually abused, more recent analysis of the CSBI has shown that sexual behaviors could also be present in non-sexually abused patients with other factors such as life stress, etc. [22]. Unfortunately the tool has thus far only been evaluated for completion by primary female caregivers.

Sexual behavior problems are those behaviors that are intrusive or developmentally inappropriate [21]. Sexual behaviors may be considered intrusive if they are affecting the child's daily life – for example, the behavior persists in school or home settings, taking away time from the child's regular activities, or if the child becomes upset when attempts are made to stop or distract from the behavior. These behaviors should be addressed and require referral for specialized care by a mental health professional. Patients with sexual behavior problems often have comorbid psychiatric diagnoses including conduct disorder, attention-deficit/hyperactivity disorder, and oppositional defiant disorder [23]. Screening tools such as the Pediatric Symptom Checklist-17 (PSC-17) may be used to assess for any comorbid mental health disorders in pediatric patients, including attention-deficit/hyperactivity disorder (ADHD), anxiety, depression, and various "externalizing" diagnoses such as conduct disorder or oppositional defiant disorder. The sensitivity of the PSC-17 ranges from 42% to 73% and the specificity 74% to 96%, depending on the mental health disorder. It should be noted with the use of such tests that while a positive screen may help guide the clinician toward a diagnosis and assist with appropriate referrals, a negative screen does not necessarily rule out any particular comorbid mental health condition. Patients with these behaviors have also sometimes been called "sexually reactive youth" to describe children and adolescents who engage in such behaviors due to prior sexual experiences including abuse, exposure to sexualized material, or witnessing sexual activity by others [21]. If suspicion for abuse is present, a referral to child protective services must be made.

It is important to note that the aforementioned "red flags" require further investigation, but they are not definitive indicators of sexual abuse. In a 1998 study, over 1000 female caregivers were asked about 38 different sexual behaviors in their children ages 2 through 12 years old who did not have a history of sexual abuse. Sexual behaviors involving exhibitionism, self-stimulation, and crossing personal boundaries were present in up to 60 percent of children, most commonly in the 2–5 year age group and declined over time. Family attitudes toward sexual behavior were an important contributor. If mothers in this study considered sexual behavior to be a normal part of development, they were more likely to report their children engaging in these behaviors [24]. In addition, children are more likely to engage in sexual behaviors if they are raised in homes where co-bathing and less privacy when dressing or going to the bathroom is common [22]. Thus, clinicians must be aware of the interplay between culture, parental attitudes, and the child's developmental stage when interpreting children's sexual behaviors.

Bullying

Bullying is a concern for both children and their caregivers, which often comes up at routine preventative visits. In particular, a child's sexual development, orientation, gender identity, and gender expression may be associated with bullying, highlighting the importance of addressing this topic within the context of sexual and reproductive health. The Centers for Disease Control and Prevention defines bullying as "any unwanted aggressive behavior(s) by another youth or group of youths who are not siblings or current dating partners that involves an observed or perceived power imbalance and is repeated multiple times or is highly likely to be repeated. Bullying may inflict harm or distress on the targeted youth including physical, psychological, or educational harm" [25]. Pediatric clinicians should ask about and address bullying for all children, but particularly for sexual and gender minority youth. In a 2014 national sample through the Youth Risk Behavior Surveillance System (YRBSS), 34.2 percent of lesbian/gay/bisexual students reported being bullied compared to only 18.8 percent of their heterosexual counterparts [26]. Bullying of sexual and gender minority youth can take various forms including verbal, physical, social/relational, and damage to property [27]. Furthermore, victimization of this population has been associated with psychological distress that lasts into adulthood [28]. According to minority stress theory, the unique stressors (i.e., bullying, etc.) that sexual and gender minority youth experience and the persistent stigma that they experience lead to physical and mental health disparities in the population, which are not the result of characteristics inherent to the individuals themselves [29]. It is therefore crucial for pediatric clinicians to be aware that the societal and social stressor placed on sexual and gender minority youth, not being an LGBTQ, is an important social determinant of health.

Clinicians should refer to evidenced-based interventions when encountered with an LGBTQ youth who has been bullied. Interventions are usually school-based and involve universal prevention programs for students, teachers, and staff as well as programs to intervene among youth who had been previously involved in LGBTQ bullying [30]. In addition, schools in which Gender and Sexuality Alliances (GSAs; also known as Gay-Straight Alliances) are present have been shown to improve the well-being of LGBTQ youth [30]. The Gay, Lesbian, and Straight Education Network is also a useful resource for pediatric clinicians for state-specific bullying policies [27]. Clinicians can refer caregivers of TGNB children to Gender Spectrum, a national resource for TGNC children and their families (https://www.genderspectrum.org/resources/parenting-and-family-2/), and to the Human Rights Campaign's national resource directory (https://www.hrc.org/resources/transgender-children-and-youth-finding-support-for-you-and-your-family.)

Special Considerations

Children Who Witness Intimate Partner Violence

Intimate partner violence (IPV) is defined as "physical, sexual, or psychological harm by a current or former partner or spouse" [31]. An estimated 10 million children in the United States witness IPV each year [32]. Given this epidemic, there are multiple consequences on the health and behavior of children. IPV-related abuse can begin even prior to birth during pregnancy. In 2000, a national survey released by the United States Department of Justice reported that 4 to 8 percent of pregnant women reported abuse at least once during their pregnancy with a higher rate among those with unintended pregnancies [33]. Abuse during pregnancy increases the risk of preterm labor, low birth weight, intracranial injury, and neonatal death [34]. Several studies have identified an increase in violent behavior among children witnesses of IPV, and this has a differential effect on boys and girls. For example, in a study of 115 children, male and female children who witness IPV were more likely than those who had not witnessed IPV to engage in violence in simulated scenarios, particularly the males [35]. Furthermore, rates of posttraumatic stress disorder (PTSD) are high among children who witness IPV (46 percent in girls and 22 percent in boys) [36]. Although most studies on this patient population are limited by small sample sizes, it is essential that pediatric clinicians are aware of the short- and long-term effects of witnessing IPV and that clinicians acknowledge and assess for such effects regardless of sex or gender of the child. Children who witness IPV also have worse educational outcomes, lower income later on in life, and higher rates of depression and engage in more risk-taking behaviors including alcohol abuse [37]. The effects of witnessing IPV are also dose-dependent, and concomitant child abuse and exposure to other forms of violence increase the negative effects on the child.

The AAP recommends that pediatric clinicians should be aware of signs of IPV and consider universal screening or case-finding screening in the office. Clinicians should also ideally have an interdisciplinary protocol in place to address IPV in the home if caregivers identify that it is going on [34]. It is important to note that, generally, exposure of a child to IPV may be considered to be a form of child abuse or neglect and therefore would fall under mandatory reporting to Child Protective Services (CPS). As of 2014, 23 states have instituted laws that protect children from exposure to domestic violence in the home, but the circumstances and details of these laws vary from state to state [38]. Additional resources include the Family Violence Prevention Fund which has a published pediatric guideline as well as a national toll-free hotline (800-799-SAFE) that providers can call to learn about local resources [34].

The co-occurrence of child abuse or maltreatment with IPV has also been well documented. In fact, IPV has been called a precursor to child maltreatment [34]. A study of over 2000 families showed that the presence of IPV in the home during the first 6 months of a child's life made it 3.4 times more likely that child abuse would occur during the child's first 5 years [39]. Thus, addressing and mitigating IPV may be an important method for intervening and preventing child abuse.

Survivors of Child Sexual Abuse

Sexual abuse of children is a common problem and may be encountered by pediatric clinicians. In 2006, an estimated 1.8 children per 1000 were survivors of sexual abuse [40]. The long-term consequences of sexual abuse include not only psychological concerns including PTSD, anxiety disorder, depression, and social phobias but also physical manifestations such as irritable bowel syndrome, fibromyalgia symptoms, sexual problems, and sexually transmitted infections [41]. In many cases, pediatric clinicians are the first to encounter reports of sexual abuse. While in many cases there are specialized clinics of child advocacy centers to which pediatricians can refer when there is suspected child sexual abuse, there are some situations when the pediatric clinician must complete the full assessment. A detailed approach to this is beyond the scope of this chapter, but additional details can be found through the AAP Clinical Report. First and foremost, a detailed history must be obtained from the caregiver and the child independently. Additionally, the five primary issues that need to be addressed are:

1. The child's safety – is the child safe to return home?
2. Reporting to child protective authorities – if no imminent danger is present, the pediatric clinician must decide whether the case should be referred to child protective services. Every state mandates professionals to report suspected child abuse and neglect.
3. The child's mental health – children should be assessed for both acute and chronic mental health concerns.
4. The need for a physical examination – a thorough examination, with special attention to the urogenital exam, should be done to rule out injury.
5. The need for forensic evidence collection – for those children with recent sexual contact, they should be referred to a specialized clinic or emergency department trained to obtain forensic evidence [41].

Many pediatric clinicians feel ill-equipped to address sexual abuse in children when the suspicion arises, but pediatric clinicians are a crucial line of defense in protecting children from sexual abuse.

Sex Trafficking

Child sex trafficking and commercial sexual exploitation of children (CSEC) are major public health concerns throughout the world. Identifying survivors of CSEC may be difficult for pediatric clinicians because victims rarely self-identify. Thus, clinicians need to maintain a high level of suspicion, particularly when certain factors on the initial presentation, history, or physical may be present. These include [42]:

- *Initial presentation*: children accompanied by domineering adult or unrelated adult, chief complaint of acute sexual or physical assault or suicide attempt, child is disoriented or appears intoxicated, or is a poor historian or frequently changes their story
- *Historical factors*: multiple STIs, frequent visits for emergency contraception, history of multiple pregnancies and/or abortions, chronic runaway behavior, involvement of child protective services, frequent substance use, or has a significantly older partner
- *Physical findings*: evidence of inflicted injury, tattoos, signs of substance misuse, poor dentition or signs of chronic lack of care, and also evidence of large amounts of cash or possession of high value items, including clothing

As with the assessment of the child with suspected sexual abuse, evaluating potential victims of sex trafficking requires mobilization of an interdisciplinary team and various resources beyond the pediatric clinician. Clinicians can educate themselves through various resources including the AAP and national anti-trafficking organizations such as HEAL Trafficking (www.healtrafficking.org, a group of multidisciplinary professionals addressing trafficking from the public health perspective) and the National Center for Missing & Exploited Children (www.missingkids.com) or the National Human Trafficking Resource Center Hotline (1-888-3737-888) [42]. The NHTRC hotline is available 24/7 and can assist clinicians in real time if they have questions and/or need resources urgently. Clinicians should be aware of their individual state laws regarding obligations as mandatory reporters; many states have recently enacted statutes, in addition to long-standing child abuse and neglect laws that specifically require reporting of the sex trafficking of minors [43].

Children with Disabilities

Addressing sexuality and sexual education should be a routine part of the care of patients with disabilities starting in childhood through adolescence. However, several barriers exist including acute medical or developmental issues that are more urgent and parents underestimating their children as sexual beings [44]. In fact, adolescents with disabilities often express desires for intimacy, marriage, and children just like their peers.

When counseling and advising caregivers, clinicians should be aware of unique issues that may arise with children with developmental disabilities. For reasons that are poorly understood, these patients are 20 times more likely to show early pubertal changes with a higher incidence of idiopathic precocious puberty [45]. In addition, while it is common in healthy children to have irregular menstrual cycles during the first 2 years after menarche, comorbid thyroid disorders, use of antiepileptics, and neuroleptic medications in patients with developmental disabilities increase the likelihood of anovulatory menstrual cycles [46]. If a pelvic examination is needed in a prepubertal patient with a developmental disability, care must be taken to explain in a developmentally appropriate manner what is to be done during the exam and to modify positioning during the exam to account for any comorbid muscular or orthopedic conditions that may limit hip abduction [44]. Furthermore, children with developmental disabilities are at higher risk for sexual behavior problems [21]. In addition, children with disabilities are twice as likely to be victims of sexual abuse due to several factors that increase their vulnerability including multiple caregivers and settings, impaired social skills, and reliance on others for self-care [44, 47]. A large study of more than 50,000 children in Nebraska using records from schools, social service databases, and police reports estimated that the rate of maltreatment (i.e., neglect, physical, emotional, and sexual abuse) for children with disabilities was 31 percent (compared to 11 percent in non-disabled children) [48].

Furthermore, in a meta-analysis of 17 studies of children with disabilities, the prevalence of sexual abuse among children with disabilities was 13.7 percent [49]. As children transition into adolescence, they should be counseled regarding sexually transmitted infections, contraception, and pregnancy.

The American Academy of Pediatrics (AAP) makes several recommendations to pediatric clinicians, including:

- Discuss issues of physical development, sexual maturity, and sexuality starting in childhood through adolescence.
- Help caregivers understand how the child's cognitive abilities affect behavior, socialization, and sexual development.
- Recognize that children with disabilities are at increased risk of sexual abuse and monitor for any indications of abuse.
- Promote developmentally appropriate sexuality education in the home, community, and school [44].

Conclusion

Sexual and reproductive health is an important aspect of caring for the well-being of children. Pediatric clinicians are charged with being a primary resource for sexual and reproductive health for patients, and caregivers and must also address the more challenging issues of potential sexual abuse and exploitation. Clinicians must educate themselves on the assessment and management of such issues as well as provide longitudinal anticipatory guidance.

References

1. Breuner CC, Mattson G, et al. Sexuality education for children and adolescents. Pediatrics. 2016;138(2).
2. Promoting healthy sexual development and sexuality. 4th ed. Elk Grove Village: American Academy of Pediatrics; 2017.
3. Haka-Ikse K, Mian M. Sexuality in children. Pediatr Rev. 1993;14(10):401–7.
4. Kellogg ND. Sexual behaviors in children: evaluation and management. Am Fam Physician. 2010;82(10):1233–8.
5. Vance SR, Ehrensaft D, Rosenthal SM. Psychological and medical care of gender nonconforming youth. Pediatrics. 2014;134(6):1184–92.
6. Steensma TD, Biemond R, de Boer F, Cohen-Kettenis PT. Desisting and persisting gender dysphoria after childhood: a qualitative follow-up study. Clin Child Psychol Psychiatry. 2011;16(4):499–516.
7. Levine SB. Facilitating parent-child communication about sexuality. Pediatr Rev. 2011;32(3):129–30.
8. Kunkel D, Eyal K, Finnerty K, Biely E, Donnerstein E. Sex on TV 4: a biennial report to the Kaiser Foundation. 2005. Available from: https://kaiserfamilyfoundation.files.wordpress.com/2013/01/sex-on-tv-4-full-report.pdf.

9. Collins RL, Strasburger VC, Brown JD, Donnerstein E, Lenhart A, Ward LM. Sexual media and childhood well-being and health. Pediatrics. 2017;140(Suppl 2):S162–S6.
10. Bickley L. Bates' guide to physical examination and history taking. 11th ed. Philadelphia: Lippincott Williams and Wilkins; 2013.
11. Pfeffer B, Ellsworth TR, Gold MA. Interviewing adolescents about sexual matters. Pediatr Clin North Am. 2017;64(2):291–304.
12. Marcell AV, Burstein GR, Committee on Adolescence. Sexual and reproductive health care services in the pediatric setting. Pediatrics. 2017;140(5).
13. Marshall WA, Tanner JM. Variations in pattern of pubertal changes in girls. Arch Dis Child. 1969;44(235):291–303.
14. Marshall WA, Tanner JM. Variations in the pattern of pubertal changes in boys. Arch Dis Child. 1970;45(239):13–23.
15. Murphy C, Allen L, Jamieson MA. Ambiguous genitalia in the newborn: an overview and teaching tool. J Pediatr Adolesc Gynecol. 2011;24(5):236–50.
16. Lee PA, Houk CP, Ahmed SF, Hughes IA. Consensus statement on management of intersex disorders. International consensus conference on intersex. Pediatrics. 2006;118(2):e488–500.
17. Wherrett DK. Approach to the infant with a suspected disorder of sex development. Pediatr Clin North Am. 2015;62(4):983–99.
18. Klein DA, Emerick JE, Sylvester JE, Vogt KS. Disorders of puberty: an approach to diagnosis and management. Am Fam Physician. 2017;96(9):590–9.
19. Sultan C, Gaspari L, Maimoun L, Kalfa N, Paris F. Disorders of puberty. Best Pract Res Clin Obstet Gynaecol. 2018;48:62–89.
20. Sexual development and behavior in children: information for parents and caregivers. September 3, 2017. Available from: http://nctsn.org/nctsn_assets/pdfs/caring/sexualdevelopmentandbehavior.pdf.
21. Kellogg ND, Committee on Child Abuse and Neglect AeAoP. Clinical report--the evaluation of sexual behaviors in children. Pediatrics. 2009;124(3):992–8.
22. Friedrich WN, Fisher JL, Dittner CA, Acton R, Berliner L, Butler J, et al. Child Sexual Behavior Inventory: normative, psychiatric, and sexual abuse comparisons. Child Maltreat. 2001;6(1):37–49.
23. Gray A, Pithers WD, Busconi A, Houchens P. Developmental and etiological characteristics of children with sexual behavior problems: treatment implications. Child Abuse Negl. 1999;23(6):601–21.
24. Friedrich WN, Fisher J, Broughton D, Houston M, Shafran CR. Normative sexual behavior in children: a contemporary sample. Pediatrics. 1998;101(4):E9.
25. Gladden RM, Vivolo-Kantor AM, Hamburger ME, Lumpkin CD. Bullying surveillance among youths: uniform definitions for public health and recommended data elements. 2014 December 12, 2017. Available from: https://www.cdc.gov/violenceprevention/pdf/bullying-definitions-final-a.pdf.
26. Kann L, Olsen EO, McManus T, Harris WA, Shanklin SL, Flint KH, et al. Sexual identity, sex of sexual contacts, and health-related behaviors among students in grades 9–12 - United States and selected sites, 2015. MMWR Surveill Summ. 2016;65(9):1–202.
27. Earnshaw VA, Bogart LM, Poteat VP, Reisner SL, Schuster MA. Bullying among lesbian, gay, bisexual, and transgender youth. Pediatr Clin North Am. 2016;63(6):999–1010.
28. Birkett M, Newcomb ME, Mustanski B. Does it get better? A longitudinal analysis of psychological distress and victimization in lesbian, gay, bisexual, transgender, and questioning youth. J Adolesc Health. 2015;56(3):280–5.
29. Meyer I. Prejudice, social stress, and mental health in lesbian, gay, and bisexual populations: conceptual issues and research evidence. Psychol Bull. 2003;129:674–97.
30. Earnshaw VA, Reisner SL, Juvonen J, Hatzenbuehler ML, Perrotti J, Schuster MA. LGBTQ bullying: translating research to action in pediatrics. Pediatrics. 2017;140(4).

31. Breiding MJ, Basile KC, Smith SG, Black MC, Mahendra RR. Intimate partner violence surveillance: uniform definitions and recommended data elements, Version 2.0. 2015 April 16, 2018. Available from: http://www.cdc.gov/ncipc/dvp/ipv_factsheet.pdf.
32. Bender E. PTSD, other disorders evident in kids who witness domestic violence. Psychiatric News [Internet]. 2014;39(11):14–50. Available from: https://doi.org/10.1176/pn.39.11.0390014a.
33. Tjaden P, Thoennes N. Full report of the prevalence, incidence, and consequences of violence against women: findings from the National Violence Against Women Survey. Publication no. NCJ-183781. 2005 July 17, 2018. Available from: https://www.ncjrs.gov/pdffiles1/nij/183781.pdf.
34. Thackeray JD, Hibbard R, Dowd MD. Intimate partner violence: the role of the pediatrician. Pediatrics. 2010;125(5):1094–100.
35. Ballif-Spanvill B, Clayton CJ, Hendrix SB. Witness and nonwitness children's violent and peaceful behavior in different types of simulated conflict with peers. Am J Orthopsychiatry. 2007;77(2):206–15.
36. Moretti M, Osbuth I, Odgers CL, Reebye P. Exposure to maternal vs. paternal partner violence, PTSD, and aggression in adolescent girls and boys. Aggress Behav. 2006;32(4):385–95.
37. Wood SL, Sommers MS. Consequences of intimate partner violence on child witnesses: a systematic review of the literature. J Child Adolesc Psychiatr Nurs. 2011;24(4):223–36.
38. Committee on Child Maltreatment Research Policy, and Practice for the Next Decade: Phase II, Board on Children, Youth, and Families, Committee on Law and Justice, Institute of Medicine, National Research Council, Peterson A, et al. New directions in child abuse and neglect research. 2014. Available from: https://www.ncbi.nlm.nih.gov/books/NBK195993/.
39. McGuigan WM, Pratt CC. The predictive impact of domestic violence on three types of child maltreatment. Child Abuse Negl. 2001;25(7):869–83.
40. Sedlak A, Mettenburg J, Basena M. Fourth National Incidence Study of Child Abuse and Neglect (NIS-4): 2004–2009. 2010 March 1, 2018. Available from: https://www.acf.hhs.gov/sites/default/files/opre/nis4_report_congress_full_pdf_jan2010.pdf.
41. Jenny C, Crawford-Jakubiak JE. The evaluation of children in the primary care setting when sexual abuse is suspected. Pediatrics. 2013;132(2):e558–67.
42. Greenbaum J, Crawford-Jakubiak JE. Child sex trafficking and commercial sexual exploitation: health care needs of victims. Pediatrics. 2015;135(3):566–74.
43. Atkinson H, Curnin K, Hanson N. U.S. state laws addressing human trafficking: education of and mandatory reporting by health care providers and other professionals. J Human Trafficking. 2016;2(2):111–38.
44. Murphy NA, Elias ER. Sexuality of children and adolescents with developmental disabilities. Pediatrics. 2006;118(1):398–403.
45. Siddiqi SU, Van Dyke DC, Donohoue P, McBrien DM. Premature sexual development in individuals with neurodevelopmental disabilities. Dev Med Child Neurol. 1999;41(6):392–5.
46. Sulpizi LK. Issues in sexuality and gynecologic care of women with developmental disabilities. J Obstet Gynecol Neonatal Nurs. 1996;25(7):609–14.
47. Crosse S, Kaye E, Ratnofsky A. A report on the maltreatment of children with disabilities; 1993.
48. Sullivan PM, Knutson JF. Maltreatment and disabilities: a population-based epidemiological study. Child Abuse Negl. 2000;24(10):1257–73.
49. Jones L, Bellis MA, Wood S, Hughes K, McCoy E, Eckley L, et al. Prevalence and risk of violence against children with disabilities: a systematic review and meta-analysis of observational studies. Lancet. 2012;380(9845):899–907.

Chapter 2
Sexual and Reproductive Health in Adolescents and Young Adults

David E. DeLaet and Scott K. Jelinek

Contents

D. E. DeLaet (✉)
Departments of Internal Medicine and Pediatrics, Icahn School of Medicine at Mount Sinai, New York, NY, USA
e-mail: david.delaet@mountsinai.org

S. K. Jelinek
Department of Pediatrics, Icahn School of Medicine at Mount Sinai, New York, NY, USA
e-mail: scott.jelinek@icahn.mssm.edu

© Springer Nature Switzerland AG 2022
J. Truglio et al. (eds.), *Sexual and Reproductive Health*,
https://doi.org/10.1007/978-3-030-94632-6_2

Introduction

Adolescence and young adulthood is a period during which individuals experience significant physical, emotional, mental, and social growth and development. Maintenance of sexual and reproductive health (SRH) is critical in assuring that such growth and development occurs appropriately. It is therefore vital that clinicians caring for adolescents and young adults (AYAs) be equipped to deliver a wide range of SRH care services. These services should focus on the overall health and well-being of the AYA and must be delivered in an inclusive, developmentally appropriate, and culturally and structurally effective manner. Health providers should be familiar with clinical guidelines and best practices for SRH care of AYAs, and they and members of their respective staffs should be competent in the care of patients of all sexual orientations, gender identities and expressions, and medical backgrounds. All SRH education and clinical guidance provided to patients should be based on the best available evidence. Finally, care should be delivered with a firm understanding of existing local legislation and standards of care regarding confidentiality and consent to care of minors.

This chapter will explore SRH care of AYAs across a broad span of topics. Though it is beyond the scope of this book to explore each subject in detail, the chapter is intended to allow primary care health providers to deliver SRH that is comprehensive in nature. Topics to be reviewed include the SRH visit, disorders of pubertal development and menstruation, sexual dysfunction, sexually transmitted infections (STIs), prevention of human immunodeficiency virus (HIV) infection, pregnancy prevention and family planning, pregnancy and abortion, immunizations, cancer screening, intimate partner violence (IPV), sexual assault, sexual exploitation, and care of sexual and gender minority youth (SGMY).

The Sexual and Reproductive Health Visit for Adolescents and Young Adults

Confidentiality and Consent

For AYAs, the delivery of SRH services that are confidential is recognized as an essential component of care by professional societies including the American Academy of Family Physicians (AAFP), the Society for Adolescent Health and Medicine (SAHM), and the American Academy of Pediatrics (AAP) [1–3]. It has been demonstrated that adolescents are more likely to access health care, disclose health risk behaviors, and return for follow-up care when confidentiality is assured and promoted, whereas, without confidentiality, necessary care is more likely to be deferred, particularly by adolescents most at risk [4, 5]. Further, obtaining confidential services does not serve as a barrier between adolescent and parental communication about reasons for seeking medical attention or the existence of a serious health problem [6].

It is recommended that providers establish explicit office policies that are consistently observed by all members of the office staff as well as posted in visible locations in the office. The SAHM and AAP recommend that these policies be discussed with patients and their families beginning during early adolescence at the outset of visits [2, 7]. To further promote autonomy of the adolescent, providers are encouraged to spend time with the adolescent alone after conducting the initial part of the medical interview with the parent in the examination room [7]. Additionally, providers should review with patients and their families instances when confidentiality would be breached, including disclosures about suicidal or homicidal ideation or suspicion about physical or sexual abuse [7].

As laws regarding confidentiality and consent vary by state, providers should be familiar with local legislation in the states in which they practice. Additionally, providers must assure that policies regarding confidential SRH services in areas such as electronic health records, clinical and laboratory billing practices, and receipt of explanation of benefits (EOBs) forms comply with the requirements of state and federal laws. In those instances when office policies or practices do not allow for adolescent confidentiality to be maintained, providers should be willing to refer patients to a health-care provider who is required to provide confidential care, such as one who participates in the Title X family planning program [8]. Finally, the presence of an intellectual disability (ID), regardless of severity, does not, in itself, justify loss of rights related to sexuality, including confidentiality, and providers should be familiar with pertinent legislation and advocate for their patients with disabilities [9]. Sexual and reproductive health in patients with intellectual disability is discussed in detail in Chap. 10.

These issues of confidentiality and consent to care will be explored in greater detail as relevant in the later discussion of topics including STIs, HIV prevention, pregnancy prevention and family planning, pregnancy and abortion, IPV, sexual assault, and sexual exploitation.

History Taking

Once the AYA and parents/guardians have been informed regarding confidentiality and consent policies as well as the overall structure of the visit, providers should initiate the medical history, typically with both the AYA and parents/guardians in the examination room, as previously noted. After discussing nonconfidential information with the patient and parents/guardians in the room, the provider should then review sensitive history questions and information with the AYA in a private setting [3]. In some instances, initially this sensitive information may in fact be more comfortably collected through the use of pre-visit paper or computer-based questionnaires [7, 10].

Best practice guidelines recommend the use of tools such as the Centers for Disease Control and Prevention (CDC) five "P"s of sexual health to guide the interviewing of AYAs. The five "P"s stand for *P*artners, sexual *P*ractices, *P*rotection from STIs, *P*ast history of STIs, and *P*revention of pregnancy [11]. Review of this information should be done with an honest, caring, nonjudgmental attitude and in a comfortable matter-of-fact approach to asking questions [12].

The use of gender-neutral language when obtaining a psychosocial history is critical. The AAP makes recommendations for interviewing techniques that may prove useful to providers when eliciting sensitive SRH information from AYAs (see Table 2.1). For those AYAs with cognitive delay, providers should ask questions in a developmentally appropriate manner.

Providers should ask all patients their preferred name and gender pronouns, ideally at the beginning of the visit and/or on an intake questionnaire. This will not only provide valuable information about the patient's identity but is also important in establishing rapport and showing respect to the patient. It can be helpful to model appropriate use of names and pronouns in the presence of parents and caregivers and to share your own pronouns with patients, asking: "Which gender pronouns do you use? For example, I use…he and him/she and hers/they and theirs."

Providers should include a discussion regarding sexual orientation, gender identity, gender expression, and sexual activity. Some questions may need to be asked at every visit, as sexual orientation and gender identity can be fluid, especially in adolescents, and providers should recall that many teens may have sexual encounters

Table 2.1 Recommended techniques for interviewing adolescents and young adults

Technique	Example
Use of open-ended questions that avoid a "yes" or "no" response	"How often do you use condoms?" rather than "Do you use condoms all of the time?"
Reflection responses that mirror the patient's feelings	"It sounds like you have a hard time getting your partner to use condoms. Tell me about that."
Restatement of the patient's feelings or summarizing the interview	"You are worried about using birth control pills because you think you will gain weight but want to be protected against pregnancy."
Clarification of a statement	"What did you mean when you said that you were worried about your partner's feelings?"
Use of questions that may give the provider insight into the patient	"What do you do outside of school?"
Offering reassuring statements	"You have made the decision to wait to have sex even though many of your friends are sexually active. It sounds like you are making the decision that is right for you."
Presenting supportive statements	"That must have been hard for you."
The use of gender-neutral language	"Have you dated/had sex with someone? If so, what was that person's name?"

[a]Adapted from Marcell et al. [3]

that may not be predicted by their declared orientation [3, 7]. Providers should not assume that sexual orientation or gender identity of patients is the same as prior visits or is based on behavior, appearance, or genders of partners. For example, many male youth do not identify as gay but have same-sex partners, and one study found that 81% of females with same-sex attraction also report having sexual experiences with males [13]. Instead, providers should ask open-ended questions and use language that is inclusive, allowing the patient to decide when and what to disclose:

- "How would you describe your sexual orientation?"
- "How would you describe your current gender identity?"
- "What are the genders of your sexual partners?"
- "What is the sex on your original birth certificate?"

Additionally, providers should base their counseling, STI screening, or contraception recommendations on sexual activities, not just sexual orientation or gender identity. A provider should refer to body parts with gender-neutral language whenever possible, such as "chest," "bottom," and "genitals," or ask the patient what terms they use for their own body parts and then utilize those terms throughout the visit [14]. Here are some examples of more targeted questions providers can ask all AYA [15]:

- "Tell me about different sexual experiences you've had. First, what are you looking for in sex? What does sex mean to you?"
- "Tell me about your sex life."
- "Are there some sexual activities more important to you than others? *(oral/anal/ vaginal; top/bottom)*"
- "When you have sex, what goes where?" *(penis, mouth, butt, anus, vagina, hands, toys and other objects)*
- "What types of sex are you having? What parts of your body do you use for sex?"

When discussing sexual activity, it is also important to inquire about the nature and patterns of sexual negotiation, such as communication and decision-making, and about condom use and STI prevention.

- "How do you feel about using condoms?"
- "In what situations do you feel you need to use condoms?"
- "Tell me about the last time you had sex and didn't use a condom."
- "How do you protect yourself from STIs? Any use of PrEP?"
- "Have you ever had sex with someone when you didn't want to?"
- "Do you use alcohol or any drugs when you have sex?"
- "Have you exchanged sex for money, drugs, or a place to stay?"

The history should include an assessment of pubertal development. Providers should not only review physical changes and inquire about menarche and menstrual cycles but should also assess the patient's comfort with these changes. Providers should additionally inquire about safety in relationships, IPV, and a history of sexual abuse or assault.

Physical Examination

Prior to the sexual health examination of an AYA, the provider should first review with the AYA and their parents/guardians the indications for the examination and describe what areas of the body will be examined. Additionally, the patient should be given the option of changing into a gown or remaining clothed and having the provider disrobe each body part as needed during the exam [3]. Reassurance should be provided that the AYA can stop the examination at any time should they become uncomfortable.

The AAP recommends the use of a chaperone when the examination of an AYA requires the inspection or palpation of anorectal or genital areas and/or the female breast, regardless of the gender of the examining physician [16]. It is further recommended that the use of a chaperone be a shared decision between the patient and physician, with patient preferences for use of and gender of a chaperone given highest priority [13]. Having an authorized member of the health-care team serve as a chaperone can not only help in making patients feel more comfortable with the examination but can also help prevent misunderstandings between patient and physician [17]. Finally, the use of a chaperone should be carefully documented in the medical record [13].

Importantly, the examination of SGMY should take into account the body parts they possess, and the provider should use the terms that the individual uses to describe their body parts. These points should be considered when reviewing the following professional society recommendations for the female and male breast and genital examinations.

As recommended by the AAP, the breast examination should include evaluation of sexual maturity rating (SMR), which should then be documented in the medical record (See Chap. 1 on "Pediatrics" for discussion of SMR) [3]. Additional assessment should be based on clinical concerns and include examination for evidence of masses or skin lesions as well as galactorrhea or nipple discharge as necessary. Using the examination as an opportunity to educate the AYA about normal and abnormal breast findings is prudent.

The AAP recommends that the external genital examination should also include an assessment and documentation of SMR for hair and genitals [3]. Evaluation for skin or vulvar lesions, vaginal or penile discharge, and evidence of soft tissue or testicular masses should be performed. As before, providers should use the examination as an opportunity to educate the AYA about normal and abnormal genital findings.

Given recent changes in recommendations for the initiation of cervical cancer screening (see section "Cervical Cancer Screening", below) as well as advances in screening tests for STIs (see section "Screening for STIs," below), fewer AYAs require a complete screening pelvic examination as part of routine care. Additionally, the American College of Obstetricians and Gynecologists (ACOG) and the AAP note that a speculum or bimanual examination is no longer considered necessary before the initiation of most forms of contraception [18, 19]. As such, an internal

Table 2.2 Indications for internal pelvic examination

Persistent vaginal discharge
Dysuria or urinary tract symptoms in a sexually active female
Dysmenorrhea unresponsive to nonsteroidal anti-inflammatory drugs
Amenorrhea
Abnormal vaginal bleeding
Lower abdominal pain
Contraceptive counseling for an intrauterine device or diaphragm
Pregnancy
Perform cervical cancer screening
Suspected/reported rape or sexual abuse

[a]Adapted from Braverman et al. [19]

pelvic examination generally is unnecessary during the initial reproductive health evaluation [18]. Rather, the decision as to whether a complete internal pelvic examination is required should be guided by clinical issues or problems discovered during the medical history [18, 19]. As outlined by the AAP, indications for an internal pelvic (bimanual and/or speculum) examination are listed in Table 2.2. As with other parts of the reproductive health examination, a thorough explanation and patient assent should always precede the procedure [18, 19]. Use of educational materials may assist in providing the patient with an understanding of the procedure to be performed [20]. For those individuals with mobility issues, accommodations may need to be made in order to perform an external genital or internal pelvic examination. As the typical pelvic exam position may increase spasticity for some patients with mobility disabilities, variations such as the knee-chest position, the diamond-shaped position, the V-shaped position, and the OB footrests position may be considered [21]. Additional details can be found in Chaps. 11 and 12 of this book.

As previously noted, the external genital examination should be performed to assess SMR of developing AYAs. Additionally, the AAP and SAHM recommend a complete examination of the male genitalia be performed annually as part of a comprehensive physical examination to evaluate for skin or hair findings, visual signs of STIs such as herpes and condyloma, asymptomatic urethral discharge, signs for genetic diseases such as firm testes or ambiguous genitalia, evidence of structural anomalies including varicocele or uncorrected hypospadias, and evidence of testicular atrophy [22, 23]. The United States Preventive Services Task Force (USPSTF) has recommended against screening by self-examination or clinical examination for testicular cancer in asymptomatic adolescent or adult men [24]. The AAP and SAHM do note that providers should be familiar with risk factors for testicular cancer and inform those with an increased risk of the potential benefits and harms associated with screening [22, 23]. Penile and testicular exams should otherwise be guided by clinical presentation. As previously noted, a thorough explanation and patient assent should always precede this portion of the sexual health examination.

Counseling and Education

Health-care professionals caring for AYAs play a critical role in providing and supporting longitudinal sexuality counseling and education to all individuals as part of preventive health care [25]. Such counseling and education should occur regardless of the presence or absence of chronic health conditions or disabilities. Those individuals with chronic health conditions and disabilities can benefit from knowledgeable and personalized anticipatory guidance, and information should be presented in a manner that is developmentally appropriate [7]. As when taking a psychosocial history, providers must maintain an open, nonjudgmental attitude and be comfortable discussing a range of SRH topics [22]. Additionally, gender-neutral language should be used by providers and their office staff when discussing SRH topics, and SGMY should be encouraged to feel comfortable talking with providers about emerging sexual and gender identities and about their sexual activities [26].

The AAFP and the SAHM emphasize the importance of providing information to AYAs and their parents/guardians that is up-to-date and evidence-based [1, 2]. Topics to be discussed should include but are not limited to anatomy, physical changes associated with pubertal development, masturbation, menstruation, nocturnal emissions, sexual fantasies, sexual orientation, gender identification and expression, abstinence, orgasms, safe sexual practices, STIs, contraception, pregnancy, abortion, and safety and legal issues pertaining to social media and SRH.

The AAP recommends that counseling of AYAs should draw on motivational interviewing approaches wherein the focus of the interview is on future goals, belief in the adolescent's capacity to change, and engagement of the adolescent in the process of adopting health-promoting behaviors. Motivational interviewing is accomplished through open-ended questions and careful listening and rooted in the following key elements [27]:

1. Expressing empathy through reflective listening (clarifying meaning of patient's statements)
2. Developing discrepancy between patients' goals or values and their current behavior
3. Avoiding argument and direct confrontation
4. Adjusting to client resistance rather than opposing it directly
5. Supporting self-efficacy and optimism in carrying out the behavior/behavioral change

Motivational interviewing relies on a provider's use of affirmation through compliments or statements of understanding, provision of summary statements to unify and reinforce discussed material, and eliciting change talk (e.g., "I will use condoms during each sexual encounter."). Providers must take into account the developmental stage of the patient when using motivational interviewing.

Finally, providers and their staff should make available to AYAs evidence-based and up-to-date brochures and other reading materials on a range of SRH topics for patient education and to promote discussion. These materials should be individualized as necessary for patients with chronic health conditions or disabilities.

Common Issues in Sexual and Reproductive Health Care of Adolescents and Young Adults

Disorders of Pubertal Development and Menstruation

A thorough discussion of disorders of pubertal development and menstruation is beyond the scope of this section. These topics have been extensively reviewed elsewhere [28–31]. However, a chapter on SRH care of AYAs would not be complete without a mention of these important topics. This brief section will instead focus on a review of clinical definitions, emphasize when clinical evaluation is indicated, and recommend a thoughtful approach to a broad but well-organized differential diagnosis.

Pubertal development in both females and males tends to progress in a predictable manner. In females, puberty typically begins with thelarche, though pubarche may occur first or simultaneously [28]. Menarche occurs on average 2.5 years after thelarche, with the average age of onset of puberty between 8 and 13 years. In most males, testicular enlargement marks the onset of puberty, typically between 9 and 14 years of age [28]. This is followed by pubarche and then spermarche, usually coincident with the growth spurt that occurs during genital stages 3 and 4.

When pubertal onset occurs before age 8 years in females and 9 years in males, it is considered precocious. Studies have observed earlier thelarche and menarche in certain racial groups [28]. However, these studies did not describe how race was ascribed to the patients included in the study, and those identified as "African American" patients made up less than 5% of the study population. As race is a social, not biologic construct, the generalizability of any such observations should be questioned. We therefore recommend using the standard definition of precocious puberty for all racial and ethnic groups, such that patients with potentially identifiable and treatable causes do not go undiagnosed. Precocious puberty was discussed previously in Chap. 1. Conversely, puberty is considered delayed when pubertal maturation has not begun by age 14 years in boys and when there is no breast development by age 13 years in girls [29]. In males, constitutional delayed puberty (CDP) accounts for the majority of cases, whereas CDP is a less common diagnosis in females, for whom a much larger number of cases are due to functional gonadotropin deficiency, typically in girls of slender build [29]. In either gender, functional gonadotropin deficiency may occur in the setting of underlying chronic disease states such as inflammatory bowel disease, cystic fibrosis, chronic renal failure, and sickle cell disease, to name a few. Primary gonadal failure is more common in females than males, with Turner syndrome accounting for the majority of these female cases.

In those adolescents with delayed puberty and poor weight gain in the setting of chronic illness, management should first focus on treatment of the underlying condition and improving nutritional status. For healthy adolescents, initial evaluation should include assessment of levels of luteinizing hormone (LH) and follicle-stimulating hormone (FSH) as well as total testosterone in boys and estradiol in girls with consideration for a hand and wrist radiograph to assess bone age [29]. Additional evaluation and management, often in consultation with an endocrinologist, will depend upon associated clinical findings and results of these initial tests.

Providers may also need to consider evaluation for endocrinological abnormalities in females with hirsutism and males with micropenis, cryptorchidism, or persistent or excessive gynecomastia. As before, initial evaluation will be guided by nutritional status of the patient, the presence or absence of associated chronic medical conditions, or clinical features suggestive of an underlying genetic disorder.

Disorders of menstruation in adolescent females are common. As previously noted, menarche typically occurs approximately 2.5 years after thelarche, with an average age between 12 and 13 years [28, 30, 31]. Primary amenorrhea is diagnosed when menarche has failed to occur by 15 years of age in the presence of normal growth and secondary sexual characteristics or within 3 years of thelarche [28, 30]. Secondary amenorrhea is defined as an absence of menses for a period of either 3 or 6 months (definition can vary by source) in females who have attained menarche, while oligomenorrhea is diagnosed when menses is infrequent and irregular [28, 30]. There is an extensive list of possible causes of amenorrhea, though pregnancy should always be the first consideration, particularly in those individuals with secondary amenorrhea. Additional initial evaluation should include assessment of levels of LH and FSH and, in cases of primary amenorrhea, consideration for abdominal and pelvic ultrasound to demonstrate normal reproductive anatomy. In those females with amenorrhea or oligomenorrhea with accompanying hirsutism, polycystic ovarian syndrome (PCOS) and late-onset congenital adrenal hyperplasia should be considered. Further work-up and management of amenorrhea and oligomenorrhea will be dictated by associated clinical symptoms and signs as well as results of initial evaluation.

Finally, menorrhagia (heavy menses) refers to menstrual loss of >80 mL, with this more practically being described by menses requiring pad or tampon changes every 1–2 hours to avoid bleeding "accidents," particularly if menses is longer than 8 days [30]. There is a broad differential diagnosis, though initial evaluation should be guided by time since last menses and other clinical symptoms and signs. PCOS is a common cause of heavy menses in women with oligomenorrhea and hirsutism, particularly if obesity is also noted. Certain medications, including nonsteroidal anti-inflammatory drugs and oral contraceptives, may cause menorrhagia. Heavy menses can also be a presenting sign of pregnancy complications, infection of the female reproductive tract, and inherited bleeding disorders.

Sexual Dysfunction

Health-care clinicians are an important source of information for AYAs and play a significant role in addressing sexual and reproductive health needs, including symptoms of and anxiety about sexual dysfunction [32]. Office visits present opportunities to educate AYAs on sexual health and development, promote healthy relationships, and screen for and address any issues or concerns related to sexual function [6].

Problems with sexual function are common for AYAs and can be a source of stress, anxiety, and shame. As a result, AYAs can be hesitant to initiate discussion of these issues. It is important for health-care providers to assess if sexually active patients are experiencing any difficulty with intercourse or problems when having sex. These problems can be related to substance use as well as certain classes of medications (e.g., selective serotonin reuptake inhibitors), anatomic differences, or lasting psychosocial impact of sexual trauma [33].

Common presentations of sexual dysfunction include lacking desire for sex, arousal difficulties (e.g., erection problems or lubrication difficulties), anxiety about performance, inability achieving or prematurely occurring of climax or ejaculation, worries about attractiveness during sex, physical pain during intercourse, not finding sex pleasurable or decreased pleasure associated with condom use, and organic performance-related issues attributable to comorbid medical conditions (e.g., diabetes, cardiac disease, neurologic deficits) or adverse effects from medication [34].

Many adolescents start to have anxieties and questions about breast or genital size and function, especially during puberty, when comparing themselves to others and after initiating sexual behavior [35]. As noted previously, adolescents are more likely to communicate about sensitive topics regarding behaviors, partners, or sexual concerns when confidentiality is promoted, and they may be more comfortable raising sensitive subjects with questionnaires or intake forms [4]. One strategy for a provider to initiate the discussion is asking, "Do you have any concerns about how your body is developing?" [3]. Another way is to ask patients "whether sex is pleasurable and/or there are problems with sexual performance" [22].

As noted previously, the physical exam provides an opportunity to educate adolescents about normal and abnormal breast and genital findings as well as to teach them about their own body and changes through puberty. Providers can also identify signs for genetic diseases such as firm testes (Klinefelter syndrome) or ambiguous genitalia (congenital adrenal hyperplasia), evidence of structural anomalies that can affect fertility including varicocele, or uncorrected hypospadias, which can cause adolescents embarrassment, problems with sexual function, and/or abnormal urine flow [36, 37].

For AYAs who are born with a disorder of sexual development or other medical conditions that affect their reproductive anatomy, providers should offer sufficient counseling and accurate information regarding perceived reproductive and anatomic differences, sexual function, and fertility [38]. If these AYAs feel unable to discuss this with their providers, then they may be more likely to obtain information from potentially less accurate sources, such as peers, media, or the Internet [39]. Because this may lead to added discomfort and confusion, these AYAs will likely benefit from professional guidance about how to disclose to others their body/sexual differences and fertility status as well as how to mitigate shame or fears of rejection [40].

Sexually Transmitted Infections

In the United States, prevalence rates of many STIs are highest among AYAs [41]. As such, health-care providers must be familiar with best practices in the evaluation and management of STIs among this young patient population. A detailed discussion of the prevention, clinical presentation, diagnosis and management of the more common STIs is presented in Chap. 6. In this section, considerations pertinent to the prevention, evaluation, and management of STIs among AYAs will be reviewed.

Confidentiality and Consent

All states and the District of Columbia allow all minors to consent to STI services. Eighteen of these states allow, but do not require, a clinician to inform a minor's parents/guardians that they are seeking or receiving STI services when the clinician deems it in the minor's best interests, though these interests vary by state and include but are not limited to the age of the minor, positive test results, and a minor's health being at risk [42]. However, many state-level legal requirements related to the mandated or presumed sending of EOBs to a policyholder whenever care is provided under his or her policy can result in loss of confidentiality for minors seeking such care [43]. Though several states have adopted regulations that could assure dependents confidentiality protection, clinicians should be familiar with legislation in their jurisdiction and refer minors to clinicians, such as health department or Title X clinics, who can provide confidential care [3, 12]. Clinicians must also be familiar with local regulations regarding those STIs such as HIV, acquired immunodeficiency disease syndrome (AIDS), syphilis, and hepatitis A, B, and C viruses that may be reportable to the state health departments and the resultant implications for confidentiality.

Counseling

Professional societies including the AAP, the AAFP, and the SAHM have guidelines recommending that health-care providers counsel adolescents on safe sexual practices that decrease the risk of STIs, provide information on the signs and symptoms of STIs, and stress the importance of routine asymptomatic STI and HIV screening for those adolescents who are sexually active [1–3]. STI education and counseling on prevention strategies should be incorporated into well-adolescent and contraception visits [3]. Such counseling should draw on motivational interviewing as previously discussed. The USPSTF recommends that, for all sexually active AYAs at increased risk for STIs, providers offer or refer to intensive behavioral counseling interventions to prevent STIs [44]. The USPSTF defines higher-risk adults as those with current STIs or infections within the past year, those who have multiple sex partners, and those who do not consistently use condoms. Interventions ranging in intensity from 30 minutes to greater than or equal to 2 hours of contact time are noted to be beneficial, with evidence of benefit increasing with intervention intensity. Most successful interventions include basic information about STIs and STI transmission, assess for risk of transmission, and provide training in pertinent skills, such as condom use, communication about safer sex, problem solving, and goal setting. The USPSTF notes that these interventions can be delivered by primary care clinicians or through referral to trained behavioral counselors [44].

As mentioned earlier, it is important for providers to obtain a comprehensive sexual history, including asking all patients which body parts they are using during sex, so providers can base their counseling, STI screening, and prevention recommendations on sexual behaviors and not identities or assumptions. For example, when compared to heterosexual youth, women who have sex with women (WSW) are almost 20 times less likely to perceive themselves at risk for STIs but are nearly as likely to have had intercourse, experience twice the rate of pregnancy, and are more likely to have had two or more pregnancies [45]. If a patient is engaging in anal sex, a provider should clarify if they are engaging in insertive ("top") or receptive ("bottom") penetration or both. Condoms should be promoted for use with sex toys and dental dams encouraged for any oral-vaginal or oral-anal contact.

Screening for STIs

Given the high prevalence of STIs among AYAs, providers should be familiar with recommendations for screening for asymptomatic infection in this patient population. The USPSTF has established guidelines for the more common STIs, and the CDC periodically summarizes recommendations for the more common STIs, as well. Recommendations of the AAP and the SAHM are in line with those of the CDC [3].

The CDC and the USPSTF recommend routine (at least annual) screening for *C. trachomatis* and *N. gonorrhoeae* in all sexually active women aged 24 years and younger [41, 46]. Both the CDC and the USPSTF also conclude that there is insufficient evidence to recommend routine screening for chlamydia and gonorrhea in sexually active young men; however, most guidelines suggest screening should be considered for young male populations considered high risk including men who have sex with men (MSM) and those with inconsistent condom use, multiple sexual partners, and sexual partners with STIs and individuals seeking care in clinical settings serving populations with high disease prevalence such as STI clinics, adolescent clinics, and correctional facilities [41, 46]. As described in the introduction to this book, such guidelines tend to conflate identity with behavior. Clearly two mutually monogamous cisgender male sexual partners are at no increased risk for STI. We therefore suggest that STI screening be informed by guidelines but be applied in the context of each individual patient after a detailed sexual history.

Infections should be diagnosed by using nucleic acid amplification tests (NAATs) given their high sensitivity and specificity and approval by the United States Food and Drug Administration (USFDA) use on urogenital sites, including male and female urine, as well as clinician-collected endocervical, vaginal, and male urethral specimens [46, 47]. Additionally, rectal and pharyngeal swabs can be collected from persons who engage in receptive anal intercourse and oral sex, although these collection sites have not been approved by the USFDA, so long as testing laboratories have met Clinical Laboratory Improvement Amendment (CLIA) and other regulatory requirements and have validated NAAT performance on swabs from these sites [41, 46].

The USPSTF recommends that clinicians screen for HIV infection in adolescents and adults aged 15–65 years as well as all pregnant women and younger adolescents at increased risk [48]. Risk factors include those previously discussed as well as those who have acquired or are requesting testing for other STIs and individuals who engage in sex for drugs or money. One-time screening with repeat screening for those at high risk is suggested. The CDC recommends HIV screening for patients aged 13–64 years in all health-care settings using an opt-out approach that is alerting individuals that testing will be performed but that they retain the option to decline or defer testing [41].

The USPSTF and CDC recommend screening for syphilis infection in all pregnant women and in non-pregnant adults and adolescents who are at high risk, including MSM, with the USPSTF additionally recommending screening of persons living with HIV and those with a history of commercial sex work [41, 49, 50]. Both the USPSPTF and CDC recommend that screening be performed using a nontreponemal test with follow-up confirmation using a treponemal test.

The USPSTF recommends screening for hepatitis B virus (HBV) infection in those who are at high risk, including but not limited to those presenting to clinics for STIs, HIV testing and treatment centers, and centers for MSM [51].

The USPSTF recommends against routine serologic screening for herpes simplex virus (HSV) infection in asymptomatic adolescents and adults, including those who are pregnant [52].

Per CDC guidelines, the routine screening of adolescents who are asymptomatic for trichomoniasis, HSV, hepatitis A virus (HAV), and HBV is not generally recommended [41].

Treatment

The SAHM recommends that health-care practitioners provide prompt, effective, and confidential STI treatment to all adolescents and their partners, recognizing the important role of expedited partner therapy (EPT), wherein sex partners of STI-infected individuals are treated without requiring the partners' prior evaluation and typically as partner-delivered therapy, in disease prevention [2]. Studies have shown that a significant number of AYAs with chlamydia and gonorrhea are reinfected within 12 months after their initial infection, with age less than 25 years and untreated partners emerging as significant risk factors for reinfection [53]. As such, EPT has been recommended for the treatment of heterosexual patients with chlamydia or gonorrhea. As described above, we recommend applying this guideline to patients regardless of their sexual orientation after an individualized assessment of additional sexually transmitted infections. The CDC and the SAHM recommend that providers who care for AYAs use EPT as an option for STI care among partners exposed within the past 60 days (or the most recent partner if the individual has not been sexually active within the last 60 days) when other treatment options are impractical or unsuccessful [53, 54]. The practice is legally permissible in 41 states and potentially allowable in 6 others yet prohibited in 2 states [54]. Clinicians should be familiar with local statutes. The AAP and the SAHM recommend that, as part of an EPT program, providers include materials detailing partner medication indication, instructions, and warnings; offer referral to a local testing center for complete STI evaluation; and review instructions to abstain from sexual intercourse for 7 days after treatment [3, 49].

HIV Prevention

According to recent data from the CDC, individuals aged 20–29 years accounted for the majority of new diagnoses of HIV infection, with more than 40% of new diagnoses of HIV infection in the year 2016 occurring in individuals less than 29 years of age [55]. As such, efforts targeting prevention of HIV infection among this young population are critical. In addition to providing routine counseling on safe sexual practices including proper condom use, providers should be familiar with guidelines for HIV pre-exposure prophylaxis (PrEP) and non-occupational post-exposure prophylaxis (nPEP).

PrEP with a fixed oral dose of tenofovir disoproxil fumarate (TDF) 300 mg and emtricitabine (FTC) 200 mg has been shown to be safe and effective in reducing the risk of sexual acquisition of HIV in adults and has been approved by the Food and Drug Administration for use in individuals at high risk. As discussed in greater detail in Chap. 6, the US Public Health Service and CDC 2014 guidelines recommend PrEP as one prevention option for sexually active adult MSM as well as for adult heterosexually active men and women at substantial risk of HIV acquisition [56]. As described in the STI screening section above, we again advise that "MSM" not be treated as a high-risk group a priori, but rather sexual practices (i.e., unprotected anal receptive sex) and number of partners be used to guide risk assessment. Additionally, it is recommended that PrEP be discussed with heterosexually active men and women whose partners are known to have HIV infection [22].

Though data on the efficacy and safety of PrEP for adolescents are limited, TDF and FTC are approved for use in combination for the treatment of HIV in individuals aged 12 years and older [57]. The CDC recommends careful consideration of the potential risk and benefits of providing PrEP for adolescents under the age of 18 years [22]. Based on the results of a single-arm, open-label clinical trial of HIV-negative individuals 15–17 years of age, the USFDA approved in May 2018 the use of once daily fixed oral dose tenofovir disoproxil fumarate (TDF) 300 mg and emtricitabine (FTC) 200 mg as PrEP among at-risk adolescents weighing at least 35 kg [58]. When prescribing PrEP for sexually active adolescents at high risk for HIV acquisition, providers must be familiar with guidelines for initiation of therapy, lab monitoring and follow-up, and potential adverse effects. Before therapy is prescribed, acute and chronic HIV infection must be excluded by symptom history and HIV testing [22]. Further, it is recommended that patients be followed for HIV infection at least every 3 months and renal function assessed at baseline and at least every 6 months while patients are on PrEP. AYAs may require even closer monitoring to assure compliance. A recent study of the safety and feasibility of antiretroviral PrEP among adolescent MSM aged 15–17 years demonstrated that while approximately one half of subjects achieved protective drug levels during monthly visits, adherence decreased as monitoring moved from monthly to quarterly visits [58]. While several studies have suggested a modest decrease in bone mineral density (BMD) among those prescribed PrEP with TDF/FTC, there is no current recommendation that BMD be monitored for those on therapy [59, 60].

The CDC recommends that health-care providers should evaluate individuals rapidly for nPEP when care is sought <72 hours after a potential non-occupational exposure that presents a substantial risk for HIV acquisition [61]. Providers must include considerations for nPEP when evaluating an individual for sexual assault. Specific recommendations regarding evaluation and management are discussed in greater detail in Chap. 6. Those individuals being offered nPEP should be prescribed a 28-day course of a fixed oral dose of TDF 300 mg and FTC 200 mg *plus* raltegravir (RAL) 400 mg twice daily or dolutegravir (DTG) 50 mg daily, though alternative regimens may be considered depending upon other patient factors [61]. Given ethical considerations, no randomized controlled trials have been conducted to test the efficacy of nPEP directly, and recommendations are therefore based on observational data. As noted previously, TDF/TFC has been approved for use in combination for the treatment of HIV in individuals aged 12 years and older, and DTG is similarly approved for children aged 12 years and older and weighing at least 40 kg [62]. RAL has been approved in combination for the treatment of HIV-1 infection in adult patients but is recommended by the CDC for off-label use as part of this nPEP regimen [61, 63].

Providers offering HIV PrEP and nPEP must be aware of local laws concerning consent, confidentiality, parental disclosure, and reporting requirements to local agencies. While no state expressly prohibits minors' access to PrEP or other HIV prevention methods, laws vary by jurisdiction as to whether consent to preventive or prophylactic services or to HIV or STI services are expressly allowed [64]. Providers considering PrEP for adolescents must include a discussion on confidentiality and consent laws and be familiar with options for confidential treatment including Title X Family Planning Program-funded clinics.

Pregnancy Prevention and Family Planning

Sexual activity is common among adolescents. Based on data from a 2015 survey of US high school students, 41% of adolescents reported having ever had sexual intercourse [65]. Among the 30% reporting having had sexual intercourse in the previous 3 months, 43% did not use a condom the last time they had sex, and 14% did not use any method to prevent pregnancy. Given these data, providers delivering care to AYAs must keep up-to-date on evidence-based best practices for pregnancy prevention and contraceptive effectiveness for adolescents [2]. Importantly, it is recommended by the AAFP, the SAHM, and the AAP that those providers who are unable or uncomfortable in providing comprehensive family planning and pregnancy prevention services to their adolescent and young adult patients identify providers in their communities to whom patients can be referred for such care [1, 2, 66]. Additionally, ACOG stresses that the initiation of sexual and reproductive health care should not be predicated on cervical cancer screening but rather begin at an age and developmental stage appropriate to the individual patient [18]. While a comprehensive discussion of pregnancy prevention and contraception across the lifespan is provided in Chaps. 5 and 17, this chapter which reviews contraceptive and family planning issues most pertinent to the AYA will be discussed. Topics to be discussed include confidentiality and consent, counseling, methods of contraception, and emergency contraception (EC).

Confidentiality and Consent

Data demonstrate that limitations on confidentiality and consent are associated with lower use of contraceptives and higher adolescent pregnancy rates [66]. Therefore, as with other areas of SRH, providers should be familiar with local legislation concerning a minor's right to consent to contraceptive services. Most states have laws explicitly allowing minors to consent to contraceptive services, at least under specific circumstances [67]. Even in those states for which there is no case law, physicians may commonly provide medical care to a mature minor without parental consent, particularly if the state allows a minor to consent to related health services [67]. As discussed previously, providers must consider the potential impact on confidentiality resulting from billing practices and legal requirements regarding the mandated or presumed sending of EOBs as well as parental access to medical record information. As before, minors should be referred as necessary to providers, such as the health department or Title X clinics, who can provide confidential care.

Counseling

The AAFP, the SAHM, and the AAP recommend that providers include counseling about pregnancy prevention and contraceptive effectiveness as part of the routine care of AYAs [1–3]. It is additionally recommended that patients be provided with up-to-date, medically accurate, and evidence-based information in all counseling efforts [1, 2]. While counseling about abstinence and the delay of sexual intercourse is an important part of sexual and reproductive health care for adolescents, such counseling should be given only in the context of providing access to comprehensive sexual health information [2, 3]. In fact, given the data demonstrating the benefits of comprehensive education about both abstinence and contraception as compared with abstinence-only interventions, the SAHM has recommended that "abstinence-only-until marriage" as a basis for adolescent health policy and programs should be abandoned [68]. Finally, parents/guardians should be viewed as potential allies to be involved when feasible in education efforts [1, 3].

Methods of Contraception

More than 80% of adolescent pregnancies are unintended, and recent data reveal that among women having abortions in the United States annually, 10.4% are accounted for by adolescents aged 15–19 years and 32.2% by young adults aged 20–24 years [69]. These data demonstrate the need for health-care providers to be actively engaged in offering nonjudgmental, evidence-based contraceptive services to their adolescent and young adult patients. While a detailed discussion of available methods of contraception will be discussed in greater detail in Chaps. 5 and 17, this section will review several critical points relevant to contraceptive services for the AYA.

Recent data reveal that among women 15–19 years of age who report ever having had sexual intercourse with a male, condoms were the most commonly used method among those reporting ever having used contraception, with 97% reporting ever having used a condom. Among this same population, reporting of "ever use" was 60% for withdrawal, 54% for oral contraceptive pills, 15% for depot medroxyprogesterone acetate (DMPA), 15% for fertility awareness (periodic abstinence), 5% for cervical ring, 3% for intrauterine device (IUD), 2% for transdermal patch, and 2% for hormonal implant [70]. Another survey demonstrates that "ever use" of contraceptive methods, however, does not necessarily correlate with consistent use. This survey found current self-reported use of at least one contraceptive measure among adolescent females aged 15–19 years as 28.2% among those surveyed [71]. Oral contraceptives, used by 15.2% of respondents, was the most commonly preferred method, with 6.4% reporting use of condoms, 2.6% use of 3-month injectable DMPA, and 1.1% or fewer use of any of the following: IUD, hormonal implant, monthly DMPA injection, transdermal patch, contraceptive ring, diaphragm, cervical cap, vaginal condom or pouch, vaginal foam, vaginal sponge, withdrawal, or periodic abstinence. Providers should be aware of these missed opportunities for pregnancy prevention and explore with their patients those barriers to more consistent contraceptive use.

In informing young patients on available options for contraception, it is recommended that providers base counseling on efficacy of typical rather than perfect use among adolescents of each option [66]. As one example, combined oral contraceptives have an increased failure rate among teens as compared to all users, suggesting that adolescent use is not consistent [71]. Additionally, providers are encouraged to counsel adolescents in order of most to least effective options [66]. As patient adherence is the greatest barrier to efficacy of any one contraceptive method, long-acting reversible contraception (LARC) methods, including hormonal implants and IUDs, should be considered first [2, 3]. Despite concerns raised due to complications associated with prior devices, currently available IUDs are not associated with an increased risk of pelvic inflammatory disease beyond a transient increase risk in infection during the first 21 days following device insertion and are, as such, now known to be safe for use in nulliparous AYAs [66]. Use of the DMPA has been associated with reductions in BMD, and the USFDA in 2004 issued a black box warning about this risk [72]. However, it has been subsequently demonstrated that there is a substantial recovery in BMD after discontinuation of DMPA. Based on currently available data, the ACOG has recommended that concerns regarding the effect of DMPA on BMD and potential fracture risk should not prevent practitioners from prescribing DMPA or continuing therapy beyond 2 years [73]. Additionally, the ACOG does not recommend routine bone densitometry monitoring in adolescents and young women using DMPA. However, the ACOG does recommend that patients should be made aware of risks and benefits and be informed of the USFDA "black box" warning as well as be counseled on other contraceptive methods that have no effect on BMD [73]. Further, caution is advisable when considering options for AYAs with other risks for osteoporosis such as metabolic bone disease, anorexia nervosa, chronic alcohol or tobacco use, and chronic use of drugs associated with reduction in bone mass such as corticosteroids and certain anticonvulsants [72]. The AAP suggests that all patients prescribed with DMPA should be counseled about measures that promote skeletal health, such as regular weight-bearing exercise and adequate intake of calcium and vitamin D [66].

Importantly, as many teens who identify as lesbian, gay, bisexual, transgender, or queer (LGBTQ) may have encounters that may not be predicted by their sexual orientation, it is important to ensure pregnancy protection to LGBTQ youth for the body parts they possess (e.g., for a transgender boy who has a uterus) [7]. A recent study of 10,000 New York City high school students showed that sexual minority students who were sexually active were about twice as likely as other students to report becoming pregnant or getting someone pregnant [74].

Providers also should assure that contraceptive services are offered universally to all AYAs, regardless of presence or absence of underlying medical conditions or physical or developmental disabilities. Data reveal that AYAs with chronic health conditions are as or even more likely to engage in high-risk sexual behavior than their healthier peers [75, 76]. Despite this, it has been shown that age- and condition-appropriate contraceptive counseling and education are not routinely provided to this patient population [77, 78]. Prevention of unintended pregnancy may be even more critical among individuals with chronic medical conditions that may be aggravated by pregnancy or in which pregnancy is contraindicated. Additionally, patients who are taking medications with known teratogenicity should be appropriately counseled about the importance of pregnancy prevention. When reviewing contraceptive options with patients, providers must consider safety concerns such as potential medication interactions as well as relative or absolute prescribing contraindications owing to underlying medical conditions. Resources are available to help guide the decision-making of clinicians in such situations. Examples include the 2016 US *Medical Eligibility Criteria for Contraceptive Use* (US MEC) and the World Health Organization *Medical Eligibility Criteria for Contraceptive Use*

(Fifth Edition) [79, 80]. Providers should also be familiar with best practices regarding use of hormonal agents for menstrual management in those patients for whom such management may be indicated for medical or hygienic reasons [81].

Emergency Contraception

As noted previously, teenage sexual activity is common, and rates of unprotected or underprotected intercourse (UPIC) are high. Recent studies have suggested that as many as nearly 1 in 4 adolescents report "ever use" of EC [70]. As such, providers should be knowledgeable about all EC options and comfortable with management of EC for their adolescent and young adult patients. Dosing, timing of dosing relative to UPIC, benefits, risks, and contraindications for each of the available EC options are discussed in greater detail in Chap. 5 on contraception and family planning. In this section, issues pertinent to the care of AYAs will be briefly discussed.

The AAP and the SAHM recommend that all AYAs, regardless of sexual orientation or gender identity, be counseled on EC as part of routine anticipatory guidance in the context of a discussion on sexual and reproductive health [82, 83]. When necessary, families of AYAs with developmental disabilities should additionally receive such counseling to augment the developmental- and age-appropriate information that has been provided to the AYA [66]. As recommended by the AAP, all reproductive health counseling or treatment encounters present an opportunity for education and counseling regarding the use and availability as well as advance prescription of EC wherever these visits occur [82]. The SAHM recommends that adolescents should be instructed to use EC as soon as possible after UPIC and to then schedule a follow-up appointment with their primary provider to address the need for STI testing and ongoing contraception. Indications for use of EC include sexual assault, UPIC (including in the setting of missed or late doses of hormonal contraceptives), and condom breakage or slippage, and EC should be offered when any of these circumstances are reported within the past 120 hours [82, 83].

The SAHM recommends that providers counsel patients about the very high efficacy, independent of patient weight, of the copper IUD for EC [79]. Additionally, it is recommended that those providers who do not insert IUDs have an established relationship with providers who do and prescribe oral EC at the time of referral for IUD insertion [82]. It is recommended that neither testing for pregnancy or STIs nor pelvic examination be required before use of EC and that advanced provision be prescribed/supplied to teenagers for future use regardless of gender identification/orientation [82, 83]. Advanced provision increases the likelihood that teenagers will use EC when needed, reduces the time to use, and does not decrease condom or other contraceptive use [82]. The USFDA ruled in 2013 to make Plan B One-Step (levonorgestrel) available over the counter (OTC) to women of childbearing potential aged 15 years and over who are in need of EC [84]. However, local legislation may limit the direct availability of OTC EC to patients, and providers should be familiar with such legislation and work with patients to eliminate barriers [85].

Finally, providers should be aware of issues pertaining to confidentiality and refer when necessary to sites such as the health department or Title X clinics to assure the provision of confidential care.

Pregnancy and Abortion

According to 2015 United States data, the birth rate was 22.3 per 1000 among women aged 15–24 years and 76.8 per 1000 among women aged 20–24 years [86].

Based on the 2011 data, 42% of pregnancies are unintended, with unintended pregnancy rates being highest among women aged 20–24 years, though actually highest among women aged 15–19 years after estimates are adjusted to include only those individuals who are sexually active [87]. Further, as previously noted, almost half of all abortions in the United States are accounted for by individuals aged 15–24 years. Accordingly, providers caring for adolescent and young adults must be prepared to diagnose, manage, and counsel young patients who are or may potentially be pregnant. While a detailed discussion of such care is beyond the scope of this text, this section will present a few concepts critical to the initial evaluation and management of the pregnant or potentially pregnant AYA. Please see Chap. 30 for additional information on the roles of the primary care clinician in management of pregnant patients in general.

Providers should be alert for symptoms or signs that may suggest pregnancy and not hesitate to pursue testing, having testing readily available, preferably on site [2, 88]. Further, providers should be able to provide or be aware of local and regional resources that provide timely, unbiased options counseling and medical services for teens choosing to continue or terminate a pregnancy [2, 88]. They should additionally offer support to teens in navigating parental consent and notification laws when parental consent is not feasible due to safety or other significant concerns [2]. Clinicians must be familiar with state laws regarding state-mandated counseling, waiting periods, and parental involvement in a minor's abortion [88, 89]. For those AYAs who are pregnant and who wish to continue pregnancy, providers should link them as soon as possible with prenatal care and assure the initiation of therapy with folic acid.

Providers should be familiar with the factors that improve outcomes for adolescent mothers and their children, including but not limited to remaining in school with no subsequent pregnancy at 26 months postpartum, having a sense of control over one's life, experiencing little social isolation, and having only 1 or 2 subsequent lifetime children after the first adolescent pregnancy [90]. As such, healthcare providers should initiate contraceptive counseling, emphasizing LARC, prior to the end of pregnancy and assure timely initiation of contraception when desired [86]. Additionally, providers should help implement a multidisciplinary and comprehensive approach to caring for parenting adolescents, utilizing available community resources that support completion of high school and minimize social isolation [90].

Immunizations

In addressing the sexual and reproductive health needs of AYAs, providers should be familiar with recommendations for immunizations effective against infectious diseases that may be transmitted through sexual contact. Transmission of human papillomavirus (HPV), HAV, and HBV can be effectively prevented through pre-exposure vaccination with widely available vaccines.

As a detailed discussion of immunization schedules, adverse effects, contraindications, and precautions is beyond the scope of this text, the reader is directed to the Advisory Committee on Immunization Practices' (ACIP) most recent recommended immunization schedules for children and adolescents aged 18 years and younger as well as for adults aged 19 years or older [91, 92]. In this section, special considerations will be reviewed. Initiation of routine vaccination against HPV is recommended for all adolescents at 11–12 years, though younger individuals with a history of sexual abuse or assault should begin the HPV immunization series at age 9 years. Though HPV vaccination is not recommended during pregnancy, there is no evidence the vaccine is harmful to the developing fetus and no intervention is needed in cases of inadvertent vaccination. For those adolescents 11–15 years of age who are unvaccinated against HBV, an alternative 2-dose schedule (with adult formulation Recombivax HB only) may be used in catch-up vaccination. Among young adults unvaccinated against HBV, vaccination is recommended for sex partners of hepatitis B surface antigen-positive persons, for sexually active persons not in a mutually monogamous relationship, for every person being evaluated or treated for an STI, and for MSM. As described above, we recommend application of this guideline to "MSM" based on an individualized risk assessment. While routine vaccination against HAV is recommended for all children, previously unvaccinated persons who should be targeted for vaccination include patients who engage in oral-anal sexual contact.

Further, providers should assure that, in the absence of any contraindication, all women of reproductive age be appropriately vaccinated with measles, mumps, and rubella as well as tetanus, diphtheria, and acellular pertussis (Tdap) vaccines. Lastly, providers should be familiar with the recommended immunization schedule for AYAs who are HIV-seropositive.

Cancer Screening

Genital HPV is the most common sexually transmitted infection in the United States. Further, HPV, most commonly HPV types 16 and 18, has been associated with malignancies of the cervix, anus, vulva, vagina, penis, and oropharynx [93]. As previously discussed, HPV vaccination is an important intervention in the prevention of HPV-associated malignancies. Consistent use of condoms and dental dams and limiting one's number of sex partners may also help in disease prevention [41].

Routine screening for infection with HPV or for HPV-associated malignancies is not recommended beyond routine health examinations except for cervical cancer screening, as to be discussed in this section [3].

Cervical Cancer Screening

In the United States, there are approximately 13,000 new cases of and 4100 deaths from cervical cancer annually [94]. The incidence for women less than 20 years of age, however, is extremely low, accounting for only approximately 0.1% of cases of cervical cancer, with a median age of diagnosis of 47 years based on recent data [95]. Additionally, though the majority of sexually active persons become infected with HPV at least once in their lifetime, most young women, especially those younger than 21 years, have an effective immune response that clears the infection in an average of 8 months, and concomitant with infection resolution, most cervical neoplasia also will resolve spontaneously in this population [95, 96]. Consistent with these facts, the ACOG, the American Cancer Society (ACS), and the USPSTF all recommend that regular cervical cancer screening with cervical cytology alone begin at age 21 years, with repeat testing every 3 years; HPV testing for screening is not recommended in those less than 21 years of age [96–98]. These recommendations apply to women at average risk of cervical cancer. This would exclude women with HIV (as discussed in the next paragraph), some cancer survivors (as discussed in Chap. 10), and some solid-organ transplant recipients. Further, these guidelines apply to all individuals with a cervix, regardless of gender identification. A discussion of the management of abnormal screening tests is beyond the scope of this text, though follow-up of abnormal results should be in line with the current recommendations of the professional societies previously referenced.

Women who are HIV-seropositive are a population for whom the above guidelines do not apply. ACOG guidelines and joint recommendations put forth by the CDC, the National Institutes of Health (NIH), and the Infectious Disease Societies of America (IDSA) both state that HIV-infected women less than 30 years of age should have screening with cervical cytology only within 1 year of onset of sexual activity, regardless of the mode of HIV transmission, but no later than 21 years of age. For those women who are found to be HIV positive between the age of 21 and 29 years, screening should occur at the time of initial diagnosis [96, 99]. Though some experts recommend follow-up cytology at 6 months after baseline, each of these guidelines recommend annual screening until three consecutive tests are normal, at which time screening can be moved to every 3 years. As before, a discussion of the management of abnormal screening tests is beyond the scope of this text, though follow-up of abnormal results should be in line with the current recommendations of the professional societies previously referenced. Data reveal missed opportunities for screening among HIV-seropositive women, with as many as nearly 1 in 4 not having had an annual Pap smear based on one recent study [100]. Women whose most recent pelvic exam was not performed at their usual source of HIV care were more likely to have not had screening, underscoring the importance of the role of the primary care clinician in the coordination of care.

Anal Cancer Screening

Anal cancer is a rare disease, with a lifetime risk of developing cancer among both men and women of 0.2%. The incidence, though, has been gradually increasing over the last several decades, with recent estimates of annual incidence of 1.8 per 100,000 persons overall, with 1.5 per 100,000 in men and 2.0 per 100,000 in women [101]. The disease is unusual before the age of 35 years, with the mean age at diagnosis of 61 years [102]. Identified risk factors include infection with HPV, HIV infection, immunosuppression, a history of having multiple sex partners, a history of receptive anal intercourse, a history of smoking, and a history of cancer of lower genital tract neoplasia among women [102]. For populations at high risk (including HIV-seropositive individuals and individuals with a history of receptive anal intercourse), some specialists recommend anal cytologic screening or high-resolution anoscopy, while others recommend annual digital anorectal examination to detect masses that could be anal cancer [99]. However, no existing national recommendations endorse routine screening for anal cancer.

Intimate Partner Violence, Sexual Assault, and Sexual Exploitation

In the care of AYAs, providers must be able to recognize instances of IPV, sexual assault, and sexual exploitation. Additionally, they must be familiar with available interventions and resources to support victims as well as local laws regarding consent and mandated reporting. Though a detailed discussion of these topics is beyond the scope of this text, this section will highlight the magnitude of these problems and present a framework for screening for and managing these issues in adolescent and young adult practices.

Intimate Partner Violence

As defined by the CDC, IPV "includes physical violence, sexual violence, stalking and psychological aggression (including coercive tactics) by a current or former intimate partner," who the CDC specifies as "a person with whom one has a close personal relationship that may be characterized by the partners' emotional connectedness, regular contact, ongoing physical contact and sexual behavior, identity as a couple, and familiarity and knowledge about each other's lives" [103]. Teen dating violence (TDV) is an emerging term that is often used to describe IPV occurring among adolescents.

Results from large, cross-sectional studies have suggested high rates of TDV as well as IPV among young adults. In a study of high school students who dated, 20.9% of females and 10.4% of males reported having experienced some form of TDV during the 12 months before the survey [104]. A US telephone survey of individuals aged 18 years or greater suggested a lifetime prevalence of contact sexual violence, physical violence, or stalking by an intimate partner of 37.3% among females and 30.9% among males [105]. Among victimized individuals, an estimated 71.1% of women and 58.2% of men first experienced these or other forms of IPV before age 25 years, with 23.2% of female victims and 14.1% of male victims reporting first victimization before age 18 years [106]. Although research has largely focused on IPV and TDV among self-described heterosexuals, recent data suggest that lesbian, gay, and bisexual youth may be at even higher risk for all types of dating violence victimization compared to heterosexual youth [107]. There are no data available regarding IPV and TDV specific to transgender and gender nonbinary AYA, so this is an area that warrants investigation.

Given these data, practitioners providing care to AYAs adults should be able to recognize and be prepared to assist in the support and management of victims of IPV. Whether assessment for IPV should occur in a universal or targeted casefinding manner is uncertain. The USPSTF makes a Grade B recommendation [108] that women of childbearing age should be screened for intimate partner violence, such as domestic violence, and provide or refer women who screen positive to intervention services [109]. The ACOG recommends that physicians screen all women for IPV at periodic intervals, including during obstetric care (at the first prenatal visit, at least once per trimester, and at the postpartum checkup), offer ongoing support, and review available prevention and referral options [110]. Though focused on the caregivers of pediatric and adolescent patients rather than adolescent patients themselves, the AAP stated in a recent clinical report that it seems reasonable to incorporate early and repeated questioning regarding IPV as part of anticipatory guidance while remaining mindful of clinical presentations that suggest risk [111]. Such presentations might include suspicious contusions, abrasions, lacerations, or fractures; injuries to the head, neck, chest, and abdomen; injuries during pregnancy; multiple sites of injury; or repeated or chronic injuries. Additionally, individuals might present with chronic pain, frequent visits with vague symptoms or complaints, gynecologic problems such as recurrent STIs, substance use or abuse, anxiety, or depression. As such, AYA presenting with such complaints should be screened for IPV and TDV.

There are a number of well-validated short surveys that are available to screen for IPV. These include but are not limited to HARK (Humiliation, Afraid, Rape, Kick) questions, HITS (Hurts, Insults, Threatens, Screams) questions, and the Woman Abuse Screen Tool (WAST) [112–114]. These instruments may be either verbally (face-to-face) administered or self-administered. One randomized clinical trial noted no difference in identification of IPV when comparing face-to-face with written or computer-based self-assessments but showed that women least preferred face-to-face questioning among the three approaches [115]. Another study evaluating use of computerized questionnaires versus face-to-face screening concluded that study participants recommended that both methods be used together [116]. Regardless of the tools or methods incorporated into practice, screening should be done in a private and safe setting with confidentiality issues and state law mandates for reporting reviewed at the outset. Clinicians should be familiar with laws regarding reporting of IPV. These vary from state to state, but generally fall into four categories: states that require reporting of injuries caused by weapons; states that mandate reporting for injuries caused in violation of criminal laws, as a result of violence, or through non-accidental means; states that specifically address reporting in domestic violence cases; and states that have no general mandatory reporting laws. Reporting requirements may also vary based on the absence or presence of a minor during the violence.

In those cases where IPV is identified, health-care providers should first assess the safety of the patient and their immediate family members as well as help in the development of a safety plan. Assessment for a history of prior IPV, estrangement, perpetrator gun ownership, threats to kill, threats with or use of a weapon, and forced sex should be made, as these are factors that have been associated with intimate partner homicide [117]. It is also important to make AYAs aware of partner behavior that aims to exert control such as limiting involvement with friends, monitoring cell phone use, and stalking/cyberstalking. Adolescent dating violence has been associated with an increase in substance use, depression, poorer educational outcomes, posttraumatic stress, unhealthy weight control, risky sexual behavior, and pregnancy [118, 119]. Providers should be prepared to assess for and manage when noted these comorbidities. Referral to community resources such as domestic violence agencies, mental health services, and social work services should be offered as appropriate. Clinicians should be familiar with resources that can assist in addressing the safety needs of AYAs. These would include but not be limited to smartphone applications such as the "Circle of 6" (https://www.circleof6app.com), a tool that allows for individuals to quickly communicate their safety needs with six trusted individuals by sending automated messages to them via quick icon buttons. Lastly, clinicians should be familiar with local legislation and report cases to the appropriate authorities as mandated [120].

Sexual Assault

Sexual assault is legally defined as any type of sexual contact or behavior that occurs without the explicit consent of the recipient and includes forced sexual intercourse, forcible sodomy, child molestation, incest, fondling, and attempted rape [121]. A 2011 US telephone survey of individuals aged 18 years or greater estimated that

19.3% of women have been raped during their lifetimes, with completed rape first experienced by an estimated 78.7% before age 25 years and an estimated 40.4% before age 18 years [103]. Additionally, an estimated 43.9% of women experienced sexual violence other than rape during their lifetimes. Among men, an estimated 1.7% have been raped and an estimated 23.4% experienced sexual violence other than rape during their lifetimes [103]. Evidence reveals that the majority of sexual assaults involve victims who were incapacitated by drugs or alcohol [122]. Further, studies have shown that two-thirds to three-quarters of adolescent sexual assault victims report the perpetrator was a relative or acquaintance [123, 124]. Providers should be aware that young adults with chronic conditions and disabilities, particularly those with intellectual disabilities, are at a greatly increased risk of sexual assault victimization [125, 126].

For an overview of pediatric sexual abuse, assault and non-accidental trauma, and the impact of intimate partner and domestic violence on children, please see Chap. 1, "Pediatrics." Here we will focus on the adolescent and young adult populations, including where there is medical and legal overlap with the pediatric population. Guidance for the screening, evaluation, and management of sexual assault among adolescents is provided in a recent clinical report from the AAP [127]. This clinical report recommends asking adolescents about exposure to sexual assault as part of a HEADSS (*H*ome, *E*ducation, *A*ctivities, *D*rug use and abuse, *S*exual behavior, *S*uicidality and depression) assessment at routine health supervision visits. In the case of the disclosure by an adolescent of an acute sexual assault, providers should offer care in a supportive and nonjudgmental manner. In addition to gathering pertinent medical and social history, adolescents should be asked about psychological and safety concerns as well as possible sexual exploitation or human traffic victimization (see section "Sexual Exploitation"). In cases in which reporting is not mandatory, patients should be made aware that a forensic evaluation does not require the victim to agree to report or press charges, but the option to do so will be available even after the acute period has passed. For those patients consenting to a forensic evaluation, the examination should be performed by the most qualified health-care provider available, preferably a child abuse specialist. In cases in which drug-facilitated sexual assault is reported or suspected, there should be timely collection of toxicology screens after patient consent. Because standard drug-screening panels do not include date rape drugs, specific testing should be requested in consultation with a toxicologist or state forensic laboratory. Providers additionally should test for pregnancy and offer EC when appropriate, evaluate for STIs and treat when clinically indicated, test for HIV and consider nPEP in accordance with CDC recommendations, test for HBV and hepatitis C virus (HCV), and offer immunizations as indicated for HBV and HPV [128]. Close follow-up should and referral to mental health and community resources should be arranged.

Physical and mental health providers, as mandatory reporters, should be familiar with local legislation and procedures for reporting. This includes instances of sex between an adult and a minor below a certain (formerly and, often still, referred to as statutory rape). Law varies by state, but each state considers legal age of consent, minimum age of the victim, age differential between victim and perpetrator, and minimum age of defendant in order to prosecute [129]. Additionally, for those individuals with intellectual disability, capacity to consent should be evaluated when considering indications for mandated reporting.

Sexual Exploitation

Commercial sexual exploitation of children (CSEC) and sex trafficking of minors are problems gaining increasing attention in recent years. Risk factors for sexual exploitation include a history of abuse or neglect, homelessness, substance misuse or abuse, a history of being involved in the foster care or criminal justice systems, and identifying as LGBTQ [130]. Though prevalence data are difficult to obtain, studies of homeless youth document rates of commercial sexual activity as high as 28% [131]. Minors who have been sexually exploited are at risk for a number of adverse physical and mental health conditions including violence-related injuries, untreated chronic medical conditions, malnutrition, sexual assault, infectious diseases including STIs, pregnancy, substance abuse, depression, anxiety, posttraumatic stress disorder, homicide, and suicidality [132].

Data reveal that minors who have been sexually exploited do seek medical attention, though they are often reluctant to reveal that they have been sexually exploited, often in fear of legal ramifications [132]. In response to this, many states have instituted "safe harbor" laws that provide legal immunity from prosecution for engaging in commercial sex and also require that specialized services such as medical and psychological treatment, emergency and long-term housing, education assistance, job training, language assistance, and legal services be provided to survivors [132, 133]. Providers should be alert for potential indicators of CSEC. A detailed list of such indicators has been compiled by the AAP Committee on Child Abuse and Neglect [132]. When evaluating potential victims, limits of confidentiality should be reviewed, including a discussion of the pediatrician's role as a mandated reporter, and the youth should be made aware that he or she is not required to answer questions. Patients need to be evaluated for safety and carefully assessed for associated physical and mental health conditions. As previously discussed under "Sexual Assault," a forensic evaluation, after obtaining patient consent, should be performed by the most qualified health-care provider available, preferably a child abuse specialist. In considering appropriate follow-up and referrals for suspected cases of CSEC/minor trafficking, providers should be familiar with local laws, including whether their state has enacted "safe harbor" laws. As recommended by the AAP, for assistance in determining how to proceed and to obtain information on relevant laws and reporting recommendations, providers are encouraged to contact organizations focused on the care of such individuals, including but not limited to the National Human Trafficking Resource Center Hotline, the Polaris Project, Shared Hope International, or National Center for Missing & Exploited Children [132].

Care of Sexual and Gender Minority Youth

Clinicians must offer affirming and inclusive care for all patients, regardless of sexual orientation or gender identity. The psychosocial, physical, and emotional well-being of SGMY is negatively impacted by lack of parental support, reported and perceived instances of discrimination, internalized negative messages, and insecurity about identity [134]. These experiences and the health system's ineffective response have created inequities and implications for future health outcomes, which make SGMY a vulnerable population in need of focused health attention. Providers must create a welcoming, supportive, confidential, and nonjudgmental environment for AYAs to talk about their emerging sexual identity and concerns about their sexual activities or feelings. Research shows LGBTQ youth value the opportunity to discuss their gender and sexuality with their primary care provider [135].

Some questions may need to be asked at every visit, as sexual orientation and gender identity can be fluid, especially in adolescents. As previously noted, using gender-neutral language when obtaining a psychosocial history is encouraged. Examples of appropriate use of gender-neutral language are listed in Table 2.3 [136]. Discussing sexuality and gender may be difficult for AYAs, and many struggle with their sexual attractions and identity formation. Some may identify as "questioning," and others might resist identifying with a label [137]. Often, patients delay disclosing their sexuality until the provider has built a trusting relationship with the patient. One study found that only 35% of SGMY reported that their physician knew that they were LGBTQ [138]. When initiating this conversation, it is important that the provider emphasize and practice confidentiality to allow for a more open discussion. It is not the role of the provider to inform parents/guardians about a teenager's sexual or gender identity, as doing so could expose the youth to harm [139].

Providers should assess patients' feelings, safety, and support when counseling about potential disclosures and "coming out." As outlined by the AAP, it is the responsibility of the provider to help adolescents identify their protective factors and strengths and build upon their existing talents [7]. Each person's "coming out" experience is unique and may be a lifelong process. For AYAs, "coming out" can be a high-risk time and expose them to family discord, abuse, and homelessness [140].

Table 2.3 Using gender-neutral terms in the psychosocial history

Heterosexist question	Instead ask
"Do you have a girlfriend?"	"Are you dating anybody?"
	"Are you involved in any romantic relationship?"
"What do you and your boyfriend do together?"	"What do the 2 of you do together?"
	"Tell me about your partner(s)."
"Are you and your girlfriend sexually active?"	"Are you having sex?"
	"Are the 2 of you in a sexual relationship?"

aReproduced from American Academy of Pediatrics, Committee on Adolescence [136]

Even for young adults, disclosing to family members can be dangerous since they may be dependent on their families financially. With this in mind, it is not the role of the provider to force the AYA to "come out," but rather to support the AYA when they feel it is the appropriate time to disclose to others. Another critical role of the provider is to assist parents/guardians of the SGMY. Parental rejection is one of the highest risk factors for suicide among transgender youth [141]. Providers can acknowledge the parents'/guardians' feelings but should provide resources and referral to parental support groups as necessary to foster parental acceptance.

Referral of SGMY for "conversion therapy" or "reparative therapy" is never indicated. The AAP notes that such therapy is not effective and may be harmful to LGBTQ individuals by increasing internalized stigma, distress, and depression [26]. The American Psychological Association's official position is that reparative therapists have not produced any rigorous scientific research to substantiate their claims and these therapists often do more harm than good by increasing stigma and fostering self-hatred [142].

It is important to note that being a SGMY is not abnormal and is not inherently a risk factor for high-risk behaviors or adverse health outcomes. As outlined above, many SGMY experience discrimination and ineffective care from the health-care system. Many of these youths are quite resilient but often are nonetheless impacted by the presence of stigma from homophobia and heterosexism. This can damage the emerging self-image of an LGBTQ AYA and result in psychological distress and an increase in high-risk behaviors. Ostracism, bullying, and parental rejection remain common and can lead to physical and emotional abuse and the possibility of home-lessness. This is often associated with health disparities and may result in poor health outcomes in the areas of mental health, substance abuse, and STIs. Studies show that with the necessary support and guidance, LGBTQ youth are quite resil-ient and are able to develop as adults with sexual and gender identities that are associated with little or no significant increase in high-risk behaviors compared with peers [136].

Women Who Have Sex with Women Youth

Women who have sex with women (WSW) are a diverse group with variations in sexual identity, sexual behaviors, sexual practices, and risk behaviors. When com-pared to heterosexual youth, lesbian and bisexual females are almost 20 times less likely to perceive themselves at risk for STIs but are nearly as likely to have had intercourse, experience twice the rate of pregnancy, and are more likely to have had two or more pregnancies [45]. In light of this data, providers should still counsel WSW youth about available methods of contraception and offer an advanced pre-scription for EC with refills [143]. Condoms should be promoted for use with sex toys and during intercourse and dental dams encouraged for any oral-vaginal or oral-anal contact.

Men Who Have Sex with Men Youth

Providers should base their STI screening recommendations for patients based on sexual activities, not sexual orientation. Unchanged for this population are the CDC annual recommendations for routine HIV screening, syphilis serologic testing, and three-site testing for chlamydia and gonorrhea with urine, pharyngeal, and rectal NAATs (see "Screening for STIs" above) [128].

Conclusion

The provision of SRH to AYAs requires a thoughtful and comprehensive approach, one that should be considered a process rather than a singular event or series of isolated interactions. Providers should be able to deliver SRH education and care services that are inclusive of all sexual orientations, gender identities and expressions, and medical backgrounds and that are developmentally appropriate and culturally sensitive. In so doing, health providers caring for AYAs help assure that their patients are able to successfully navigate this challenging period of physical, mental, emotional, and social development while maintaining the highest possible level of general health and well-being.

References

1. American Academy of Family Physicians. Adolescent health care, sexuality, and contraception. 2017. Available at: https://www.aafp.org/about/policies/all/adolescent-sexuality.html. Accessed 2 Mar 2018.
2. The Society for Adolescent Health and Medicine. Sexual and reproductive health: a position paper of the Society for Adolescent Health and Medicine. J Adolesc Health. 2014;54(4):491–6.
3. Marcell AV, Burstein GR; Committee on Adolescence. Sexual and reproductive health care services in the pediatric setting. Pediatrics. 2017;140(5):87–99.
4. Ford CA, Millstein SG, Halpern-Felsher BL, Irwin CE. Influence of physician confidentiality assurances on adolescents' willingness to disclose information and seek future health care. JAMA. 1997;278(12):1029–34.
5. Lehrer JA, Pantell R, Tebb K, Shafer MA. Forgone health care among U.S. adolescents: associations between risk characteristics and confidentiality concern. J Adolesc Health. 2007;40(3):218–26.
6. Lerand SJ, Ireland M, Boutelle K. Communication with our teens: associations between confidential service and parent-teen communication. J Pediatr Adolesc Gynecol. 2007;20(3):173–8.
7. Hagan JF, Shaw JS, Duncan PM, editors. Bright futures: guidelines for health supervision of infants, children, and adolescents. 4th ed. Elk Grove Village: American Academy of Pediatrics; 2017.
8. Office of Population Affairs. Program requirements for title X funded family planning projects. Washington, D.C.: Department of Health and Human Services; 2014. Available

    at: https://www.hhs.gov/opa/sites/default/files/ogc-cleared-final-april.pdf. Accessed on 21
    Mar 2018.
 9. The Arc of the United States. Position statement-- sexuality. Washington, D.C.: The Arc of
    the United States; 2008. Available at: http://www.thearc.org/who-we-are/position-statements/
    life-in-the-community/sexuality. Accessed 16 Jan 2018.
10. Gutiérrez JP, Torres-Pereda P. Acceptability and reliability of an adolescent behavior
    questionnaire administered with audio and computer support. Rev Panam Salud Publica.
    2009;25(5):418–22.
11. Centers for Disease Control and Prevention. A guide to taking a sexual history. Atlanta; 2006.
    Available at: https://www.cdc.gov/std/treatment/sexualhistory.pdf. Accessed on 25 Mar 2018.
12. Ott MA, Sucato GS; Committee on Adolescence. Technical report: contraception for adoles-
    cents. Pediatrics. 2014;134(4):1257–81.
13. Diamant AL, Schuster MA, McGuigan K, Lever J. Lesbians' sexual history with men: impli-
    cations for taking a sexual history. Arch Intern Med. 1999;159(2):2730–6.
14. Samuel L, Zaritsky E. Communicating effectively with transgender patients. Am Fam
    Physician. 2008;78(5):649–50.
15. Center for AIDS Prevention Studies, University of California San Francisco. Sexual nego-
    tiations among young adults in the era of AIDS. Available at: https://prevention.ucsf.edu/
    uploads/goodquestions/section3/3c6_men.html Accessed on 1 May 2018.
16. Curry ES, Hammer LD, Brown OW, Laughlin JJ, Lessin HR, Simon GR, Rodgers CT;
    Committee on Practice and Ambulatory Medicine. Use of chaperones during the physical
    examination of the pediatric patient. Pediatrics. 2011;127(5):991–3.
17. American Medical Association. Code of medical ethics opinion 1.2.4: use of chaperones.
    Available at: https://www.ama-assn.org/delivering-care/use-chaperones. Accessed on 19
    Mar 2018.
18. The American College of Obstetricians and Gynecologists; Committee on Adolescent Health
    Care. The initial reproductive health visit. Committee Opinion No. 598. Obstet Gynecol.
    2014;123(5):1143–7.
19. Braverman PK, Breech L; Committee on Adolescence. Clincal report – gynecologic exami-
    nation for adolescents in the pediatric setting. Pediatrics. 2010;123(6):583–90.
20. The American College of Obstetricians and Gynecologists. ACOG patient education FAQ,
    "Your first gynecologic visit, especially for teens." Washington, D.C. 2017. Available at:
    https://www.acog.org/Patients/FAQs/Your-First-Gynecologic-Visit-Especially-for-Teens.
    Accessed on 29 Mar 2018.
21. Simpson KM, editor. Table manners and beyond: the gynecological exam for women with
    developmental disabilities and other functional limitations. Oakland: Women's Wellness
    Project; 2001. Available at: http://lurie.brandeis.edu/pdfs/TableMannersandBeyond.pdf.
    Accessed on 21 Mar 2018.
22. Marcell AV, Wibbelsman C, Seigel W; Committee on Adolescence. Clinical report – male
    adolescent sexual and reproductive health care. Pediatrics. 2011;128(6):e1666–76.
23. Society for Adolescent Health and Medicine. The male genital examination: a position paper
    of the Society for Adolescent Health and Medicine. J Adolesc Health. 2012;50(4):425.
24. The United States Preventive Services Task Force. Testicular cancer: screening. Rockville;
    2011. Available at: https://www.uspreventiveservicestaskforce.org/Page/Document/
    UpdateSummaryFinal/testicular-cancer-screening. Accessed 21 Mar 2018.
25. Breuner CC, Mattson G; AAP Committee on Adolescence and Committee on Psychosocial
    Apsects of Child and Family Health. Sexuality education for children and adolescents.
    Pediatrics. 2016;138(2):e1–11.
26. Committee on Adolescence. Policy statement: office-based care for lesbian, gay, bisexual,
    transgender, and questioning youth. Pediatrics. 2013;132(1):198–203.
27. Erickson SJ, Gerstle M, Feldstein SW. Brief interventions and motivational interviewing
    with children, adolescents, and their parents in pediatric health care settings: a review. Arch
    Pediatr Adolesc Med. 2005;159(12):1173–80.

28. Bordini B, Rosenfield RL. Normal pubertal development: part II: clinical aspects of puberty. Pediatr Rev. 2011;32(7):281–92.
29. Kaplowitz PB. Delayed puberty. Pediatr Rev. 2010;31(5):189–95.
30. Peacock A, Alvi NS, Mushtaq T. Period problems: disorders of menstruation in adolescents. Arch Dis Child. 2012;97(6):554–60.
31. Jamieson MA. Disorders of menstruation in adolescent girls. Pediatr Clin N Am. 2015;62(4):943–61.
32. Hoover KW, Tao G, Berman S, Kent CK. Utilization of health services in physician offices and outpatient clinics by adolescents and young women in the United States: implications for improving access to reproductive health services. J Adolesc Health. 2010;46(4):324–30.
33. Marcell AV; Male Training Center for Family Planning and Reproductive Health. Preventive male sexual and reproductive health care: recommendations for clinical practice. Philadelphia: Male Training Center for Family Planning and Reproductive Health; 2014. Available at: http://www.maletrainingcenter.org/wp-content/uploads/2014/09/MTC_White_Paper_2014_V2.pdf. Accessed on 26 Mar 2018.
34. Greydanus DE, Pratt HD, Baxter T. Sexual dysfunction and the primary care physician. Adolesc Med. 1996;7(1):9–26.
35. Bell DL. Adolescent male sexuality. Adolesc Med. 2003;14(3):583–94, vi.
36. Marcell AV. Making the most of the adolescent male health visit. Part 2: the physical exam. Contemp Pediatr. 2006;23(6):38–46.
37. Adelman WP, Joffe A. The adolescent male genital examination: what's normal and what's not. Contemp Pediatr. 1999;16(7):76–92.
38. Lee PA, Houk CP, Ahmed SF, Hughes IA; International Consensus Conference on Intersex organized by the Lawson Wilkins Pediatric Endocrine Society and the European Society for Paediatric Endocrinology. Consensus statement on management of intersex disorders. Pediatrics. 2006;118(2):e488–500.
39. Sanders C, Carter B, Lwin R. Young women with a disorder of sex development: learning to share information with health professionals, friends and intimate partners about bodily differences and infertility. J Adv Nurs. 2015;71(8):1904–13.
40. Nahata L, Quinn GP, Tishelman A. A call for fertility and sexual function counseling in pediatrics. Pediatrics. 2016;137(6). pii: e20160180. https://doi.org/10.1542/peds.2016-0180.
41. Frieden TR, Jaffe HW, Cono J, Richards CL, Iademarco MF; Centers for Disease Control and Prevention. Sexually transmitted diseases treatment guidelines, 2015. Morb Mortal Wkly Rep. 2015;64(3):1–137.
42. Guttmacher Institute. An overview of minors' consent law. New York; 2018. Available at: https://www.guttmacher.org/state-policy/explore/overview-minors-consent-law. Accessed on 2 Mar 2018.
43. Levine J, Gold RB, Nash E, English A. Confidentiality for individuals insured as dependents: a review of state laws and policies. New York; 2012. Available at: https://www.guttmacher.org/report/confidentiality-individuals-insured-dependents-review-state-laws-and-policies. Accessed on 2 Mar 2018.
44. LeFevre M, U.S. Preventive Services Task Force. Behavioral counseling interventions to prevent sexually transmitted infections: U.S. preventive services task force recommendation statement. Ann Intern Med. 2014;161(12):894–901.
45. Saewyc EM, Bearinger LH, Blum RW, Resnick MD. Sexual intercourse, abuse, and pregnancy among adolescent women: does sexual orientation make a difference? Fam Plan Perspect. 1999;31(3):127–31.
46. U.S. Preventive Services Task Force. Final recommendation statement, chlamydia and gonorrhea: screening. Rockville; 2014. Available at: https://www.uspreventiveservices-taskforce.org/Page/Document/RecommendationStatementFinal/chlamydia-and-gonorrhea-screening#consider. Accessed on 2 Mar 2018.

47. Centers for Disease Control and Prevention. Recommendations for the laboratory-based detection of chlamydia trachomatis and Neisseria gonorrhoeae— 2014. MMWR Wkly Rep. 2014;63(RR02):1–19.
48. United States Preventive Services Task Force. Final recommendation statement: human immunodeficiency virus (HIV) infection: screening. Rockville; 2013. Available at: https://www.uspreventiveservicestaskforce.org/Page/Document/RecommendationStatementFinal/human-immunodeficiency-virus-hiv-infection-screening. Accessed 2 Mar 2018.
49. U.S. Preventive Services Task Force. Syphilis infection in pregnancy: screening. Rockville; 2009. Available at: https://www.uspreventiveservicestaskforce.org/Page/Document/ClinicalSummaryFinal/syphilis-infection-in-pregnancy-screening. Accessed on 2 Mar 2018.
50. U.S. Preventive Services Task Force. Screening for syphilis infection in non-pregnant adults and adolescents. JAMA. 2016;315(21):2321–7.
51. U.S. Preventive Services Task Force. Final recommendation statement. Hepatitis B virus infection: screening. Rockville; 2014. Available at: https://www.uspreventiveservicestaskforce.org/Page/Document/RecommendationStatementFinal/hepatitis-b-virus-infection-screening-2014. Accessed on 2 Mar 2018.
52. U.S. Preventive Services Task Force. Final recommendation statement. Genital herpes infection: serologic screening. JAMA. 2016;316(23):2525–30.
53. Society for Adolescent Medicine. Expedited partner therapy for adolescents diagnosed with chlamydia or gonorrhea: a position paper of the Society for Adolescent Medicine. J Adolesc Health. 2009;45(3):303–9.
54. Centers for Disease Control and Prevention. Legal status of expedited partner therapy (EPT). Atlanta; 2017. Available at: https://www.cdc.gov/std/ept/legal/default.htm. Accessed on 7 Mar 2018.
55. Centers for Disease Control and Prevention. HIV surveillance report, 2016, vol. 28. Atlanta; 2017. Available at: http://www.cdc.gov/hiv/library/reports/hiv-surveillance.html. Accessed 8 Mar 2018.
56. U.S. Public Health Service. Preexposure prophylaxis for the prevention of HIV infection in the United States – 2014; A clinical practice guideline. 2014. Available at: https://www.cdc.gov/hiv/pdf/prepguidelines2014.pdf. Accessed on 8 Mar 2018.
57. U.S. Food and Drug Administration. Truvada. Highlights of prescribing information. Silver Spring; 2018. Available at: https://www.accessdata.fda.gov/drugsatfda_docs/label/2018/021752s055lbl.pdf https://www.accessdata.fda.gov/drugsatfda_docs/label/2012/021752s030lbl.pdf. Accessed on 8 Mar 23 May 2018.
58. Hosek SG, Landovitz RJ, Kapogiannis B, et al. Safety and feasibility of antiretroviral pre-exposure prophylaxis for adolescent men who have sex with men aged 15 to 17 years in the United States. JAMA Pediatr. 2017;171(11):1063–71.
59. Mulligan K, Glidden DV, Anderson PL, et al. Effects of Emtricitabine/Tenofovir on bone mineral density in HIV-negative persons in a randomized, double-blind, placebo-controlled trial. Clin Infect Dis. 2015;61(4):572–80.
60. Liu A, Vittinghoff E, Sellmeyer DE, et al. Bone mineral density in HIV-negative men participating in a tenofovir pre-exposure prophylaxis randomized clinical trial in San Francisco. PLoS One. 2011;6(8):e23688.
61. Centers for Disease Control and Prevention. Updated guidelines for antiretroviral post exposure prophylaxis after sexual, injection drug use, or other nonoccupational exposure to HIV— United States, 2016. Atlanta; 2016. Available at: https://www.cdc.gov/hiv/pdf/programresources/cdc-hiv-npep-guidelines.pdf. Accessed on 12 Mar 2018.
62. U.S. Food and Drug Administration. Tivicay. Highlights of prescribing information. Silver Spring; 2013. Available online at: https://www.accessdata.fda.gov/drugsatfda_docs/label/2014/204790s001lbl.pdf. Accessed on 12 Mar 2018.
63. U.S. Food and Drug Administration. Isentress. Highlights of prescribing information. Silver Spring; 2007. Available online at: https://www.accessdata.fda.gov/drugsatfda_docs/label/2011/022145s018lbl.pdf. Accessed on 12 Mar 2018.

64. Culp L, Caucci L. State adolescent consent laws and implications for HIV pre-exposure prophylaxis. Am J Prev Med. 2013;44(1S2):S119–24.
65. Centers for Disease Control and Prevention. Youth risk behavior surveillance— United States, 2015. MMWR Wkly Rep. 2016;65(6):1–174.
66. Committee on Adolescence. Contraception for adolescents. Pediatrics. 2014;134(4):e1244–56.
67. The Guttmacher Institute. Minors' access to contraceptive services. New York; 2018. Available at: https://www.guttmacher.org/print/state-policy/explore/minors-access-contraceptive-services. Accessed on 12 Mar 2018.
68. The Society for Adolescent Health and Medicine. Abstinence-only-until-marriage policies and programs: an updated position paper of the Society for Adolescent Health and Medicine. J Adolesc Health. 2017;61(3):400–3.
69. Jatlaoui TC, Shah J, Mandel MG, et al. Abortion surveillance— United States, 2014. MMWR Surveill Summ. 2017;66(24):1–48.
70. Martinez G, Copen CE, Abma JC. Teenagers in the United States: sexual activity, contraceptive use, and childbearing, 2006-2010 national survey of family growth. Vital Health Stat. 2011;23(31):1–35.
71. Mosher WD, Jones J. Use of contraception in the United States: 1982-2008. Vital Health Stat 23. 2010;(29):1–44.
72. U.S. Food and Drug Administration. Highlights of prescribing information: depo-Provera contraceptive injection. Silver Spring; 2010. Available at: https://www.accessdata.fda.gov/drugsatfda_docs/label/2010/020246s036lbl.pdf. Accessed on 13 Mar 2018.
73. American College of Obstetricians and Gynecologists; Committee on Adolescent Health Care and Committee on Gynecologic Practice. Committee opinion number 602: depot medroxyprogesterone acetate and bone effects. Obstet Gynecol. 2014;123(6):1398–402.
74. Lindley LL, Walsemann KM. Sexual orientation and risk of pregnancy among New York City high-school students. Am J Public Health. 2015;105(7):1379–86.
75. Choquet M, Du Pasquier FL, Manfredi R. Sexual behavior among adolescents reporting chronic conditions: a French national survey. J Adolesc Health. 1997;20(1):62–7.
76. Valencia LS, Cromer BA. Sexual activity and other high-risk behaviors in adolescents with chronic illness: a review. J Pediatr Adolesc Gynecol. 2000;13(2):53–64.
77. Hinze A, Kutty S, Sayles H, Sandene EK, Meza J, Kugler JD. Reproductive and contraceptive counseling received by adult women with congenital heart disease: a risk-based analysis. Congenit Heart Dis. 2013;8(1):20–31.
78. Vigl M, Kaemmerer M, Seifert-Klauss V, et al. Contraception in women with congenital heart disease. Am J Cardiol. 2010;106(9):1317–21.
79. Curtis KM, Tepper NK, Jatlaoui TC, et al. U.S. medical eligibility criteria for contraceptive use, 2016. MMWR Recomm Rep. 2016;65(RR-3):1–104.
80. Berry-Bibee E, Curtis K, Dragoman M, et al. Medical eligibility criteria for contraceptive use. Fifth ed. Geneva: The World Health Organization; 2015. Available at: http://apps.who.int/iris/bitstream/10665/181468/1/9789241549158_eng.pdf. Accessed on 19 Mar 2018.
81. Quint EH. Adolescents with special needs: clinical challenges in reproductive health care. J Pediatr Adolesc Gynecol. 2016;29(1):2–6.
82. Committee on Adolescence. Policy statement: emergency contraception. Pediatrics. 2012;130(6):1174–82.
83. The Society of Adolescent Health and Medicine. Position paper: emergency contraception for adolescents and young adults: guidance for health care professionals. J Adolesc Health. 2016;58(2):245–8.
84. Center for Drug Evaluation and Research, United States Food and Drug Administration. Approval package for: Application number: NDA 021998/S-002. Silver Spring; 2013. Available at: https://www.accessdata.fda.gov/drugsatfda_docs/nda/2013/021998Orig1s002.pdf. Accessed on 15 Mar 2018.

85. The Guttmacher Institute. Emergency contraception. New York; 2018. Available at: https://www.guttmacher.org/state-policy/explore/emergency-contraception. Accessed on 15 Mar 2018.
86. Martin JA, Hamilton BE, Osterman MJK, Driscoll AK, Mathews TJ. Births: final data for 2015. National vital statistics report. Atlanta: National Center for Health Statistics; 2017. 66(1). Available at: https://www.cdc.gov/nchs/data/nvsr/nvsr66/nvsr66_01.pdf. Accessed on 15 Mar 2018.
87. The Guttmacher Institute. Fact sheet: unintended pregnancy in the United States. New York; 2016. Available at: https://www.guttmacher.org/fact-sheet/unintended-pregnancy-united-states#8. Accessed on 15 Mar 2018.
88. Hornberger LL; Committee on Adolescence. Clinical report: diagnosis of pregnancy and providing options counseling for the adolescent patient. Pediatrics. 2017;140(3):e20172273.
89. The Guttmacher Institute. An overview of abortion laws. New York; 2018. Available at: https://www.guttmacher.org/state-policy/explore/overview-abortion-laws. Accessed on 15 Mar 2018.
90. Pinzon JL, Jones VF, Committee on Adolescence and Committee on Early Childhood. Care of adolescent parents and their children. Pediatrics. 2012;130(6):e1743–56.
91. Advisory Committee on Immunization Practices. Recommended immunization schedule for children and adolescents aged 18 years or younger, United States, 2018. Atlanta: Centers for Disease Control and Prevention; 2018. Available at: https://www.cdc.gov/vaccines/schedules/hcp/child-adolescent.html. Accessed on 27 Feb 2018.
92. Advisory Committee on Immunization Practices. Recommended immunization schedule for adults aged 19 years or older, United States, 2018. Atlanta: Centers for Disease Control and Prevention; 2018. Available online at: https://www.cdc.gov/vaccines/schedules/hcp/adult.html. Accessed on 27 Feb 2018.
93. Cogliano V, Baan R, Straif K, Grosse Y, Secretan B, El Ghissassi F; WHO International Agency for Research on Cancer. Carcinogenicity of human papillomaviruses. Lancet Oncol. 2005;6(4):204.
94. U.S. Cancer Statistics Working Group. United States cancer statistics: 1999–2014 incidence and mortality web-based report. Atlanta: Department of Health and Human Services, Centers for Disease Control and Prevention, and National Cancer Institute; 2017. Available at: http://www.cdc.gov/uscs. Accessed on 28 Feb 2018.
95. Viens LJ, Henley SJ, Watson M, et al. Human papillomavirus-associated cancers—United States, 2008-2012. MMWR Wkly Rep. 2016;65(26):661–6.
96. American College of Obstetricians and Gynecologists. Practice bulletin no. 168: cervical cancer screening and prevention. Obstet Gynecol. 2016;128(4):e111–30.
97. Saslow D, Solomon D, Lawson HW, et al.; American Cancer Society; American Society for Colposcopy and Cervical Pathology; American Society for Clinical Pathology. American Cancer Society, American Society for Colposcopy and Cervical Pathology, and American Society for Clinical Pathology screening guidelines for the prevention and early detection of cervical cancer. Am J Clin Pathol. 2012;137(4):516–42.
98. Moyer VA; U.S. Preventive Services Task Force. Screening for cervical cancer: U.S. preventive services task force recommendation statement. Ann Intern Med. 2012;156(12):880–91.
99. Panel on Opportunistic Infections in HIV-Infected Adults and Adolescents. Guidelines for the prevention and treatment of opportunistic infections in HIV-infected adults and adolescents: recommendations from the Centers for Disease Control and Prevention, the National Institutes of Health, and the HIV Medicine Association of the Infectious Diseases Society of America. Available at: https://aidsinfo.nih.gov/contentfiles/lvguidelines/adult_oi.pdf. Accessed on 18 Mar 2018.
100. Oster AM, Sullivan PS, Blair JM. Prevalence of cervical cancer screening of HIV-infected women in the United States. J Acquir Immune Defic Syndr. 2009;51(4):430–6.
101. National Cancer Institute. SEER cancer statistics fact sheet: anal cancer. Bethesda; 2014. Available at: https://seer.cancer.gov/statfacts/html/anus.html. Accessed 1 Mar 2018.

102. American Cancer Society. Key statistics for anal cancer. Atlanta; 2017. Available at: https://www.cancer.org/cancer/anal-cancer/about/what-is-key-statistics.html. Accessed on 1 Mar 2018.
103. Breiding MJ, Basile KC, Smith SG, Black MC, Mahendra RR. Intimate partner violence surveillance: uniform definitions and recommended data elements, version 2.0. Atlanta: National Center for Injury Prevention and Control, Centers for Disease Control and Prevention; 2015. Available at: https://www.cdc.gov/violenceprevention/pdf/intimatepartnerviolence.pdf. Accessed on 18 Feb 2018.
104. Vagi KJ, Olsen EO, Basile KC, Vivolo-Kantor AM. Teen dating violence (physical and sexual) among US high school students: findings from the 2013 National Youth Risk Behavior Survey. JAMA Pediatr. 2015;169(5):474–82.
105. Smith SG, Chen J, Basile KC, et al. The national intimate partner and sexual violence survey (NISVS): 2010–2012 state report. Atlanta: National Center for Injury Prevention and Control, Centers for Disease Control and Prevention; 2017. Available at: https://www.cdc.gov/violenceprevention/pdf/NISVS-StateReportBook.pdf. Accessed on 18 Feb 2018.
106. Breiding MJ, Smith SG, Basile KC, et al. Prevalence and characteristics of sexual violence, stalking, and intimate partner violence victimization — National Intimate Partner and Sexual Violence Survey, United States, 2011. MMWR. 2014;63(SS08):1–18.
107. Dank M, Lachman P, Zweig JM, Yahner J. Dating violence experiences of lesbian, gay, bisexual, and transgender youth. J Youth Adolesc. 2014;43(5):846–57.
108. The USPSTF recommends the service. There is high certainty that the net benefit is moderate or there is moderate certainty that the net benefit is moderate to substantial.
109. U.S. Preventive Services Task Force. Final update summary: intimate partner violence and abuse of elderly and vulnerable adults: screening. Rockville; 2016. Available at: https://www.uspreventiveservicestaskforce.org/Page/Document/UpdateSummaryFinal/intimate-partner-violence-and-abuse-of-elderly-and-vulnerable-adults-screening. Accessed on 2 Feb 2018.
110. Committee on Health Care for Underserved Women. Committee opinion-- intimate partner violence. Washington, D.C.: The American College of Obstetricians and Gynecology; 2012. (Number 518). Available at: https://www.acog.org/Clinical-Guidance-and-Publications/Committee-Opinions/Committee-on-Health-Care-for-Underserved-Women/Intimate-Partner-Violence. Accessed on 16 Feb 2018.
111. Thackeray JD, Hibbard R, Dowd MD; The Committee on Child Abuse and Neglect, and the Committee on Injury, Violence, and Poison Prevention. Clinical report – intimate partner violence: the role of the pediatrician. Pediatrics. 2010;125(5):1094–100.
112. Sohal H, Eldridge S, Feder G. The sensitivity and specificity of four questions (HARK) to identify intimate partner violence: a diagnostic accuracy study in general practice. BMC Fam Pract. 2007;8:49.
113. Sherin KM, Sinacore JM, Li XQ, Zitter RE, Shakil A. HITS: a short domestic violence screening tool for use in a family practice setting. Fam Med. 1998;30(7):508–12.
114. Brown JB, Lent B, Brett PJ, Sas G, Pederson LL. Development of the Woman Abuse Screening Tool for use in family practice. Fam Med. 1996;28(6):422–8.
115. MacMillan HL, Wathen CN, Jamieson E, et al.; McMaster Violence Against Women Research Group. Approaches to screening for intimate partner violence in health care settings: a randomized trial. JAMA. 2006;296(5):530–6.
116. Chang JC, Dado D, Schussler S, et al. In person versus computer screening for intimate partner violence among pregnant patients. Patient Educ Couns. 2012;88(3):443–8.
117. Campbell JC, Glass N, Sharps P, Laughon K, Bloom T. Intimate partner homicide: review and implications of research and policy. Trauma Violence Abuse. 2007;8(3):246–69.
118. Silverman JG, Raj A, Clements K. Dating violence and associated sexual risk and pregnancy among adolescent girls in the United States. Pediatrics. 2004;114(2):e220–5.
119. Holmes K, Sher L. Dating violence and suicidal behavior in adolescents. Int J Adolesc Med Health. 2013;25(3):257–61.

120. Durborow N, Lizdas KC, O'Flaherty AO, Marjavi A; Family Violence Prevention Fund. Compendium of state statutes and policies on domestic violence and health care. Washington, D.C.: The Administration for Children and Families, Administration on Children, Youth, and Families, U.S. Department of Health and Human Services; 2010. Available at: https://www. acf.hhs.gov/sites/default/files/fysb/state_compendium.pdf. Accessed on 18 Feb 2018.
121. The United States Department of Justice. Sexual assault. Washington, D.C.; 2017. Available online at https://www.justice.gov/ovw/sexual-assault#sa. Accessed on 16 Feb 2018.
122. Senn CY, Eliasziw M, Barata PC, Thurston WE, Newby-Clark IR, Radtke HL, Hobden KL, SARE Study Team. Sexual violence in the lives of first-year university women in Canada: no improvements in the 21st century. BMC Womens Health. 2014;14:135.
123. Muram D, Hostetler BR, Jones CE, Speck PM. Adolescent victims of sexual assault. J Adolesc Health. 1995;17(6):372–5.
124. Peipert JF, Domagalski LR. Epidemiology of adolescent sexual assault. Obstet Gynecol. 1994;84(5):867–71.
125. Nixon M, Thomas SDM, Daffern M, Ogloff JRP. Estimating the risk of crime and victimization in people with intellectual disability: a data-linkage study. Soc Psychiatry Psychiatr Epidemiol. 2017;52(5):617–26.
126. Suris JC, Resnick MD, Cassuto N, Blum RW. Sexual behavior of adolescents with chronic disease and disability. J Adolesc Health. 1996;19(2):124–31.
127. Crawford-Jakubiak JE, Alderman EM, Leventhal JM, Committee on Child Abuse and Neglect, Committee on Adolescence. Care of the adolescent after an acute sexual assault. Pediatrics. 2017;139(3):e20164243.
128. Centers for Disease Control and Prevention. 2015 sexually transmitted diseases treatment guidelines: sexual assault and abuse and STDs. Atlanta; 2015. Available at: www.cdc.gov/ std/tg2015/sexual-assault.htm. Accessed on 18 Feb 2018.
129. U.S. Department of Health and Human Services. Statutory rape: a guide to state Laws and reporting requirements. Washington, D.C.; 2014. Available at: https://aspe.hhs.gov/report/ statutory-rape-guide-state-laws-and-reporting-requirements. Accessed 18 Feb 2018.
130. Clayton EW, Krugman RD, Chaffee T, Diaz A, English A, et al.; Institute of Medicine and National Research Council of the National Academies. Confronting commercial sexual exploitation and sex trafficking of minors in the United States: a guide for the health care sector. Washington, D.C.; 2014. Available at: http://www.nationalacademies.org/hmd/~/media/ Files/Resources/SexTrafficking/guideforhealthcaresector.pdf/. Accessed on 19 Feb 2018.
131. Greene JM, Ennett ST, Ringwalt CL. Prevalence and correlates of survival sex among runaway and homeless youth. Am J Public Health. 1999;89(9):1406–9.
132. Greenbaum J, Crawford-Jakubiak JE, Committee on Child Abuse and Neglect. Child sex trafficking and commercial sexual exploitation: health care needs of victims. Pediatrics. 2015;135(3):567–74.
133. American Bar Association, Commission on Youth at Risk. Child trafficking. Chicago; 2011. Available at: http://www.americanbar.org/groups/youth_at_risk/commission_policyresolu- tions/child_trafficking.html. Accessed on 19 Feb 2018.
134. Higa D, Hoppe MJ, Lindhorst T, et al. Negative and positive factors associated with the wellbeing of lesbian, gay, bisexual, transgender, queer, and questioning (LGBTQ) youth. Youth Soc. 2014;46:663–87.
135. Hoffman ND, Freeman K, Swann S. Healthcare preferences of lesbian, gay, bisexual, transgender and questioning youth. J Adolesc Health. 2009;45(3):222–9.
136. Levine DA; AAP Committee on Adolescence. Technical report: office-based care for lesbian, gay, bisexual, transgender, and questioning youth." Pediatrics. 2013;132(1):198–203.
137. Spigarelli MG. Adolescent sexual orientation. Adolesc Med State Art Rev. 2007;18(3):508–18, vii.
138. Meckler GD, Elliott MN, Kanouse DE, Beals KP, Schuster MA. Nondisclosure of sexual orientation to a physician among a sample of gay, lesbian, and bisexual youth. Arch Pediatr Adolesc Med. 2006;160(12):1248–54.

139. Arreola S, Neilands T, Pollack L, Paul J, Catania J. Childhood sexual experiences and adult health sequelae among gay and bisexual men: defining childhood sexual abuse. J Sex Res. 2008;45(3):246–52.
140. Cianciotto J, Cahill S. Education policy: issues affecting lesbian, gay, bisexual, and transgender youth. New York: The National Gay and Lesbian Task Force Policy Institute; 2003. Available at: http://www.thetaskforce.org/static_html/downloads/reports/reports/EducationPolicy.pdf. Accessed on 29 Mar 2018.
141. Klein A, Golub S. Family rejection as a predictor of suicide attempts and substance misuse among transgender and gender nonconforming adults. LGBT Health. 2016;3(3):193–9.
142. Anton BS. Proceedings of the American Psychological Association for the legislative year 2009: resolution on appropriate affirmative responses to sexual orientation distress and change efforts. Am Psychol. 2010;65(5):385–475.
143. Herrick AL, Matthews AK, Garofalo R. Health risk behaviors in an urban sample of young women who have sex with women. J Lesbian Stud. 2010;14(1):80–92.

Chapter 3
Sexual and Reproductive Health for Adults

Joan Bosco, Kevin Yan, and Jose Cortes

Contents

J. Bosco
Icahn School of Medicine at Mount Sinai, New York, NY, USA

Division of General Internal Medicine, Department of Medicine at Mount Sinai Beth Israel, New York, NY, USA
e-mail: Joan.Bosco@mountsinai.org

K. Yan
Icahn School of Medicine at Mount Sinai, New York, NY, USA

Division of General Internal Medicine, Department of Medicine at Mount Sinai West and Mount Sinai Morningside), New York, NY, USA
e-mail: Kevin.Yan@mountsinai.org

J. Cortes (✉)
Icahn School of Medicine at Mount Sinai, New York, NY, USA

© Springer Nature Switzerland AG 2022
J. Truglio et al. (eds.), *Sexual and Reproductive Health*,
https://doi.org/10.1007/978-3-030-94632-6_3

Introduction

Sexual and reproductive health (SRH) is a critical yet often averted component of the overall health of adults. Talking about sexual and reproductive health can be difficult both for the patient and the healthcare provider – due to apprehension, feeling unprepared, embarrassment, and time constraints. In some surveys, as few as 35% of primary care physicians report they often or always take a sexual history [1]. These findings have been consistent on other medical specialties. In a 2012 survey of US obstetrician and gynecologists, only 40% of the surveyed physicians routinely ask about sexual health [2]. On the other hand, patients do want to talk about their SRH concerns with their healthcare providers. Surveys have found that two-thirds (73%) of patients do want to discuss their sexual concerns as they find them important to their overall health/wellness and would prefer their health provider bring up the sexual health topic [3]. In contrast, 74% of providers rely on their patients to initiate a discussion about sexual health [4].

This chapter will address the approach to obtaining a sexual health history, common sexual health issues in adults, and the care of sexual and gender minority adults. For this chapter, we define adults as those age 18–65 years of age.

The Sexual and Reproductive Health Visit for Adults

Confidentiality and Consent

Confidentiality and consent are the cornerstones to building trust with a patient, particularly when we seek sensitive personal sexual history information. Open, transparent, and honest communication is essential to achieving a trusting clinician-patient relationship. Patients need to be able to trust that clinicians will protect information shared in confidence during their interaction, particularly their sexual history. Patients should feel they can fully disclose sensitive personal information to enable their healthcare provider to most effectively provide needed services. Healthcare providers are bound by ethical standards to preserve the confidentiality of information gathered in association with the care of the patient. The knowledge and promise of confidentiality cement the trust patients place on healthcare workers.

In general, clinicians should ensure patients of the confidentiality of the information they discuss. There are limited exceptions to confidentiality, many of which vary by state. For example, intimate partner violence (IPV) is generally not reportable without the consent of the survivor; however, some states have mandated reporting laws for all cases of IPV, cases involving certain weapons, or cases in which children are present and witness the violence. Clinicians should be aware of the laws regarding confidentiality and mandated reporting where they practice and inform patients of any limitations to confidentiality at the start of the history.

As will be discussed below, confidentiality also mandates that the sexual history is conducted without other family members, caregivers, or partners in the room. However, there may be clinical scenarios in which caregivers participate in the sexual and reproductive health decisions of patients, including but not limited to adults with specific developmental delays, severe mental illness, or cognitive impairments, depending on the severity of each condition. Developmental delay and cognitive impairment are discussed in more detail in Chap. 11.

History Taking

Despite the central role of sexual and reproductive health in the overall care of a patient, many clinicians feel unprepared to obtain an effective sexual history. In a 2003 study of 200 primary care physicians in Belgium, almost 1 in 5 physicians responded that they regularly felt uncomfortable taking a sexual history, and 30.6% were worried that questions about sexually transmitted infections (STIs) would be considered intrusive by their patients [5]. A 2012 survey of 1154 American obstetricians and gynecologists showed that only 40% routinely asked about sexual problems, with even fewer asking about sexual satisfaction (28.5%), sexual orientation/identity (27.7%), or pleasure (13.8%) [6].

Before taking a sexual history, it is essential to create an environment of confidentiality and trust. History taking should take place in a private setting with limited distractions or interruptions. Many patients come to their appointments with other people, be it a family member, spouse, or partner. While a 2002 study characterizing patient accompaniment to medical appointments actually found that physicians and patients both largely felt that having a companion at the appointment favorably influenced patient and physician understanding [7], the situation becomes a bit more difficult to navigate in terms of discussing more sensitive issues such as sexual history. While the literature on this is scarce, a 2007 article from a publication of the American Academy of Family Physicians (AAFP) broaches the topic, emphasizing "thoughtful assessment of the situation and mindfulness of the patient's needs." It is important to discuss with the patient alone whether or not they want their companion in the exam room and, if the patient wants the companion to be present, to "consider this request in light of the situation at hand." For example, is the patient agreeable to allowing the companion to be present at the visit due to fear of later repercussions from the companion if he or she is not allowed to partake in the visit? Are there cultural or religious reasons why the companion must be present? One potential compromise is to allow the companion in the room for the discussion but not for the exam. Regardless, with a companion in the exam room, the provider should still speak directly to the patient, avoid taking sides in any conflict, and assess all parties' understanding of the management plan [8].

The provider should "set the stage" by emphasizing that sexual history questions are a part of the overall history and are asked of all patients. Clinicians can develop their own style or routine of transitioning to the sexual history. While there is no "one-size-fits-all" approach to the sexual history, the below framework can be modified to nearly any clinical situation. The basic principles of this approach (see Table 3.1 for examples of language to use) are (1) ask permission, (2) give permission, (3) ensure confidentiality, (4) make no assumptions, (5) stay non-judgmental, (6) use inclusive terminology, (7) be professional, and (8) understand your own biases.

The first principal, "asking permission" to discuss sexual health with the patient, creates an environment of mutual respect between patient and provider and lets the patient engage in a conversation that is well within his or her level of comfort. "Giving permission" ensures the patient that questions about or concerns regarding their sexual health are welcome, now or in the future. "Ensuring confidentiality" will further put the patient at ease. "Making no assumptions" about a patient's sexual orientation, gender identity, gender expression, or sexual practices is essential for developing open and honest dialogue between the provider and patient, as is "staying non-judgmental" by avoiding the use of descriptive terms like "wrong," "bad," "promiscuous," or "sleep around" to describe behaviors. Using neutral and "inclusive terminology" such as "partner" rather than "boyfriend/girlfriend" and mirroring the patient's own language and terminology again creates a trusting environment and nourishes the therapeutic relationship. "Being professional" and "understanding your own biases" are essential steps for effective communication. For example, taking some time to think about how one might respond if he or she learns a patient has same-sex partners or identifies as lesbian, gay, bisexual, or transgender (LGBT) can help the provider become more comfortable discussing these issues and maintain a consistent level of professionalism by taking inventory and ownership of his or her own feelings and biases.

There are several established models in place to help guide providers in beginning to take a sexual history. The CDC proposes the "5 P's" [9] as a way to jump into an initial risk assessment: partners (number of, preferred genders), practices (such as exchanging sex for money or drugs, using substances while having sex, specific sexual practices), past history of sexually transmitted infections (STIs), protection from STIs (what is the patient doing to protect himself against infection?), and pregnancy plans. To these "5 P's" we add "pronouns" to discuss a patient's gender identity if not already done at the start of the encounter, "patient concerns" to center the discussion around what is most pressing for the patient, and "parts" to ensure an inclusive history that affirms a patient's understanding of and language used to describe their sex organs. Table 3.2 "The 6 P's" provides some sample language for each of these domains.

Table 3.1 Basic principles of an effective sexual history

Basic principle	Sample language
Ask permission:	"Sexual health is paramount to overall health, I always ask my patients about their sexual history. If it's ok, I would like to ask some questions about your sexual health."
Give permission:	Using open-ended questions gives the patient permission to talk about their sexual concerns. State that any and every question is valid and it should be asked by the patient any time deemed necessary
Ensure confidentiality[a]	"I am going to ask you a few personal questions about your life including sexual history. I ask these questions at least once a year of all my patients because they are vital for your overall health. Everything you tell me is confidential*. Your medical history will not be shared it with anyone without your permission. Do you have any questions or concerns before we start?"
Make no assumptions	Ask about patient's sexual orientation, and use the terms such as partner instead of boyfriend, girlfriend, etc. "Are you sexually active?" "What are the genders of your sexual partners?" "Do you have a partner, significant other, or spouse?" or "Are you currently in a relationship? What do you call your partner?"
Stay non-judgmental	Avoid asking questions in a way that implies there is a right or wrong answer, such as: "Do you always use condoms?" or "You don't have partners outside your marriage, do you?" Instead, open-ended questions that are specific to the health impact of behaviors: "How often do you use condoms?" or "How many partners do you have?"
Use inclusive terminology	Instead of: "Do you have a wife/husband or boy/girlfriend?" Ask: "Do you have a partner?" or "Are you in a relationship?" "What do you call your partner?" Pay attention to the descriptors your patients use to talk about themselves and their partners and try to use the same words (if you feel comfortable using them). If you don't understand something they have said, ask them to explain
Be professional	It is essential not to let your beliefs interfere with providing the best care. Check your nonverbal communication clues such as posture, facial expressions, etc. – you may be sending unintended nonverbal messages. For example, are you shaking your head "no"? Are you rolling your eyes? Are you maintaining eye contact? If you ever slip up or use the wrong term, practice professional humility by asking the patient for guidance in understanding. "Please help me understand…"
Understand your own biases	It takes time and practice to feel completely comfortable communicating with patients about their sexual health, identities, and behaviors. Part of the process of becoming comfortable is taking inventory of your own biases or preconceived ideas. What stereotypes do you carry? Negative feelings? Try to be honest about your feelings and reactions. Explore them and evaluate how they might impact your ability to care for all patients

[a]Exceptions to the rule of confidentiality discussed above in the "Confidentiality and Consent" section

Table 3.2 "The 6 P's"

"P"	Sample language
Pronouns (gender identity)	"How would you describe your current gender? What sex were you assigned at birth?" "What pronouns do you use? For example I use he, him and his."
Patient concerns	"Before I get started, do you have any concerns around your sexual health you would like us to address today?"
Partners	"What are the genders of your sexual partners?" "How many partners have you had in the past year? What were their genders?"
Practices/parts	"So I can provide the best possible care, what parts (organs) do you have? What do you call your parts? Are those the names you would like me to use?" "What sexual practices do you participate in? What types of sex do you have? What does that mean to you?"
Protection from/past history of sexually transmitted infections	"Have you ever been told that you had a sexually transmitted infection in the past?" "What kind of things are you doing now to lower your risk of getting an infection from sex?"
Pregnancy plans	"Are you currently trying to become pregnant?" "What concerns do you have about yourself or your partner becoming pregnant?" "What information can I provide you with regarding birth control/contraceptive options?"

The National LGBT Health Education Center recommends asking three key screening questions and then adapting your discussion from there based on the patients' responses and overall risk: (a) Have you been sexually active in the past year? (b) What are the genders of your sexual partners? and (c) How many people have you slept with in the past year? (including a gender breakdown) [10].

After the initial screening questions are asked, more detailed questioning can take place based on the patients' responses [10]. For example, patients who endorse multiple partners or a new partner should be asked about protection from STIs and STI history, while a patient who endorses a long-term monogamous partner may benefit more from questions about pregnancy/reproductive plans and general sexual function/satisfaction (although these questions are not always exclusive to one group and should be asked of all patients as appropriate). A patient who is not sexually active should still be asked about past partners and overall questions/concerns. Questions appropriate for most patients include history of substance use as well as trauma/violence.

Getting into specific practices (the second "P" of the CDC's "5 P's") is a crucial part of the sexual history. The key is asking these questions in a conversational and open-ended manner (e.g., "What kind of sex are you having?" rather than "You don't practice anal sex, do you?") [10]. This gives the patient a chance to explain what kind of sex they are engaging in (anal, oral, vaginal, etc.) and open the door for asking about other practices such as sharing sex toys. This can also be the opportunity to ask about substance use or exchanging sex for drugs, commodities, or money. In this case, direct, simple questions are often the most effective. ("Have you or any of your partners ever received or given money, shelter, or drugs for sex?") See Table 3.3 for additional questions that could be asked if a basic history is positive.

Table 3.3 Comprehensive sexual history questions

Topic	Additional questions [11]
Sexual orientation	How do you self-identify your sexual orientation? What have been the genders of your sexual partners? What are the genders of your current sexual partners? Do you have any questions or concerns about your sexual orientation?
Sexuality	How important is sexuality in your life? Toward whom are your sexual attractions directed? Are you happy with your sexual life right now? What would make things better? How is your medical illness/health affecting your sexuality?
STI risk	Have you ever been told you had a sexually transmitted infection? Have you ever been diagnosed/told you had HIV? (Review other STIs as well) Have any of your partners ever been told they had an STI? What do you do to prevent STIs when you have sex? (Can follow up with more detailed questioning re frequency of use of barrier protection with different types of sex, adherence to pre-exposure prophylaxis for HIV, etc. as indicated). How many total sexual partners have you had in your life? Have you ever had sex for money, food, or housing? Have you ever paid anyone for sex?
Sexual functioning	What types of sexual activities do you participate in? Do you have any difficulties or problems with any of these activities: libido, arousal, erectile functioning, vaginal dryness, pain with intercourse, orgasm? How long have you struggled with this issue? Do you always have the problem or is it situational? Other ways of expressing sexuality
Sexual abuse	Has anyone ever touched you sexually or forced you to have sex when you didn't want to? Assess safety of current situation (see section below on IPV)

Physical Exam

The physical examination serves as an opportunity for primary care providers to promote sexual and reproductive health by educating patients about anatomy, function, and health maintenance. Office policies regarding the presence of appropriate chaperones must always be followed prior to the initiation of any breast or genital examination. Every effort should be made to maintain patient safety, comfort, dignity, and autonomy during examination.

Becoming familiar with your exam room and its resources helps ensure an efficient office visit and is one of the most important steps for any new provider or providers who are less comfortable with performing genital exams. This includes familiarity and comfort with the operation of tools such as adjustable lights, speculums, and footrests. Additionally, have quick and easy access to resources such as patient gowns, examination lubricants or jellies, and diagnostic swabs.

As with any type of physical examination, communication is key. Remember that patients' knowledge of and comfort with their bodies can vary greatly. Prior to starting examination, first inform the patient which exams you plan to perform and the reasons for performing them. This helps to alleviate patient discomfort by allowing them to anticipate your actions and creating an opportunity for questions to be asked, which is particularly important if patients are not familiar with the exams or procedures you will be performing. Likewise, it is best to avoid the overuse of medical terminology and to adopt patients' terms when possible. This will help facilitate patient understanding during examination and comprehension when educating patients regarding anatomy and function.

Remember that a genitourinary exam is part of an annual comprehensive physical exam, and it is also indicated when patients present with genital symptoms such as dysuria, vaginal or penile discharge, or pelvic, lower abdominal, or rectal pain. Providers should keep in mind that all body parts involved in sexual activity should be examined and tested if indicated, such as rectal and pharyngeal swabs to check for gonorrhea and chlamydia. Additionally, patients presenting with sexual and reproductive health related complaints often require physical examination beyond only a genital exam. For instance, a patient reporting irregular menses should have their thyroid examined, or a patient presenting with a genital ulcer should have their skin examined to check for rash involving the palms or soles. More details on screening for sexually transmitted infections can be found below and in Chap. 6.

Counseling and Education

The healthcare provider is in a unique and privileged position to positively influence a patient's choices and decision-making regarding their sexual health. The National LGBT Health Education Department's 2015 "Sexual History Toolkit" publication emphasizes counseling patients from the approach of risk reduction [10]. The initial step is to assess a patient's interest or willingness to engage in a discussion about risk reduction. If the patient is agreeable, a discussion of ways to decrease potential harm can unfold, with suggestions such as a reduction in the number of partners or the number of anonymous partners, engaging only in lower-risk sexual activities such as oral sex or mutual masturbation, and carrying condoms at all times (and using them as consistently as possible).

One exercise proposed in this toolkit [10] is to ask patients to write down ideas about how to better protect themselves and their partners. Invite patients to self-reflect on times where they perhaps engaged in riskier sexual behavior, and ask them what could have been done differently. While counseling patients on risk reduction, it is important to have appropriate resources or referrals on hand in order to further educate and engage patients. For example, giving an in-office demonstration of proper condom use, discussing a brochure or advertisement about pre-exposure prophylaxis (PrEP), or browsing a website that discusses various contraception options. Having samples of supplies like male and female condoms, dental dams, and water-based lubricants provides patients with direct access to harm reduction strategies and establishes the healthcare provider as an ally willing to engage in candid discussions about sex.

A key aspect of counseling is providing patients with the knowledge and tools to make informed decisions about their sexual and reproductive health. Therefore, the primary care provider must rectify common misconceptions that may exist even into adulthood. Examples include the fact that oral contraceptives cannot protect against sexually transmitted infections, or that sexually transmitted infections such as gonorrhea or chlamydia can be contracted during oral sex if barrier protection is not used. If a patient states incorrect information, such as a belief that two people with HIV do not need to use condoms when having sex, the provider must correct the misconception in a swift and non-judgmental manner, with referral to appropriate resources such as websites, classes, or a specialist if necessary.

Knowledge of and access to organizations or resources that can provide evidence-based interventions to particular patient populations, such as older adults, men who have sex with men, members of a racial minority group, etc., is crucial [10]. The overarching goal is to empower patients and provide them with the tools to make risk-reducing decisions on their own.

Common Issues in Sexual and Reproductive Healthcare in Adults

Disorders of Menstruation

Here, we will discuss disorders of menstruation that occur in nonpregnant, reproductive-age patients with female sex organs.

Amenorrhea and Oligomenorrhea

"Typical" menstruation is defined as having a cycle every 24–38 days, occurring at fairly regular intervals (variation in cycle intervals of less than 7–9 days). Oligomenorrhea is defined as fewer than nine menstrual cycles per year or cycle length greater than 35 days. Amenorrhea can be divided into primary amenorrhea, which is no menstrual cycle by age 15 and secondary amenorrhea, which is defined as no menses for at least 3 months in those with previously regular cycles. Both amenorrhea and oligomenorrhea require evaluation.

The initial evaluation includes ruling out pregnancy. A thorough history includes asking about recent stressors, weight changes, changes in diet or exercise patterns, illness, and new medications (specifically, androgenic drugs, OCPs or other progestin-containing drugs, metoclopramide, antipsychotics). Symptom-specific questions can help to narrow the diagnosis, such as asking about hirsutism or acne if there is concern for hyperandrogenism/polycystic ovary syndrome (PCOS), headaches or visual field changes in the case of a pituitary tumor, hot flashes, vaginal dryness, and decreased libido in the case of primary ovarian insufficiency. In addition to a thorough history and physical exam, the laboratory workup for secondary amenorrhea typically includes checking follicle-stimulating hormone (FSH), estradiol, thyroid-stimulating hormone, prolactin, and, if signs of hyperandrogenism, testosterone levels [12]. A stepwise approach would start with prolactin levels. If elevated on more than one occasion, a pituitary MRI would be indicated. If prolactin levels are normal, TSH, FSH, and E2 levels would be considered.

Treatment goals include correcting underlying pathology, preserving fertility if desired, and preventing secondary complications of amenorrhea (such as osteoporosis from low estrogen states seen in primary ovarian insufficiency). Primary care clinicians may need to co-manage with appropriate subspecialists (endocrinology, gynecology) depending on their comfort and experience managing each condition.

Abnormal Uterine Bleeding

A "typical" menstrual cycle involves a volume of blood loss between 5 and 80 mL, does not significantly interfere with day-to-day life, and lasts 4.5–8 days long [13]. An abnormal uterine bleeding pattern is any deviation from this and is a common complaint that primary care clinicians face. In the United States, the annual prevalence rate of abnormal uterine bleeding is about 53 per 1000 patients aged 18–50 years old [14]. In nonpregnant, premenopausal patients with abnormal uterine bleeding (AUB), initial questioning should be focused on determining the pattern and severity of bleeding. Questions about menstrual history, sexual history, history of obstetric or gynecological surgery, and contraceptive/hormone history are all warranted, as is a complete pelvic exam, to determine if a structural or nonstructural cause is more likely. The role of the primary care clinician is, predominantly, to start the initial evaluation and to determine if referral is necessary or if this is the manifestation of a primarily non-gynecological systemic process.

In 2011, the International Federation of Gynecology and Obstetrics renamed the various descriptions of abnormal uterine bleeding (AUB). Terms such as menorrhagia, or heavy menstrual bleeding, are now classified using the PALM-COEIN system [15]. For a summary of common causes of AUB, refer to Table 3.4.

Other causes not mentioned in Table 3.4 include uterine arteriovenous malformation, an uncommon cause of AUB. This can be congenital or acquired after failed pregnancies, uterine curettage, or cesarean delivery. Abnormal bleeding can also be from an extrauterine source, such as the vagina/vulva (infection, benign growths, malignancy), from trauma/injury such as accrued during sexual intercourse, or systemic processes such as Crohn's disease, chronic liver disease, lymphoma, and thyroid disease.

Table 3.4 Causes of abnormal uterine bleeding [15]

Structural causes of AUB: PALM	
AUB-P: Polyp	Endometrial or cervical
AUB-A: Adenomyosis	Often accompanied by painful menstruation or chronic pelvic pain
AUB-L: Leiomyomas	Categorized as submucosal (AUB-LSM) or other (AUB-LO)
AUB-M: Malignancy and Hyperplasia	Endometrial hyperplasia or carcinoma or uterine sarcoma. Typically presents as irregular postmenopausal bleeding
Non-structural causes of AUB: COEIN	
AUB-C: Coagulopathy	Includes local disorders of hemostasis at the endometrial level
AUB-O: Ovulatory dysfunction	Causes irregular bleeding. Can be seen in the extremes of reproductive age (i.e., postmenarchal, perimenopausal) as well as, among others, with PCOS and other endocrine disorders such as hyperprolactinemia and thyroid dysfunction
AUB-E: Endometrial	Primary disorders of the endometrium such as endometritis, endometriosis, or pelvic inflammatory disease. Typically presents as intermenstrual bleeding
AUB-I: Iatrogenic	Examples include Cesarean-section scar defect, contraception (in particular, the copper IUD), anticoagulation
AUB-N: Not yet classified	

When inquiring about deviations from "typical" bleeding, there are certain patterns and clues that point toward one etiology over another. Regular menstrual bleeding that is heavy or prolonged, previously referred to as "menorrhagia" and now commonly referred to as "heavy menstrual bleeding" or "HMB," indicates cyclic (ovulatory) menses. HMB with an enlarged uterus or uterine masses felt on exam may indicate a uterine leiomyoma; painful menses, chronic pelvic pain, and/ or an enlarged, boggy uterus on exam may indicate adenomyosis. Both of these etiologies require a pelvic ultrasound for initial evaluation and possible referral for a saline infusion sonography (SIS) or hysteroscopy if an intracavitary lesion is suspected. Cyclic, postmenstrual bleeding in a patient with a history or one or more cesarean sections may have a cesarean scar defect. A family history of bleeding disorders or other symptoms of a bleeding diathesis warrant a coagulopathy workup, and a patient with risk factors for uterine malignancy (see below) should be referred to a gynecologist to consider endometrial biopsy (although the typical pattern is intermenstrual or postmenopausal bleeding).

Regular menstrual periods with intermenstrual bleeding is suggestive of an endometrial or cervical polyp, warranting imaging with a pelvic ultrasound. A recent history of uterine or cervical procedure, including childbirth, raises concern for endometritis, diagnosed by endometrial biopsy. Irregular periods are more indicative of ovulatory dysfunction. Consider PCOS in a patient with hirsutism, acne, or obesity, and check total testosterone levels, hyperprolactinemia if there is galactorrhea, and thyroid disease in a patient with weight changes, heat/cold intolerance, or a family history of thyroid disease. Contraception-induced AUB can result in both irregular bleeding and heavy or prolonged regular bleeding. A patient with no menses for 3 months (who previously had regular cycles) is considered to have secondary amenorrhea; see above section for evaluation.

According to the American College of Obstetricians and Gynecologists, primary care clinicians should have increased concern regarding endometrial malignancy in patients 45 years old or older. After age 45, any AUB including intermenstrual bleeding, cycles less than 21 days, heavy bleeding, or cycles longer than 5 days is an indication for an endometrial biopsy as the first step in working up the AUB. In those younger than 45, biopsy is indicated only if the AUB is persistent (6 months or more), there is a history of unopposed estrogen exposure (such as obesity, chronic ovulatory dysfunction), or the patient has risk factors for endometrial cancer such as tamoxifen use or Lynch syndrome [13, 16]. Suspicion for endometritis is another indication for biopsy. Transvaginal ultrasound assessment of endometrial thickness is not an appropriate substitution for biopsy in premenopausal patients given normal variation throughout the menstrual cycle.

Premenstrual Syndrome and Premenstrual Dysphoric Disorder

One other topic primary care clinicians should be familiar with is that of premenstrual syndrome (PMS) and premenstrual dysphoric disorder (PMDD). Both of these syndromes are comprised of physical and behavioral symptoms that occur in the second half of the menstrual cycle, with PMDD being a more severe form with prominent symptoms of anger and irritability that interfere with daily functioning. PMS symptoms include depression, anxiety, irritability, labile mood, and increased appetite as well as somatic symptoms such as fatigue, abdominal bloating, breast pain, headaches, hot flashes, and dizziness. The symptoms impair functioning in some way and resolve with menses (or shortly after). In both PMS and PMDD, patients are symptom-free during the follicular phase of their cycles. A validated method for diagnosing PMDD is to ask patients to record their symptoms through at least one (ideally, two) menstrual cycle using the Daily Record of Severity of Problems (DRSP) questionnaire [17]. Treatment goals for both syndromes are to relieve symptoms and improve functionality. First-line therapies for mild symptoms include exercise and relaxation techniques. For symptoms that include cause social dysfunction, selective serotonin reuptake inhibitors (SSRIs) are first-line treatment, with fluoxetine and sertraline being the most extensively studied and approved for use in premenstrual disorders. However, citalopram and escitalopram have been shown to also be effective [18]. Additional treatment may include oral contraceptives, gonadotropin-releasing hormone agonists, and, potentially, surgery (such as oophorectomy) for severe, refractory symptoms.

Sexual Dysfunction

Sexual problems and dysfunction are common in adults. Please see Chaps. 7 and 14 for more in-depth exploration into the diagnosis and treatment of these problems.

The three most common sexual concerns for which individuals with which male sex organs will present to their primary care clinician include (1) diminished libido, (2) erectile dysfunction, and (3) abnormal ejaculation. Sexual complaints become more common as individuals turn 40 years old and increases with advancing age [19, 20].

1. Decreased libido: The prevalence of decreased libido in cisgender men is esti-mated to be 5–15 percent, increasing with age [21]. There are several causes, including medications (commonly, selective serotonin reuptake inhibitors (SSRIs), anti-androgens, 5-alpha reductase inhibitors, and opioids), alcohol or drug abuse, and testosterone deficiency. Depression, hypoactive sexual disorder, sexual aversion disorder, and relationship problems should also be considered when organic causes have been ruled out.

2. Erectile dysfunction (ED): This disorder is defined as the inability to acquire or sustain an erection sufficient for sexual intercourse and is the most common sexual complaint in cisgender men, with an overall prevalence of about 16 per-cent and increasing with age [22]. Common causes of ED include diabetes, sed-entary lifestyle, hypertension, obesity, dyslipidemia, cardiovascular disease, smoking, and use of medications including antihypertensives (clonidine, meth-yldopa; thiazide diuretics), antidepressants (particularly SSRIs), antipsychotics, and antiandrogens (spironolactone). Other causes of ED include ketoconazole, cimetidine, alcohol, recreational drugs (e.g., cocaine and heroin) obstructive sleep apnea, restless legs syndrome, scleroderma, hyperprolactinemia, thyroid dysfunction, Peyronie's disease, and prostate cancer treatment [23]. Psychosocial factors such as depression, stress, or relationship problems should also be con-sidered, as well as neurologic causes such as stroke, spinal cord injury, multiple sclerosis, or pelvic trauma. Avid cyclists may be more likely to experience ED, although the etiology of this relationship is controversial [24]. Testosterone defi-ciency usually impacts libido more than erectile function, but can still be associ-ated with ED; testosterone replacement can restore erections in hypogonadal men.

3. Abnormal ejaculation: Premature ejaculation occurs in about 4–30 percent of males and is defined as ejaculation that is nearly always within 1 minute of pen-etration, the inability to delay ejaculation, and having negative feelings such as stress, frustration, or anxiety regarding this [25, 26]. The etiology is often uncer-tain or multifactorial and may be related to penile hypersensitivity, negative con-ditioning, genetics, and/or psychosocial factors.

There is also a spectrum of disorders that range from delayed ejaculation to male anorgasmia. The etiology is often similar to those disorders and conditions associated with ED. Retrograde ejaculation occurs commonly after surgery for benign prostatic hyperplasia; anejaculation can be associated with radical prostatectomy or cystoprostatectomy. Drugs such as alpha-blockers (tamsulosin) or SSRIs can cause decreased ability to orgasm or ejaculate.

Sexual dysfunction in individuals with female sex organs is a broad and often multifactorial spectrum of complaints and disorders, very commonly seen in the primary care setting, with an estimated 40% of cisgender women who have endorsed having "sexual concerns." [27] It is important for clinicians to initiate conversations on sexual function. In a study of over 1000 women, 98% reported at least one sexual concern, but only 18% reported that their primary care provider had asked about their sexual health [20]. An open-ended question can be asked while taking the sexual history, such as "In terms of your sexual life, is anything bothering you?"

Female sexual dysfunction can refer to a problem occurring at any stage of the sexual response cycle, which includes desire (libido), excitement (arousal), plateau, orgasm, and resolution. Notably, this cycle is individualized for each person, and the stages may overlap, repeat, or not occur at all. The major categories of female sexual dysfunction are (1) female sexual interest/arousal disorder, (2) female orgasmic disorder, (3) genitopelvic pain disorder, (4) substance- or medication-induced sexual dysfunction, and (5) other or unspecified sexual dysfunction disorders.

Female sexual dysfunction can be secondary to a number of both physical and psychosocial causes. Psychosocial factors such as depression, anxiety (and the medications used to treat these), and a history of sexual abuse or trauma are associated with sexual dysfunction. Women should be asked about their relationship with their partner and be assessed for emotional well-being within the relationship, as several studies have shown this to be a key marker for sexual satisfaction and overall function. Patients should also be screened for intimate partner violence and provided with appropriate resources and referrals if positive.

Women who are peri- or post-menopause will often present with complaints regarding sexual function in the setting of lowered estrogen levels. This is known as the genitourinary syndrome of menopause and can result in decreased libido, less lubrication and vasocongestion during arousal, vaginal atrophy, and perhaps painful intercourse. Surgical menopause results in greater dysfunction than natural menopause [27].

In the postpartum period, many women report decreased libido and dyspareunia (improving with time post-delivery) [28, 29]. Pelvic floor dysfunction (such as pelvic organ prolapse), urinary incontinence, and interstitial cystitis are also associated with increased risk of sexual complaints [30, 31]. Deep dyspareunia can be a sign of endometriosis or uterine fibroids. Prolactinemia can lead to decreased sexual desire, arousal/lubrication, orgasm, and overall sexual satisfaction. Neurologic conditions such as multiple sclerosis are associated with sensory dysfunction [32]. Additionally, seizure disorder itself can lead to hyposexuality, although some of the antiepileptics used to treat seizure disorder such as gabapentin and topiramate can also contribute to anorgasmia [33, 34, 35]. Interestingly, partner sexual dysfunction (such as ED in a male partner) is a significant risk factor for or cause of female sexual dysfunction [36].

As introduced earlier, many medications can cause sexual dysfunction. Aromatase inhibitors used for breast cancer can result in profoundly low estrogen levels thus impacting sexual desire and arousal. Antidepressants such as SSRIs can cause decreased libido and anorgasmia. It is controversial whether or not hormonal contraception can affect libido and sexual function, and there is no randomized trial to support this [37]. Nicotine and alcohol abuse can also lead to decreased arousal [38, 39].

Sexually Transmitted Infections

A common sexual health complaint primary care providers will encounter is signs or symptoms of a sexually transmitted infection (STI). A detailed discussion of the prevention, clinical presentation, diagnosis, and management of STIs and HIV is presented in Chap. 10, "Sexually Transmitted Infections." Here we provide an overview of the approach to STIs in adults. According to the annual 2016 CDC Sexually Transmitted Disease Surveillance Report, more than two million cases of chlamydia, gonorrhea, and syphilis occurred in the United States during this period, the highest number ever. The vast majority were new cases of chlamydia (1.6 million), followed by 470,000 cases of gonorrhea and 28,000 cases of syphilis [40]. These diseases, if undiagnosed and untreated, could have severe associated morbidity and mortality including infertility, neurological and cardiovascular sequelae (syphilis), life-threatening ectopic pregnancy, stillbirth in infants, and increased risk for HIV transmission among others.

While young women of reproductive age account for almost half of all diagnosed chlamydia infections, the incidence of syphilis and gonorrhea is increasing, particularly in men who have sex with men. In 2016, syphilis rates increased by nearly 18 percent overall in one year – there was a 36 percent increase among women and a 28 percent increase among newborns (congenital syphilis). The disease is easily diagnosable and preventable through routine screening of all pregnant women (and women in reproductive age) and timely treatment.

Gonorrhea infections increased among men and women with the largest increase seen among men (22%). In general, ulcer-forming diseases and rectal and genitourinary STIs are known to increase the risk of HIV acquisition [40]. Additionally, the surging of resistant strains of gonococcal and *Mycoplasma genitalium* infections possess a challenge to currently available treatments.

To help change this trend, primary care clinicians should remember to obtain an appropriate sexual history and physical exam (see above section) on all patients to evaluate for STIs and treat them promptly. Providers should also follow state and local surveillance, treatment, and reporting guidelines from reliable resources such as the CDC [41].

HIV infection and its sequelae remain a severe health problem in the United States. There are health disparities in the risk and rates of HIV infection as per CDC HIV surveillance report of 2015 – infections in the heterosexual population declined by 24%, patients who use injection drugs had a 31% decline, and men who have sex with men had no change in HIV prevalence since 2010 [42]. The overall lifetime risk of HIV in the United States is 1:99, but this varies by race and gender [43]. The highest reported lifetime risk is in men who have sex with men population group, with African American and Hispanic men who have sex with men having a 1:2 and 1:4 lifetime risk, respectively [44]. Current estimates suggest 25% of transgender women are living with HIV, while more than half of the African American transgender women are living with HIV [45]. In interpreting these widely cited data, it is critical to understand that sexual orientation, self-identified race, and gender identity are not themselves risk factors for HIV or other STIs. Rather, they represent communities and individuals that have been placed at risk by broader structural drivers of inequities including racism, homophobia, and transphobia. It is critical that primary care clinicians recognize the complex interactions of gender, risk factors, race, social factors, and intersectionality in screening and counseling patients about HIV risk.

Patients often ask about the particular risk of HIV infection associated with a specific sexual act. The knowledge of relative risk informs the clinician and the patient on the potential need for preventive, diagnostic, or therapeutic intervention. Refer to Table 3.5 for the risk of HIV infection per 10,000 exposures as described by Patel et al. [46] (assuming no condom use) according to exposure type.

HIV prevention takes several forms in a continuum of care of sexually active patients. A comprehensive approach to HIV prevention incorporates multiple interventions for both HIV-positive and HIV-negative individuals. These include behavioral, biomedical, and structural interventions [47, 48]. . The behavioral interventions (directed at those who are not infected with HIV) include the following: educate people about prevention, encourage access to services such as treatment for sexually transmitted infections or drug abuse, delay onset of first intercourse, increase condom use, and reduce the number of sexual partners and/or sharing of syringes and needles. The biomedical interventions include (1) PrEP (pre-exposure prophylaxis) – the use of daily antiretroviral (ARV) medications to help reduce the risk of HIV infection in HIV-negative individuals at high risk for acquiring HIV-1. It should be used as part of a comprehensive HIV prevention plan (2). PEP (post-exposure prophylaxis) – the use of ARV medications after an uninfected person has come into contact with bodily fluids that represent a substantial HIV risk. (3) TasP (treatment as prevention) – the use of ARV treatment by an HIV-positive individual to suppress viral load in bodily fluids, thereby reducing the chances that HIV will be transmitted to an HIV-negative partner. Structural interventions include scaling up effective,

Table 3.5 Risk of HIV infection per type of exposure

Type of exposure	Risk per 10,000 exposures
Receptive anal intercourse	138
Insertive anal intercourse	11
Receptive vaginal intercourse	8
Insertive vaginal intercourse	4
Receptive fellatio/oral sex	Low
Insertive fellatio/oral sex	Low

evidence-based programs that address social determinants of health; providing new, sterile syringes and other injection equipment to persons who inject drugs; community outreach programs with point-of-care HIV testing; and prevention education.

The components of a comprehensive STI/HIV prevention approach for all patients include:

1. Initiating a sexual history discussion during the initial patient visit, at routine prevention exams, and at the first signs of STIs.
2. Perform regular STI and HIV testing on sexually active and at-risk patients. At-risk individuals should be tested for STIs every 3–6 months, depending on their risk factors. Test for chlamydia and gonorrhea at least annually for sexually active at-risk patients at the site of contact (urethra, pharynx, and rectum) regardless of condom use.
3. Provide sexual health and prevention education with up-to-date information about STIs, HIV, and safer-sex practice options, including discussing the appropriate use of barrier protection (e.g., condoms) with every sexually active individual.

Pregnancy Prevention and Family Planning

Patients will present throughout the reproductive spectrum and have greatly varying reproductive desires and plans. As a primary care clinician, it is crucial to have a basic understanding of various forms of contraception to effectively counsel your patients looking for protection against pregnancy. For details on contraception and family planning, please see Chaps. 5 and 14 (for overview and family planning specific to the TGNB population, respectively).

Unintended Pregnancy

As a primary care provider, you may be faced with diagnosing a patient with a new pregnancy. In 2011, nearly half of pregnancies in the United States were unintended [49]. Unintended pregnancies can occur at any age. Despite fertility decreasing by about 50% after age 40 for women, unintended pregnancies in the perimenopausal period are still possible. Some sources estimate that nearly half (about 48%) of pregnancies from age 40 to 44 are unintended [50]. In a 2011 survey of 7800 American women with unintended pregnancies, the top reason for not using protection was that they believed they could not get pregnant at the time of conception (33%) [51]. However, it is important to avoid making assumptions about the patient's reproductive goals/desires, especially in sexually and gender diverse patients, and engage in patient-centered decision-making.

The Reproductive Health Access Project [52] has proposed an effective, 5-step approach for counseling patients on their pregnancy options. Refer to Table 3.6 for a summary of the 5-step approach.

Table 3.6 5-Step approach for counseling on pregnancy options

1. Clarify	Clarify the actual timing of pregnancy
2. Normalize	Normalize any feelings of uncertainty patient may be experiencing
3. Acknowledge	Acknowledge and address common feelings such as "shame, disappointment, guilt, and regret"
4. Reframe	Reframe the situation – perhaps not continuing the pregnancy is the most responsible decision for the patient and her present situation
5. Reassure and encourage	Reinforce the patient's confidence in her own decisions

For patients who express ambivalence around their pregnancy, one might suggest the following exercise. On Day 1 (usually the day the patient finds out about her pregnancy), they should write a pro/con list about keeping the pregnancy. On Day 2, the patient should focus solely on feelings and not make any decisions. On Day 3, they should write a pro/con list about *not* keeping the pregnancy. On Day 4, the patient should be scheduled for a follow-up appointment to discuss the two pro/con lists and thoughts and feelings on the current situation [52].

If a patient chooses to electively terminate the pregnancy, it is important, as the primary care provider, to have basic knowledge of the patient's options in order to effectively counsel and refer the patient to the appropriate provider. While this may vary state by state, there are two primary options [53].

Medication termination of pregnancy: This option can be used up to 10 weeks from the first day of the patient's last period. The patient will come for an appointment and will be given mifepristone (one pill), which can be taken at the patient's convenience. The main side effect is nausea. 6 to 72 hours later, the patient will insert four misoprostol pills into the vagina, which will induce cramps and heavy bleeding (usually starting 1–4 hours after insertion and lasting a few hours). This method is 98–99% effective. Cramps can be painful, and patients may have bleeding on and off for a few weeks after the termination. This method is generally considered to be safe but does involve more bleeding and cramps than with a surgical termination.

Surgical termination of pregnancy: The "surgical" option, known as an aspiration, can be performed up to 12 weeks from the first day of the patient's last period. The procedure must be done in a medical office and takes about 5–10 minutes. This can also result in cramps and residual bleeding, although usually less so than with a medication termination. This method is 99% effective and is safe; both abortion methods are considered to be at least 10 times safer than continuing a pregnancy.

Fertility

Primary care clinicians may encounter patients who come to them to discuss infertility or challenges becoming pregnant. Here we present an overview and approach to fertility issues in patient with a variety of genders and medical conditions. Please see the family planning chapters in parts 2 and 3 of this book for additional details.

Infertility in Cisgender Patients/Heterosexual Couples

While a discussion of the various etiologies and treatments for infertility is beyond the scope of this chapter, it will often be the primary care clinician who initiates the workup for infertility. According to the CDC, about 12% of cisgender women aged 15–44 years old in the United States have struggled with difficulty getting pregnant or carrying their pregnancy to term [54]. First, workup should not be started unless a couple has been unable to conceive after trying consistently for 12 months. Some sources suggest initiating evaluation for infertility after 6 months of unprotected and frequent intercourse for women aged 35–40 years old, or less than 6 months for women over 40 years old or with factors in their medical history such as oligo or amenorrhea, history of chemotherapy or radiation therapy or endometriosis, or known or suspected uterine or tubal disease [55]. Additionally, if her male partner has a history of chemotherapy or radiation therapy, groin/testicular surgery, adult mumps, or sexual dysfunction, workup should also be started after less than 6 months of trying to conceive.

Aside from supportive care for patients' emotions during this often stressful time, initial evaluation should include a complete history and physical examination as the etiology of infertility is often multifactorial. The first steps include a thorough menstrual history, as well as measurement of the luteinizing hormone (LH) in urine prior to ovulation, thyroid-stimulating hormone, and a semen analysis. Education can be provided regarding how to track ovulation (there are various smartphone apps that can be used for this). The functioning of the ovary can be assessed with Day 3 serum follicle-stimulating hormone, estradiol, and anti-Mullerian hormone levels. Antral follicle count can also be performed via ultrasound. It is advisable at this point to refer to a gynecologist or fertility specialist for additional workup, as a hysterosalpingogram can look for tubal patency and visualizing the uterus may be needed.

Fertility and Family Planning in Same-Sex Couples and Patients Without Sexual Partners

Many options exist for same-sex couples or patients without sexual partners who wish to have children [56]. Referral to a specialist will be necessary for many of these options. However the primary clinician should be able to have a supportive, affirming, and informed conversation with patients about family planning.

Adoption is one option, and it is important to have resources for this in the office. One option when both partners have female sex organs is intrauterine insemination (IUI) with donor sperm. IUI uses sperm that is washed (to eliminate any prostaglandins that can cause uterine cramping with direct insertion) and concentrated; it is then inserted directly into the uterus via a catheter. In vitro fertilization (IVF) with a sperm donor is another option and is unique in that, if desired, both partners can participate in the pregnancy (one partner's fertilized egg can be implanted into the other partner's uterus, known as "reciprocal IVF" or "egg sharing"). Additionally, eggs from both partners can be used, allowing the couple to not know which egg was fertilized. For gay male couples, there are also several options including using IUI or IVF with a surrogate (can use the sperm from one or both partners). Special counseling should also be given to TGNB patients regarding egg or sperm cryo-preservation prior to starting hormonal transitioning.

Fertility and Family Planning in Patients with HIV

It is also important to reassure patients living with HIV or serodiscordant couples that reproduction can be done safely [57]. It is advised to achieve maximal viral suppression before attempting conception in order to avoid transmission among partners in serodiscordant couples and, in the case of women with HIV, to avoid transmission to the fetus. Patients should be screened for genital tract infections before attempting to conceive. It is recommended to limit sex without a condom only to the days of peak fertility. Assisted insemination or using donor sperm may also be used. The HIV-negative partner can use PrEP to further reduce the risk of transmission when engaging in unprotected sex.

For fertility considerations in other populations, please see the relevant chapters in parts 2 and 3 of this book.

Immunizations

Ensuring that patients are up to date with all recommended vaccinations are a routine part of comprehensive primary care. Providers should remember to offer the appropriate vaccinations for all indicated populations, including immunocompromised patients, pregnant women, and men who have sex with men. This is especially important as new vaccine recommendations are regularly released by the CDC that change clinical practice in the primary care setting, such as the ability to protect immunocompromised patients against herpes zoster infection with Shingrix (GSK) [58]. Clinicians should refer to the CDC guidelines to obtain the most up-to-date recommendations regarding immunizations. For a brief summary of vaccine recommendations related to patients' sexual and reproductive health, see Table 3.7.

According to a review in *JAMA Pediatrics*, HPV vaccination rates in the United States are low compared to other recommended vaccines [59]. Barriers included patients or their parents not understanding the prevalence of HPV infection and clinicians not routinely ensuring that their patients are up to date with HPV vaccination. While typically recommended for patients aged 11–12, clinicians should offer catch-up vaccination to eligible patients. If not previously vaccinated, female patients may receive the vaccine age 13–45. Unvaccinated male patients may receive

Table 3.7 Vaccination guidelines

Vaccine	Population	Recommendation
Human papillomavirus (HPV) [62]	All genders age 9–45	9-Valent HPV Initiating age < 15: 2 doses (0, 6–12 months) Initiating age ≥ 15: 3 doses (0, 1–2, and 6 months) Patients with HIV or are immunocompromised should receive 3 doses
Hepatitis A [63]	Unvaccinated adults Men who have sex with men (MSM) Intravenous drug use (IVDU)	HAVRIX 2 doses (0 and 6–12 months) or VAQTA 2 doses (0 and 6–18 months)
Hepatitis B [64]	Age < 19 without prior vaccination Adults at increased risk (multiple sexual partners, MSM, IVDU, HIV, HCV, healthcare workers, high-risk travel, chronic liver disease) Adults requesting vaccination	Twinrix (HAV and HBV) 3 doses (0, 1, and 6 months) Twinrix – accelerated schedule 4 doses (0, 7, and 21–30 days, followed by one dose at 1 year)
Meningococcal A, C, W, and Y [61]	Adults with HIV, complement deficiency, or functional/anatomic asplenia	Menactra or Menveo 2 doses (0 and 8 weeks), then every 5 years if risk remains
	Military recruits College students in residence halls	Menactra or Menveo Dose once, then every 5 years if risk remains
Measles, mumps, rubella (MMR) [65]	Women of reproductive age without evidence of immunity	MMR Dose once
Tetanus, diphtheria, pertussis (Tdap) [66]	Women in 3rd trimester of every pregnancy	Tdap Dose once every pregnancy
Varicella [67]	Age 13 and older without prior immunity	Varivax 2 doses (0 and 4–8 weeks)
	Age > 8 with HIV and CD4 count ≥200 cells/µL	Varivax 2 doses (0 and 3 months)

the vaccine age 13–21. Guidelines describe that men who are gay, bisexual, or have sex with men, patients who are immunocompromised, those living with HIV, and transgender individuals may be vaccinated through age 26. We recommend individualizing each patient's risk assessment. Remind patients and parents of the importance of receiving HPV vaccination prior to the onset of sexual activity in order to gain protection prior to exposure of HPV [60].

Administration of the meningococcal conjugate vaccine provides protection against meningococcal serogroups A, C, W, and Y [61]. Determining patients of increased risk requires a discussion with patients regarding their personal risk factors, which involves obtaining a thorough sexual and reproductive history (refer to sections above). According to the CDC, these risk factors include persistent complement deficiencies, functional or anatomic asplenia, infection with HIV, first-year college students living in residence halls, travel to countries with endemic meningococcal disease, microbiologists routinely exposed to *Neisseria meningitidis*, and patients at risk during a community outbreak [61]. Please refer to the CDC for the most up-to-date guidelines regarding indications for meningococcal vaccination.

Cancer Screening

The introduction of cervical cancer screening in the United States in the 1950s and 1960s has decreased the incidence and associated mortality of cervical cancer; however there have been challenges in defining the optimal methods and timing of routine screening [68, 69]. Current USPSTF recommendations begin routine screening in patients with a cervix at age 21 until age 65 unless otherwise indicated. Also, use of testing for high-risk HPV has lengthened the recommended intervals between screenings in populations at average risk for cervical cancer. Note that the guidelines presented in Table 3.8 apply to patients at average risk for cervical cancer. Patients with HIV and solid organ transplants and other patients at higher risk for cervical cancers should follow condition-specific screening guidelines.

Similarly, patients with a history of treated cervical cancer will require more frequent surveillance. It is recommended that a pelvic examination and Pap smear for cytology evaluation be repeated every 3–6 months for the first 2 years after treatment of cervical cancer, then repeated every 6 months until 5 years after diagnosis, and finally repeated annually [70]. However, retrospective studies have suggested that the majority of recurrences are detected by physical exam and reported symptoms (such as pelvic pain or vaginal bleeding), whereas cytologic evaluation has been low yield [71].

In both men and women, HPV infection increases the risk of anal cancer. While there are no general consensus guidelines regarding anal cancer screening, one strategy is to perform an anal Pap with cytology evaluation annually for high-risk patients (e.g., patients with HIV) in clinics where referral for high-resolution anoscopy is available to further evaluate abnormal results [72]. Systematic reviews have shown that some high-risk populations, such as men having anal receptive sex with multiple partners, have an increased risk of anal HPV and anal cancer precursor lesions [73]. Guidelines from the HIV Medicine Association of the Infectious Diseases Society of America in 2013 offered a weak recommendation for MSM, women with a history of receptive anal intercourse or an abnormal cervical Pap test, and all patients with HIV to undergo screening with anal Pap testing [74]. Anal cytology sampling should be done prior to a digital rectal exam or other examination in which lubricant will be applied to the anus or rectum because lubricants may interfere with cytology analysis [72].

Table 3.8 Cancer screening recommendations

Topic	Recommendation
Cervical cancer screening [68]	Age < 21: Screening not recommended Age 21–29: Pap smear with cytology without HPV testing every 3 years Age 30–65: Pap smear with cytology every 3 years, Pap smear with high-risk HPV testing every 5 years, or Pap smear with cytology and HPV testing (co-testing) every 5 years Age > 65: Screening not recommended if patient has had 3 consecutive negative cytology results or 2 consecutive negative cotesting results within 10 years before stopping screening, with the most recent test occurring within 5 years Precancerous lesions: Screen for 20 years after spontaneous regression or appropriate management Post-hysterectomy: Screening not recommended if patient had cervix removed and no prior result of HSIL or greater Patients with HIV: Age < 21: Initial pap smear within 1 year of onset of sexual activity. Repeat in 6 months and if normal then screen annually. If 3 consecutive pap smears are normal, repeat every 3 years. HPV co-testing not recommended Age 21–29: Initial pap smear at time of HIV diagnosis. Repeat in 6 months and if normal then screen annually. If 3 consecutive Pap smears are normal, repeat every 3 years. HPV co-testing not recommended Age ≥ 30: Pap smear annually, if 3 consecutive Pap smears normal then repeat every 3 years. Alternatively, may do Pap smear with HPV co-testing every 3 years. Continue screening for patient's lifetime
Anal cancer screening [72]	No guidelines are available regarding target high-risk populations or screening intervals. Common practices include screening high-risk patients (MSM with HPV, patients with HIV and anogenital condylomas, or patients with HIV and abnormal cervical histology) Anal cytology done annually if referral for high-resolution anoscopy is available. Digital anal exam as part of annual physical is done after cytology sampling because lubricants may interfere with cytology analysis
Breast cancer screening [75]	Women age 40–49: Individual discussion regarding risks and benefits as well as patient's individual risk factors Women age 50–74: Screening mammogram every 1–2 years based on shared decision-making Women age ≥ 75: Insufficient evidence for routine screening; based on shared decision-making
Prostate cancer screening [76]	USPSTF recommends that men aged 55–69 years make an individual decision about whether to be screened after a conversation with their clinician about the potential benefits and harms. For men 70 years and older, the potential benefits do not outweigh the expected harms, and these men should not be routinely screened for prostate cancer No controlled studies have shown a reduction in the morbidity or mortality of prostate cancer when detected by digital rectal exam (DRE) at any age, and therefore we do not recommend DRE for screening of prostate cancer

Note that while some guidelines for cancer screening may specify target populations such as "male" or "female" for their recommendations, these screening recommendations should be applied based upon the organs present in the patient regardless of gender. For instance, a patient who identifies as a transgender male may have a cervix and should therefore have cervical cancer screening according to current guidelines. Maintaining an open communication style and adopting a patient's language when referring to their anatomy during examinations and procedures can help maintain patient comfort. For a more detailed discussion, refer to Part 3.

Intimate Partner Violence, Sexual Assault, and Sexual Exploitation

One increasingly relevant and extremely important topic in the health and well-being of the adult patient is that of intimate partner violence (IPV). IPV is defined as actual or threatened harm by a current or former partner or spouse. This harm can be physical, psychological, or sexual and can be found in heterosexual and same-sex couples. IPV is underdiagnosed due to a combination of patient hesitation to reveal and physician hesitation to ask. More than 32 million Americans are affected by IPV, with women more likely to be affected than men [77]. It is estimated that 22–39% of American women will experience IPV in their lifetime [78], with the estimate expanding to 10–69 percent when considering women worldwide [79]. It is unclear if aforementioned statistics are only including cisgender women or also include TGNB women. There is limited data on IPV in transgender people or couples; however, a few studies suggest that TGNB people may be affected by similar, if not higher, levels of IPV than cisgender people. One source estimates lifetime IPV among transgender people ranges from 31.1% to 50.0% [80].

This brings into question who should be screened and when. Different organizations propose varying recommendations. For example, in 2013 the United States Preventive Services Task Force (USPSTF) recommended screening all women of childbearing age (14–46 years old) [81, 82], as a 2012 systematic review showed that screening is minimally harmful and potentially very beneficial [78]. The World Health Organization (WHO), however, recommend against routine screening and only women who are deemed to be at high risk or with possible signs or symptoms of IPV be screened, noting there is a lack of evidence that screening asymptomatic patients improves overall health outcomes in the general population [83].

Using the approach of screening only when there are signs or symptoms to raise suspicion of IPV poses a difficult challenge, as IPV spans all demographics including socioeconomic class, race, and sexual orientation. Certain demographic subsets are at potentially higher risk for IPV (namely, being female, pregnant, younger, of lower socioeconomic status, and/or having a personal or family history of violence), but certain features should raise suspicion, such as an inconsistent explanation of injuries, delay in seeking treatment, frequent emergency department or urgent care visits, frequent missed appointments, inappropriate affect, and reluctance to allow a genital or rectal exam or undress [84]. Common presenting complaints include chronic pelvic pain or gynecological conditions such as premenstrual syndrome, sexually transmitted infections, and unintended pregnancy; somatic complaints such as dizziness, headaches, chronic pain including headaches, and irritable bowel syndrome; and psychological conditions such as depression, anxiety, substance abuse, eating disorder, posttraumatic stress disorder, and dissociative disorders.

There are several resources available to screen patients for IPV, as demonstrated in Table 3.9. Unfortunately there is no "gold standard" screening tool so that the specificity and sensitivity of these various surveys cannot be compared or

Table 3.9 Screening tools for intimate partner violence

Name of IPV screening tool	Questions
SAFE Questionnaire [85]	*S: Stress/safety:* Do you feel safe in your relationship? *A: Afraid/abused:* Have you ever been in a relationship where you were threatened, hurt, or afraid? *F: Friend/family:* Do your loved ones know you have been hurt? *E: Emergency plan:* Do you have a safe place to go or the necessary resources in the case of an emergency? *2+ affirmative answers raise high index of suspicion for IPV*
Massachusetts Medical Society Committee on Violence Recommendation [86]	Ask a single question routinely to a patient, such as "I see patients in my practice who have been hurt or threatened by a loved one. Has this ever happened to you?"
Abuse Assessment Screen (AAS) [87] for identifying abuse in pregnancy	1. Within the last year, have you been hit, slapped, kicked, or otherwise physically hurt by someone? 2. Since you've been pregnant, have you been hit, slapped, kicked, or otherwise physically hurt by someone? 3. Within the last year, has anyone forced you to have sexual activities? *An affirmative answer to any of these is considered a positive screen*

HITS Questionnaire [88], where each question is scored on a 5-point Likert scale ("never, rarely, sometimes, fairly often, frequently")	How often does your partner:
	    Hurt you physically?
	    Insult or talk down to you?
	    Threaten you with harm?
	    Scream or curse at you?
	Each item is scored from 1–5. A score of 10+ is positive

Partner Violence Scale [89], used in emergency room and urgent care settings	1. Have you ever been hit, kicked, punched or otherwise hurt by someone within the past year? If so, by whom? 2. Do you feel safe in your current relationship? 3. Is there a partner from a previous relationship making you feel unsafe now? *An affirmative answer to any of these is considered a positive screen*
HARK Questionnaire [90]. A point is given to every "yes" answer	Within the past year have you been: *H: Humiliated:* Humiliated or emotionally abused in other ways by your partner or ex-partner? *A: Afraid:* Afraid of your partner or ex-partner? *R: Raped:* Raped or forced to have any kind of sexual activity by your partner or ex-partner? *K: Kicked:* Kicked, hit, slapped, or otherwise physically hurt by your partner or ex-partner? *An affirmative answer to any of these is considered a positive screen*

(continued)

Table 3.9 (continued)

Name of IPV screening tool	Questions
STaT Questionnaire [91]	Have you ever been in a relationship where your partner has: *S: Slapped:* Pushed or slapped you? *T: Threatened:* Threatened you with violence? *T: Thrown things:* Thrown, broken or punched things? *One affirmative answer is considered a positive screen, with a sensitivity of 96% and a specificity of 75% for IPV*
Women Abuse Screening Tool (WAST) [92]	In general, how would you describe your relationship? A lot of tension, some tension, no tension Do you and your partner work out arguments with: Great difficulty, some difficulty, no difficulty? Do arguments ever result in you feeling down or bad about yourself? Often, sometimes, never Do arguments ever result in hitting, kicking or pushing? Often, sometimes, never Do you ever feel frightened by what your partner says or does? Often, sometimes, never Has your partner ever abused you physically? Often, sometimes, never Has your partner ever abused you emotionally? Often, sometimes, never Has your partner ever abused you sexually? Often, sometimes, never *Each question is answered with a: 1 (never or none), 2 (sometimes), 3 (a lot or often). Total scores range from 8 to 24, with a cutoff of 13 recommended to indicate presence of IPV*

determined. One tool is called the 39-item Conflict Tactics Scale-Revised (CTS-2) and is widely used in the literature as a reference standard; however, many providers feel this lengthy survey to be unreasonable and impractical for day-to-day clinic use. In general, we recommend primary care clinicians become familiar and comfortable with multiple screening tools and use the tool that seems most appropriate for the individual patient.

Providers should assess the patient's safety and refer to appropriate resources if a patient screens positive for IPV. According to the Massachusetts Medical Society Committee on Violence Recommendation, "the most important determinants in assessing risk are the patient's level of fear and his or her own appraisal of both immediate and future safety needs." However, it is common for patients to downplay or even deny the severity of their danger, so the following are potential red flags for escalating danger: increased frequency or severity of threats or assaults, new or increasing homicidal or suicidal ideation by the partner, new access to firearms, or new or increasing violence outside of the relationship by the partner [86].

The next step should be to develop a safety plan with the patient. This plan should include a safe place to go (a family member or friend's house, or a shelter, with appropriate resources and referrals provided). If the patient has filed an order of protection (restraining order), he or she should carry a copy on their person at all times. The patient should also pack an emergency bag with money, legal documents such as ID cards and passports, car keys, and a change of clothing (for the patient and his or her children). The patient should be referred to a local, state, or national domestic violence program, which provides free and confidential services. According to the Massachusetts Medical Society Committee on Violence Intervention and Prevention, "trained advocates from these programs can provide information regarding...legal rights, police and court procedures for protective orders, emergency shelter and safe house availability, support groups and other valuable support resources." [86] The National Domestic Violence Hotline at (800) 799-SAFE is another resource for additional information. Other than providing practical and logistical information, another important role of the provider is to provide support and validation to the patient who is facing IPV [86].

The decision to report IPV must balance the desire to remove the survivor from a dangerous environment with the potential for acute increase in risk of violence as the result of reporting. As primary care clinicians, it is crucial to become familiar with local mandatory reporting laws. As of 2012, only a minority of states had laws requiring mandatory reporting of IPV in adults. Chapter 1, and Chap. 2, outline the legal issues surrounding sexual violence in the pediatric and adolescent populations. Situations that would commonly require reporting include use of certain weapons, abuse of a person who is disabled, or IPV witnessed by children. As per the Massachusetts Medical Society Committee on Violence, "a physician who fails to comply with his or her mandated reporting responsibilities may be subject to disciplinary action, fines, or civil liability." [86]

Care of Sexual and Gender Minority Adults

The care of the sexual and gender minority adult must aim to amend the inequities in healthcare that these groups have experienced and continued to endure. These inequities have its root in homo- and transphobia and their effects on society and the healthcare system. Barriers to healthcare have yielded serious morbidity and mortality with higher rates of depression, attempted suicide, substance abuse, lower rates of screening and prevention interventions, higher cardiovascular risk (bisexuals), overweight and increased cardiovascular disease risk in lesbians, and high drinking and IPV among bisexual women among other [93].

Clinicians and healthcare workers, in general, have the responsibility to provide quality care to all patients and to attain the necessary skills to achieve this goal. They must recognize that a sizeable portion of the population are LGBQ or TGNB and understand that they are in the normal range of human sexuality. Validating their experiences, connecting at a personal level, and learning and practicing professional humility as one learns the effects of minority stress on patients are critical. Clinicians should partner with their patients to attain a higher state of health while respecting, reaffirming, and supporting their identity. Asking the patient about their sexual orientation and gender identity, inquiring about pronoun use and preferred name, and utilizing this information in an affirming way for further interactions represent measures of acceptance and respect. Clinicians should use the same identifier the patient prefers for sexual and/or love relationships (e.g., partner, wife, spouse, etc.).

For TGNB patients, it is important to provide a safe environment and to perform a physical examination by anatomical region, exposing only the region to be examined. Refrain from using anatomical names unless the anatomical description is gender reaffirming. For example, in a male who was assigned female at birth, state "We will be examining your chest or top" instead of using the term breasts or for a male to female patient that has undergone gender affirming surgery, refer to their vagina rather than their "neo-vagina."

In general, screening follows age-related recommendations and the concept of "if you have it or use it, we should test it." Providers must be aware of the patient's anatomy and practices to provide appropriate screening. For further information sexual and reproductive health in TGNB patients, please refer to Part 3 of this book.

Conclusion

When caring for the adult patient, it is critical to recognize that sexual and reproductive health is central to overall health. The role of healthcare workers is to enhance understanding of SRH by educating, guiding, and promoting a positive and respectful approach to sex. The transformation must happen first when providers can confidentially and safely discuss and assess patients' sexual practices in an open, non-judgmental, and supportive way. Clinicians must address the physical, social, emotional, and mental health needs of their patients and promote safe sexual behavior that is free of intimidation, violence, or coercion.

References

1. McCone KL, Moser R Jr, Smith KR. A survey of physicians' knowledge and application of AIDS prevention capabilities. Am J Prev Med. 1991;7:141–5.
2. Sobecki JN, et al. What We Do not Talk about When We Don't Talk about Sex: Results of a National Survey of US Obstetrician/Gynecologists. J Sex Med. 9(5):1285–94.
3. The Women's Sexual Health Foundation. Sexual health discussion survey. Retrieved from www.twshf.org/survey.html.
4. Association of Reproductive Health Professionals and the National Women's Health Resource Center. 2009. Women's sexual health: provider survey. Retrieved from www.arph.org/Publications-and-Resources.
5. Verhoeven V, Bovijn K, Helder A, Peremans L, Hermann I, Van Royen P, Denekens J, Avonts D. Discussing STIs: doctors are from Mars, patients from Venus. Fam Pract. 2003;20:11–5.
6. Sobecki JN, Curlin FA, Rasinski KA, Lindau ST. What we don't talk about when we don't talk about sex: results of a national survey of U.S. obstetrician/gynecologists. J Sex Med. 2012;9:1285–94.

7. Schilling LM, Scatena L, Steiner JF, et al. The third person in the room: frequency, role and influence of companions during primary care medical encounters. J Fam Pract. 2002;51:685–90.
8. Hull SK, Karen B. How to manage difficult patient encounters. Fam Pract Manag. 2007;14(6):30–4.
9. Centers for Disease Control and Prevention. A guide to taking a sexual history. Retrieved from https://www.cdc.gov/std/treatment/sexualhistory.pdf.
10. National LGBT Health Education Center & National Association of Community Health Centers. November 2015. Taking routine histories of sexual health: a system-wide approach for health centers. Retrieved from http://www.lgbthealtheducation.org/wp-content/uploads/COM-827-sexual-history_toolkit_2015.pdf.
11. Nussbaum MRH, et al. The proactive sexual history. Am Fam Physician. 2002;66:1705–12.
12. UpToDate, Inc. 2018. Evaluation of secondary amenorrhea. Retrieved from https://www.uptodate.com/contents/image?imageKey=ENDO%2F109616&topicKey=ENDO%2F7402&source=see_link.
13. Committee on Practice Bulletins—Gynecology. Practice bulletin no. 128: diagnosis of abnormal uterine bleeding in reproductive-aged women. Obstet Gynecol. 2012;120:197. Reaffirmed 2016.
14. Kjerulff KH, Erickson BA, Langenberg PW. Chronic gynecological conditions reported by US women: findings from the National Health Interview Survey, 1984 to 1992. Am J Public Health. 1996;86:195.
15. Munro MG, Critchley HO, Broder MS, et al. FIGO classification system (PALM-COEIN) for causes of abnormal uterine bleeding in nongravid women of reproductive age. Int J Gynaecol Obstet. 2011;113:3.
16. Committee on Practice Bulletins—Gynecology. Practice bulletin no. 136: management of abnormal uterine bleeding associated with ovulatory dysfunction. Obstet Gynecol. 2013;122:176. Reaffirmed 2018
17. Endicott J, Nee J, Harrison W. Arch Womens Ment Health. 2006;9:41. Retrieved from. https://doi.org/10.1007/s00737-005-0103-y.
18. Marjoribanks J, Brown J, O'Brien PM, Wyatt K. Selective serotonin reuptake inhibitors for premenstrual syndrome. Cochrane Database Syst Rev. 2013;2013:CD001396.
19. Feldman HA, Goldstein I, Hatzichristou DG, et al. Impotence and its medical and psychosocial correlates: results of the Massachusetts Male Aging Study. J Urol. 1994;151:54.
20. Araujo AB, Mohr BA, McKinlay JB. Changes in sexual function in middle-aged and older men: longitudinal data from the Massachusetts Male Aging Study. J Am Geriatr Soc. 2004;52:1502.
21. Laumann EO, Paik A, Rosen RC. Sexual dysfunction in the United States: prevalence and predictors. JAMA. 1999;281:537.
22. Rosen RC, Fisher WA, Eardley I, et al. The multinational Men's attitudes to life events and sexuality (MALES) study: I. Prevalence of erectile dysfunction and related health concerns in the general population. Curr Med Res Opin. 2004;20:607.
23. Cocores JA, Miller NS, Pottash AC, Gold MS. Sexual dysfunction in abusers of cocaine and alcohol. Am J Drug Alcohol Abuse. 1988;14:169.
24. Schwarzer U, Sommer F, Klotz T, et al. Cycling and penile oxygen pressure: the type of saddle matters. Eur Urol. 2002;41:139.
25. Patrick DL, Althof SE, Pryor JL, et al. Premature ejaculation: an observational study of men and their partners. J Sex Med. 2005;2:358.
26. Rosen RC, McMahon CG, Niederberger C, et al. Correlates to the clinical diagnosis of premature ejaculation: results from a large observational study of men and their partners. J Urol. 2007;177:1059.
27. Shifren JL, Monz BU, Russo PA, et al. Sexual problems and distress in United States women: prevalence and correlates. Obstet Gynecol. 2008;112:970.
28. Aydin M, Cayonu N, Kadihasanoglu M, et al. Comparison of sexual functions in pregnant and non-pregnant women. Urol J. 2015;12:2339.

29. Barrett G, Pendry E, Peacock J, et al. Women's sexual health after childbirth. BJOG. 2000;107:186.
30. Achtari C, Dwyer PL. Sexual function and pelvic floor disorders. Best Pract Res Clin Obstet Gynaecol. 2005;19:993.
31. Handa VL, Whitcomb E, Weidner AC, et al. Sexual function before and after non-surgical treatment for stress urinary incontinence. Female Pelvic Med Reconstr Surg. 2011;17:30.
32. Hulter BM, Lundberg PO. Sexual function in women with advanced multiple sclerosis. J Neurol Neurosurg Psychiatry. 1995;59:83.
33. Grant AC, Oh H. Gabapentin-induced anorgasmia in women. Am J Psychiatry. 2002;159:1247.
34. Newman LC, Broner SW, Lay CL. Reversible anorgasmia with topiramate therapy for migraine. Neurology. 2005;65:1333.
35. Carey JC. Pharmacological effects on sexual function. Obstet Gynecol Clin North Am. 2006;33:599.
36. Lindau ST, Schumm LP, Laumann EO, et al. A study of sexuality and health among older adults in the United States. N Engl J Med. 2007;357:762.
37. Boozalis A, Tutlam NT, Chrisman Robbins C, Peipert JF. Sexual desire and hormonal contraception. Obstet Gynecol. 2016;127:563.
38. Harte CB, Meston CM. The inhibitory effects of nicotine on physiological sexual arousal in nonsmoking women: results from a randomized, double-blind, placebo-controlled, cross-over trial. J Sex Med. 2008;5:1184.
39. Van Thiel DH, Gavaler JS, Eagon PK, et al. Alcohol and sexual function. Pharmacol Biochem Behav. 1980;13(Suppl 1):125.
40. Centers for Disease Control and Prevention. Sexually transmitted diseases surveillance 2016. Atlanta: Department of Health and Human Services; 2017. Retrieved from https://www.cdc.gov/std/stats16/CDC_2016_STDS_Report-for508WebSep21_2017_1644.pdf.
41. Centers for Disease Control and Prevention. 2015 Sexually transmitted diseases treatment guidelines. Retrieved from https://www.cdc.gov/std/tg2015/default.htm.
42. Centers for Disease Control and Prevention. November 2016. HIV Surveillance Report, 2016; vol 27. Retrieved from https://cdc.gov/hiv/library/reports/hiv-surveillance.html.
43. Hess K., Hu X., Lansky A., Mermin J., & Hall H. I. 2016. Estimating the lifetime risk of a diagnosis of HIV infection in the United States. Conference on retroviruses and opportunistic infections 2016. Boston MA #52.
44. Herbst JH, et al. Estimating HIV prevalence and risk behaviors of transgender persons in the United States: a systematic review. AIDS Behav. 2008;12(1):1–17.
45. Clark H, et al. Diagnosed HIV infection in transgender adults and adolescents: results from the National HIV Surveillance System 2009-2014. AIDS Behav. 2017;21(9):2774–83.
46. Patel P, et al. Estimating per-act HIV transmission risk: a systematic review. AIDS. 2014;28(10):1509–19. https://doi.org/10.1097/QAD.0000000000000298.
47. Rotheram-Borus MJ, et al. The past, present and future of HIV prevention:integrating behavioral, biomedical, and structural intervention strategies for the next generation HIV prevention. Annu Rev Clin Psychol. 2009;5:143–67.
48. Bekker L-G, Beyrer C, Quinn TC. Behavioral and biomedical combination strategies for HIV prevention. Cold Spring Harb Perspect Med. 2012;2(8):a007435. https://doi.org/10.1101/cshperspect.a007435.
49. Finer LB, Zolna MR. Declines in unintended pregnancy in the United States, 2008-2011. N Engl J Med. 2016;374:843.
50. Johnson-Mallard et al. Women's midlife health. 2017; 3:8. 10.1186/s40695-017-0027-5.
51. Nettleman MD, Chung H, Brewer J, et al. Reasons for unprotected intercourse: analysis of the PRAMS survey. Contraception. 2007;75:361.
52. Reproductive Health Access Project. December 2014. Pregnancy options counseling model. Retrieved from https://www.reproductiveaccess.org/resource/pregnancy-options-counseling-model/.

53. Reproductive Health Access Project. June 2016. Early abortion options. Retrieved from https://www.reproductiveaccess.org/wp-content/uploads/2014/12/early_abortion_options.pdf.
54. Centers for Disease Control and Prevention. April 2018. Infertility FAQs. Retrieved from https://www.cdc.gov/reproductivehealth/infertility/index.htm.
55. American College of Obstetricians and Gynecologists Committee on Gynecologic Practice and Practice Committee. Female age-related fertility decline. Committee Opinion No. 589. Fertil Steril. 2014;101:633.
56. Southern California Reproductive Center. May 2016. Fertility treatment options for LGBT couples. Retrieved from https://blog.scrcivf.com/fertility-treatment-options-for-lgbt-couples.
57. AIDSinfo. November 2017. Recommendations for use of antiretroviral drugs in pregnant HIV-1-infected women for maternal health and interventions to reduce perinatal HIV transmission in the United States. Retrieved from https://aidsinfo.nih.gov/contentfiles/lvguidelines/glchunk/glchunk_153.pdf.
58. Centers for Disease Control and Prevention. August 2018. Shingles vaccination. Retrieved from https://www.cdc.gov/vaccines/vpd/shingles/public/shingrix/index.html.
59. Holman DM, Benard V, Roland KB, Watson M, Liddon N, Stokley S. Barriers to human papillomavirus vaccination among U.S. adolescents: A systematic review of the literature. JAMA Pediatr. 2014;168(1):76–82.
60. Meites E, Kempe A, Markowitz LE. Use of a 2-dose schedule for human papillomavirus vaccination — updated recommendations of the advisory committee on immunization practices. MMWR Morb Mortal Wkly Rep. 2016;65:1405–8. https://doi.org/10.15585/mmwr.mm6549a5.
61. Centers for Disease Control and Prevention. Prevention and control of meningococcal disease. MMWR. 2013;62(RR-2):1–26.
62. Centers for Disease Control and Prevention. May 2018. HPV Vaccine information for clinicians. Retrieved from https://www.cdc.gov/hpv/hcp/need-to-know.pdf.
63. Centers for Disease Control and Prevention. May 2006. Prevention of hepatitis A through active or passive immunization: recommendations of the advisory committee on immunization practices (ACIP). Retrieved from https://www.cdc.gov/mmwr/preview/mmwrhtml/rr5507a1.htm.
64. Schillie S, Vellozzi C, Reingold A, et al. Prevention of hepatitis B virus infection in the United States: recommendations of the advisory committee on immunization practices. MMWR Recomm Rep. 2018;67(RR-1):1–31. https://doi.org/10.15585/mmwr.rr6701a1.
65. Centers for Disease Control and Prevention. June 2013. Prevention of measles, rubella, congenital rubella syndrome, and mumps, 2013: Summary Recommendations of the advisory committee on immunization practices (ACIP). Retrieved from https://www.cdc.gov/mmwr/preview/mmwrhtml/rr6204a1.htm.
66. Centers for Disease Control and Prevention. April 2018. Prevention of pertussis, tetanus, and diphtheria with vaccines in the United States: recommendations of the advisory committee on immunization practices (ACIP). Retrieved from https://www.cdc.gov/mmwr/volumes/67/rr/rr6702a1.htm.
67. Centers for Disease Control and Prevention. November 2016. Routine Varicella Vaccination. Retrieved from https://www.cdc.gov/vaccines/vpd/varicella/hcp/recommendations.html.
68. U.S. Preventive Services Task Force. August 2018. Final recommendation statement: cervical cancer: Screening. Retrieved from https://www.uspreventiveservicestaskforce.org/Page/Document/RecommendationStatementFinal/cervical-cancer-screening2.
69. Vesco KK, Whitlock EP, Eder M, Lin J, Burda BU, Senger CA, Holmes RS, Fu R, Zuber S. Screening for cervical cancer: a systematic evidence review for the U.S. preventive services task force. Evidence Synthesis No. 86. AHRQ Publication No. 11-05156-EF-1. Rockville: Agency for Healthcare Research and Quality; 2011.
70. Elit L, Fyles AW, Devries MC, et al. Follow-up for women after treatment for cervical cancer: a systematic review. Gynecol Oncol. 2009;114:528.

71. Salani R, Backes FJ, Fung MF, et al. Posttreatment surveillance and diagnosis of recurrence in women with gynecologic malignancies: Society of Gynecologic Oncologists recommendations. Am J Obstet Gynecol. 2011;204:466.

72. Salit I, Lytwyn A, Raboud J, et al. The role of cytology (pap tests) and human papillomavirus testing in anal cancer screening. AIDS. 2010;24(9):1307–13. https://doi.org/10.1097/QAD.0b013e328339e592.

73. Machalek DA, Poynten M, Jin F, et al. Anal human papillomavirus infection and associated neoplastic lesions in men who have sex with men: a systematic review and meta-analysis. Lancet Oncol. 2012;13(5):487–500. https://doi.org/10.1016/S1470-2045(12)70080-3. Epub 2012 Mar 23

74. Aberg JA, Gallant JE, Ghanem KG, Emmanuel P, Zingman BS, Horberg MA. Executive summary: primary care guidelines for the management of persons infected with HIV: 2013 Update by the HIV Medicine Association of the Infectious Diseases Society of America. Clin Infect Dis. 2014;58(1):1–10. https://doi.org/10.1093/cid/cit757.

75. Siu AL, Bibbins-Domingo K, Grossman DC, et al. Screening for breast cancer: U.S. preventive services task force recommendation statement. Ann Intern Med. 2016;164:279–96. https://doi.org/10.7326/M15-2886.

76. U.S. Preventive Services Task Force. May 2018. Final recommendation statement: prostate cancer: Screening. Retrieved from https://www.uspreventiveservicestaskforce.org/Page/Document/RecommendationStatementFinal/prostate-cancer-screening1.

77. Tjaden P, Thoennes N. Extent, nature, and consequences of intimate partner violence: findings from the National Violence Against Women Survey. Washington, DC: Publication No. NCJ-181867, US Department of Justice; 2000.

78. Nelson HD, Bougatsos C, Blazina I. Screening women for intimate partner violence: a systematic review to update the U.S. Preventive Services Task Force recommendation. Ann Intern Med. 2012;156:796.

79. World Health Organization. Violence by intimate partners. Retrieved from http://www.who.int/violence_injury_prevention/violence/global_campaign/en/chap4.pdf.

80. Brown T. N. T. and Herman J. L. November 2015. The Williams Institute. Intimate partner violence and sexual abuse among LGBT people: A Review of Existing Research. Retrieved from https://williamsinstitute.law.ucla.edu/wp-content/uploads/Intimate-Partner-Violence-and-Sexual-Abuse-among-LGBT-People.pdf.

81. Moyer VA, U.S. Preventive Services Task Force. Screening for intimate partner violence and abuse of elderly and vulnerable adults: U.S. preventive services task force recommendation statement. Ann Intern Med. 2013;158:478.

82. U.S. Preventive Services Task Force. Screening for intimate partner violence and abuse of vulnerable adults: U.S. Preventive Services Task Force recommendation. Ann Intern Med. 2013;158:I.

83. World Health Organization. Responding to intimate partner violence and sexual violence against women. WHO clinical and policy guidelines. 2013. http://www.who.int/reproductive-health/publications/violence/9789241548595/en/. Accessed on 29 Aug 2013.

84. American College of Physicians. In: Ryden J, Blumenthal PD, Charney P, editors. Intimate Partner violence in practical gynecology: a guide for the primary care physician. 2nd ed. Philadelphia: American College of Physicians; 2009.

85. Ashur ML. Asking about domestic violence: SAFE questions. JAMA. 1993;269:2367.

86. Alpert, EJ. Intimate Partner Violence. The clinician's guide to identification, assessment, intervention, and prevention. 5th Edition. Massachusetts Medical Society, 2010. http://www.massmed.org/AM/Template.cfm?Section=Home6&CONTENTID=36015&TEMPLATE=/CM/ContentDisplay.cfm.

87. McFarlane J, Parker B, Soeken K, Bullock L. Assessing for abuse during pregnancy. Severity and frequency of injuries and associated entry into prenatal care. JAMA. 1992;267:3176.

88. Sherin KM, Sinacore JM, Li XQ, et al. HITS: a short domestic violence screening tool for use in a family practice setting. Fam Med. 1998;30:508.

89. Feldhaus KM, Koziol-McLain J, Amsbury HL, et al. Accuracy of 3 brief screening questions for detecting partner violence in the emergency department. JAMA. 1997;277:1357.
90. Sohal H, Eldridge S, Feder G. The sensitivity and specificity of four questions (HARK) to identify intimate partner violence: a diagnostic accuracy study in general practice. BMC Fam Pract. 2007;8:49.
91. Paranjape A, Liebschutz J. STaT: a three-question screen for intimate partner violence. J Womens Health (Larchmt). 2003;12:233.
92. Brown JB, Lent B, Schmidt G, Sas G. Application of the woman abuse screening tool (WAST) and WAST-short in the family practice setting. J Fam Pract. 2000;49:896.
93. Conron KJ, Mimiaga MJ, Landers SJ. A population-based study of sexual orientation identity and gender differences in adult health. Am J Public Health. 2010;100(10):1953–60. https://doi.org/10.2105/AJPH.2009.174169. Epub 2010 Jun 1.

Chapter 4
Sexual Health in the Older Adults

Noelle Marie Javier and Rainier Patrick Soriano

Contents

N. M. Javier (✉)
Brookdale Department of Geriatrics and Palliative Medicine, Mount Sinai Hospital,
New York, NY, USA
e-mail: noelle.javier@mssm.edu

R. P. Soriano
Brookdale Department of Geriatrics and Palliative Medicine and Department of Medical
Education, Icahn School of Medicine at Mount Sinai, New York, NY, USA

Brookdale Department of Geriatrics and Palliative Medicine, The Mount Sinai Hospital,
New York, NY, USA
e-mail: rainier.soriano@mssm.edu

© Springer Nature Switzerland AG 2022
J. Truglio et al. (eds.), *Sexual and Reproductive Health*,
https://doi.org/10.1007/978-3-030-94632-6_4

Introduction

As of 2014, older adults account for about 14.5% of the population in the USA. This translates to about 46.2 million adults 65 years of age and older [1]. With advancing technology and better health care, it is expected that the older adult population will continue to rise. By 2060, about 98 million people will belong to the 65 years old and over age group. There is an ongoing need to provide high-quality and comprehensive primary geriatric care. Sexual health is part of this holistic care. The World Health Organization (WHO) views sexuality as a central aspect of being human throughout life, while sexual health is a state of physical, emotional, mental, and social well-being related to sexuality, not merely the absence of disease, dysfunction, or infirmity. It requires a positive and respectful approach to sexuality and sexual relationships, as well as the possibility of having pleasurable and safe sexual experiences, free of coercion, discrimination, and violence [2]. There is a growing body of evidence that older adults across the life course have sexual needs similar to their younger cohorts [3]. However despite the evidence, there persists a misconception that people become asexual as they get older and that they lose their interest in sex and their capacity for sexual behavior [4, 5]. Consequentially, clinicians do not address sexual health as proactively as they do other aspects of clinical care. Hence sexual health surveillance continues to be underemphasized in routine care. Therefore, healthcare professionals should be trained not only in eliciting relevant history taking and conducting physical examinations but also managing sexual health concerns and including it as part of the standard of care for all patients of various backgrounds.

This chapter underscores the value of bringing sexual health to the forefront of comprehensive geriatric care. It provides guidance for clinicians in knowing common barriers to sexual health care and effective strategies in mitigating them through effective history taking and physical examination thereby allowing for sound management plans. Furthermore, the scope of this chapter includes specific considerations in sexual health surveillance such as screening for sexually transmitted infections (STIs) and HIV, immunization recommendations, and targeted cancer screening guidelines. Additionally, an overview for an all-inclusive and gender-affirming care for the LGBTQ population will also be highlighted towards the end of this chapter.

Significance of Sexual Health

Adults remain sexually active until their later years. Only a few report discussing sexual health with a physician after age 50 [6]. Furthermore the available research that exists continues to be limited by challenges such as embarrassment during interviews, self-report biases, and poor response rates to survey questionnaires [7]. Having said that, the existing literature supports the findings that as people age, there is an overall decline in sexual interest while a significant proportion of older adults gave it at least some importance [8, 9]. A study by Gott and Hinchliff in the United Kingdom noted that older adults aged 70 years and above placed less importance on sex than the younger participants [10]. This is somewhat consistent with the study by Lindau et al. using a national probability sample of more than 3000 adults in the United States where 59% of the 75- to 85-year-old age groups still attributed some importance to sex [11]. Across genders, older adult cisgender males have a higher prevalence in sexual interest compared to their cisgender female counterparts [12]. A 2010 study by Schick et al. focused on the sexual behavior, condom use, and sexual health of older Americans 50 years of age and over. They concluded that many older adults continue to be sexually active well into their 80s. This highlights the need for providers to be attentive to the diverse sexual needs of their older adult patients [13]. In a 2012 study by Trompeter et al. looking at the sexual activity and satisfaction of healthy community-dwelling older cisgender women ($n = 1303$) whose median age is 67 years old, half of these women were sexually active with arousal, lubrication, and orgasm that carried through old age despite low libido in a one-third. Sexual satisfaction increased with age and did not require sexual activity [14]. A recent 2017 cross-sectional study looked at the prevalence of sexual activity and tenderness in older adults. Of a sample of more than 2000 dementia-free and community-dwelling older adults aged 65 years and above, almost half of partnered older adults engaged in sexual activity and more than two-thirds engaged in physical tenderness. Furthermore, the study showed that the biggest barrier to sexual activity is a lack of partner especially among older cisgender, heterosexual women. Therefore, sexuality is an important aspect of active aging [15]. With that said, it is also a known fact that healthcare professionals contribute to minimal exploration of sexual health issues by virtue of their own discomfort asking questions related to this topic and the underestimate of sexual health needs and concerns in comparison to their younger cohort of patients. Furthermore, the providers' stereotypes on aging and sexuality provide an additional challenge to comprehensive care [16]. Therefore sexual history taking remains suboptimal [17, 18]. Along with other barriers to care as explored later in this chapter, there is an immediate call to action to create changes in how healthcare professionals conduct comprehensive health visit examinations by improving what constitutes standard medical care afforded to all patients across age and settings.

Aging Considerations in Sexual Physiology

The human sexual response cycle is mediated by the complex interplay of psychological, environmental, and physiological factors (hormonal, vascular, muscular, and neurological) [19]. The hormonal levels of both estrogen and testosterone are important considerations in the human sexual response. As a function of aging, the levels change over time. The reduction in estrogen level is associated with changes in the structural integrity of the female genitalia resulting in vaginal dryness and atrophy, dyspareunia, and urinary tract symptoms. The reduction of testosterone levels after the fifth decade results from testicular aging, increased sex hormone binding globulin (SHBG), and testosterone binding. Furthermore, there is a relative failure of the hypothalamic-pituitary-adrenal (HPA) axis. [19] Per Masters and Johnson, the speed and intensity of the vaso-congestive responses to sexual stimulation tend to be reduced in the aging genders. Bancroft describes the changes for individuals with female genitalia as follows: decreased sexual desire, increased time for sexual arousal, slower vaginal lubrication response, less intense orgasms, increased need for stimulation towards orgasms, no change in the ability to have orgasms, less likely to have multiple orgasms, and more rapid resolution following orgasms [20]. For those with male genitalia, the changes are as follows: decreased sexual desire, longer time for erections, shorter period of time to sustain erection, less frequent nocturnal erections and emissions, less marked scrotal and testicular changes to arousal, production of less pre-ejaculatory mucus, less powerful erections, reduction of seminal fluid, challenges associated with the inevitability of ejaculation, more rapid resolution, and longer refractory period [20].

The Sexual Health Visit

Consent, Privacy, and Confidentiality

Since sexual history is an important aspect of overall medical care, obtaining information pertaining to this should be given the same importance for confidentiality in comparison to other aspects of comprehensive medical histories. Therefore, information reflected on the medical records should be treated with utmost respect for privacy and confidentiality. Healthcare professionals should observe HIPAA (Health Insurance Portability and Accountability Act) compliance. This should be adhered to at all times especially when sharing information with other medical providers. Informed consent should be obtained prior to sharing sensitive information [21]. This should be laid out on any given patient visit. Furthermore, from an institutional standpoint, offices should show visible signs of confidentiality and privacy. This should include patient waiting areas, staff spaces, restrooms, and patient rooms.

When obtaining relevant information for sexual health, the healthcare professional should obtain consent from patients to ask questions as well as formal documentations on the medical records. The reassurance for privacy and utmost confidentiality could not be overemphasized before eliciting further information. One strategy involves normalizing the conversation regarding overall sexual health and concerns as part of the standard of health care. During the actual visit, patients should be afforded privacy before eliciting questions pertaining to sexual health especially if they have accompanying family members or caregivers. Additionally, patients should also be asked their consent regarding sexual history taking when there are other learners, trainees, and staff members in the room. It is important to highlight that obtaining sexual history as standard of care should not make the patient feel as though they have to answer questions related to this. They should be offered an opportunity to defer and refuse further conversations.

It is also important to underscore that laws regarding confidentiality and consent vary by state. Therefore, healthcare professionals should be familiar with local legislation in the states they practice especially around the aspects of the electronic medical records, clinical and laboratory billing practices, explanation of benefits forms, and sharing and delivery of medical information with other providers and institutions [22].

The issues of consent, privacy, and confidentiality will be explored further as it remains relevant to subsequent topics such as sexual health screening, STI and HIV prevention, and sexual abuse among others.

History Taking

A proper sexual health assessment starts with a comprehensive history taking of sexual function, needs, and concerns. By doing so, healthcare professionals serve to enhance the quality of life of older adult patients by bringing out in the open sexual health as an integral domain of humanistic medical care. Risen [23], Tomlinson [24], and Kingsberg [25] provide ideas in the conduct of proper history taking. The strategies are outlined below.

1. Understand the barriers to taking a sexual history including lack of knowledge other than one's own experience, fear of the effects generated by taking a sexual history, use of sexual vocabulary, and ageism.
2. Ensure comfortable seating by the patient in a private room and free from interruptions.
3. Assure patient confidentiality.
4. Interview both partners when available. However, offer the option for the patient to discuss separately from an accompanying partner(s).
5. The ideal time for taking a sexual history is when the clinician collects information about the psychosocial aspect of care. The advantage of taking a sexual history at an early stage, regardless of whether or not a sexual problem exists, is that it gives the patient permission to speak of sexual issues in the future.

6. Use open and non-threatening questions. Avoid judgmental questions. These encourage patients to tell their sexual history using their own language. Examples include:
   (a) What is the role of sexuality in your life right now?
   (b) Are you experiencing any sexual problems or concerns?
7. Obtain a thorough psychosocial history when time allows for it. Components that could be included are childhood to adulthood history; role of religion; quality of relationships with family, friends, and others; family attitudes towards sexuality and gender; and current relationships among others.
8. Obtain a thorough medical and psychiatric history.
9. Elicit information about use of medical and recreational chemical substances.
10. Formulation and summation of problems identified in the context of predisposing, precipitating, and maintaining factors as well as developing a management plan and discussed with patients and their partner(s).

The components of sexual history taking are shown in Table 4.1 [7, 26–28].

Physical Examination

Following a thorough sexual history is a comprehensive physical examination with attention to areas of concern and potential factors that may cause the problems. It is important to maintain confidentiality and privacy while examining patients. Moreover, it is essential obtain proper consent before conducting an exam. It is helpful to have another staff member (of the same gender as your patient) to be present in the room as part of care. Asking patients if their family members or caregivers should be asked to leave or stay in the room is consistent with good bedside manners. At all times, the healthcare provider should practice utmost competence and professionalism. Avoidance of premature judgments and insensitive remarks should be upheld consistently throughout the process. By doing so, there is mutual trust between the patient and the provider. It will be helpful to have the patients take the lead in identifying issues in the genital areas as these relate to perceived problems. For the medical provider, explaining what is being examined will be highly appreciated by patients thereby strengthening collaboration and therapeutic alliance.

For older adult patients endorsing problems with erection, attention should be paid to signs of vascular or neurologic disease. Other parts to be considered include palpation of peripheral pulses, checking for orthostasis, and examination of the bulbocavernosus reflex. Additionally, palpation of the penis and testicles is mandatory when men present with erectile dysfunction (ED) and hypogonadism. Examination of the breasts to look for gynecomastia should not be overlooked.

When examining breasts and pelvic organs in older adult patients, one may observe gross abnormalities that can narrow down possible diagnoses. Asking and/or confirming prior surgeries will aid in a more targeted examination. Since older adult patients are prone to developing vaginal dryness leading to dyspareunia once menopause hits, a focused exam is warranted. Palpating the walls for suspicious growths, vaginal wall lining abnormalities, and spasms can help narrow down sexual dysfunction issues among women. Additionally, women are prone to developing urinary tract infections (UTI).

Table 4.1 Components of sexual history taking (adapted from multiple references with additional modifications)

Component	Sample questions
Status of sexual activity of the patient (to include frequency)	Are you currently sexually active? When was the last time you had sex? How often do you have sex?
Number of current partners (current, specific time period, and in a lifetime)	How many partner(s) do you have sex with at the current time? In the last 6 months? In the past year? In your lifetime since the start of sexual activity?
Gender identities of current and former sexual activity partners	What is/are the gender identity(−ies) of your current sexual partner(s)? What is/are the gender identity(−ies) of your former sexual partner(s)? What is/are the gender identity(−ies) of your sexual partner(s) over your lifetime?
Type(s) of sexual behavior and practice(s)	What type(s) of sexual practices do you engage in? e.g., oral sex (penis/clitoris in the mouth), anal sex (penis in the anus/rectum), mutual masturbation (aka hand job), vaginal sex (penis inside the vagina), combination, use of toys other(s)?
Safety in sexual practices	When engaging in sex, do you use any type of protection such as condoms, OCPs, etc. If so, how often do you use protection such as condoms, oral contraceptives (OCPs), etc.? In what sexual practices do you use protective barriers, medications, etc.? Are you taking prophylactic medications such as PrEP at the current time? Have you taken this medication in the past?
Sexually transmitted infection (STI) screening to include sexual partner STI screening	Have you ever had an STI in the past? Have you been treated for an STI in the past Do you currently have an STI? Are you taking any medications for it? Has your partner(s) been treated for an STI in the past What do you know of your partner(s)' sexual history? What is your HIV status? Have you ever been tested for HIV? How often? When was the last time you were tested for HIV? What is your hepatitis status? Have you ever been tested for hepatitis B and C? When was the last time you were tested for hepatitis B and C? Is/are there specific STI(s) that your medical provider need to know?
Birth control	What are you doing to prevent pregnancy? Do you use barrier protection such as condoms, or take medications such as oral contraceptives, some combination, or others?

Table 4.1 (continued)

Component	Sample questions
State of sexual being	Do you have any concerns about your state of sexual being? Are you experiencing any problems in your sexual life? Are you satisfied or dissatisfied overall with sex? Sometimes when people feel very low or depressed, they lose interest in sex. Do you think that is an issue for you? Do you have any concerns about keeping yourself sexually healthy and safe?
State of sexual performance	Have you been satisfied with the frequency and nature of your sexual activities? Do you have any concerns or issues regarding sexual performance? Are there challenges achieving arousal, erection, ejaculation, lubrication, orgasm(s), etc.? Do you currently experience sexual performance anxiety? Have you had sexual performance anxiety in the past? For cisgender women-identified: Often cisgender women around the time of menopause can suffer not only with the hot flushes you have described but also with sexual problems such as vaginal dryness. Is that something you have experienced?
History of sexual abuse	Have you ever been sexually abused in the past? Are you currently being sexually abused? Do you worry about being sexually abused? Have you sought treatment regarding sexual abuse? Has anyone ever coerced or forced you to have sex? Have you ever been touched in a sexual way against your consent?
High-risk sexual behavior associated with use of chemical substance(s)	Do you currently engage in use of street drugs? What type of drug(s) have you used in the past when engaging in sex? How do you use these chemicals? Shooting, skin popping, injecting, snorting, smoking, etc.? Do you currently drink? What types of drink(s)? How often do you drink? Do you mix alcohol with another chemical substance while having sex? Have you ever been treated for drug addiction, alcohol abuse, both, etc.? Are you interested in seeking treatment for drug addiction, alcohol abuse, etc.? Do your partner(s) use illicit substances when having sex with you?
Other sexual concerns	Do you have other sexual concerns not covered during this or past visit?

References: Taylor et al. [7]; Granville et al. [26]; Ports et al. [27]; Sexually Transmitted Diseases Treatment Guidelines CDC [153]

Counseling and Education

Healthcare professional knowledge about sexuality at older ages should improve patient education, counseling, and the ability to recognize the spectrum of health-related and potentially treatable sexual problems. A big part of education is normalizing the conversation about sexuality with colleagues and patients. Using an open and empathic language when eliciting information on sexual health can go a long way to establish trust and provide holistic care. Since the 1960s, experts in sexuality and aging have emphasized the need for information dissemination regarding sexual physiology and the acceptability of sexual feelings and behaviors well into old age. The preparation and distribution of educational pamphlets and brochures as well as promoting wellness sessions to include sexual health are avenues for information sharing. Educating the older adult about safe sexual practices is equally important. Extending this information towards the patients' partners may be helpful in promoting safe and better sexual health.

Common Sexual Health Issues Among Older Adults

Barriers to Sexual Health

Sexuality is broadly defined as the dynamic outcome of physical capacity, motivation, attitudes, opportunity for partnership, and sexual conduct [29]. As people age over time, there may be external and internal forces or stressors that may affect the definition and expression of sexuality. Physical illnesses such as atherosclerosis and diabetes mellitus can affect sexual function directly by interfering with endocrine, neural, and vascular processes that mediate the sexual response. The indirect consequence is a manifestation of distressing symptoms such as weakness, pain, and psychological destabilization such as loss of self-esteem and changes in body image [30]. Other examples of diseases that alter the human sexual response cycle include hypertension, prostate cancer, urinary tract infection, obesity, pelvic surgery, stroke, hemodialysis patients, arthritis, depression, thyroid dysfunction, and Parkinson's disease among others [31–33]. Furthermore, having multiple medical problems and chronic conditions raises the odds of low sexual desire, less than monthly sexual activity, and low sexual satisfaction [34]. As a result, many older adults are on multiple medications for these chronic medical issues. Drug-induced sexual dysfunction may occur from taking certain medications such as antidepressants, antipsychotics, benzodiazepines, antihypertensives, anticonvulsants, and statins [35–37]. The barriers to seeking treatment for sexual problems include attributing concerns towards aging, embarrassment of the issue, fears, lack of knowledge about services, and perceptions of a healthcare provider's negative attitudes towards sex in later life [26]. Chapter 7 of this book covers sexual dysfunction in detail. Here we focus on sexual dysfunction in older adults. The terminology used below (i.e. male and female sexual dysfunction) reflects the gender-binary state of contemporary literature on the topic. Clinicians should extrapolate the pertinent data for transgender and gender diverse patients.

Male Sexual Dysfunction

One of the most prevalent causes for male sexual dysfunction is erectile dysfunction [38]. Erectile dysfunction (ED) in the older adults is a significant health problem affecting more than 75% of men over 70 years of age in the United States. There is a linear correlation of ED with age, with older men reporting more severe symptoms than younger men [39]. Furthermore in a national study of sexuality and health among older adults in the United States, Lindau found that 37% of men who were sexually active experienced difficulty in achieving or maintaining an erection [11]. Albraugh's study showed that the loss of the ability to engage in penetrative sex adversely affected quality of life [40].

ED is defined as the persistent inability to achieve or maintain an erection sufficient for sexual penetration [41]. The cause for ED is maybe a combination of organic and/or psychological factors. Organic causes include neurogenic, vascular, medication-related, anatomic, and surgical complications, while psychological causes include anxiety, stress, depression, mental illness, or dementia. As men age the more likely precipitants for ED are the organic causes [42]. Hypertension, coronary artery disease, diabetes mellitus, obesity, androgen deficiency, and dyslipidemia are typical organic causes that place men at higher risk for developing erectile dysfunction. A 2006 prospective study of risk factors for erectile dysfunction among men aged 40–75 years showed a positive correlation with obesity and smoking, while physical activity showed an inverse relationship [43]. Furthermore a 2007 study of medication use related to coexisting morbidities among men aged 40 years and above showed a positive correlation of ED with selected antihypertensives, namely, thiazides and diuretics and antidepressants mainly selective serotonin reuptake inhibitors [44]. Therapies for ED include a combination of non-pharmacological and pharmacological modalities of treatment. Examples of non-pharmacological approach include counseling and education about ED; lifestyle modifications such as diet, exercise, and smoking cessation; medication changes; and regular intercourse and penile stimulation. The cornerstones for oral pharmacological therapy are phosphodiesterase inhibitors such as sildenafil, tadalafil, and vardenafil. There is data to support the use of alprostadil which is a synthetic vasodilator administered as an intraurethral suppository or as an intracavernosal injection. This is recommended as second-line pharmacological treatment [45].

Female Sexual Dysfunction

The prevalence of sexual dysfunction occurring in women is disparate in a range of 15% or less to more than 90% in part because of how research questions are phrased and how sexual dysfunction is defined [46, 47]. Female sexual dysfunction (FSD) is an umbrella term comprising a range of common disorders to include hypoactive sexual desire, reduced subjective and/or physical genital arousal (poor sensation, vasocongestion, lubrication), sexual pain, and inability to achieve orgasm/satisfaction which are multidimensional in nature and often coexisting [48].

As women age and reach perimenopausal and menopausal status, they experience more genitourinary symptoms primarily related to vulvovaginal atrophy as a result of reduced estrogen levels. This leads to vaginal itching, soreness, dryness, and painful sex. Furthermore, menopause is accompanied by decreased sexual responsiveness and coital frequency. This therefore leads not only to sexual dysfunction but also emotional well-being, interpersonal relationships, body image perceptions, and day-to-day activities such as bike riding and prolonged sitting [49, 50]. One of the main implications of urogenital atrophy on sexual function is painful sexual intercourse or dyspareunia. As estrogen levels decline, the vaginal epithelium becomes thinner, and the pH rises from a premenopausal value of 3.5–4.5 to a post-menopausal range of 5–7.5. This will then lead to increased microbial colonization and urinary tract infections. About 45% of postmenopausal women experience urogenital atrophy [51]. Apart from the endocrine effects, dyspareunia also results from inadequate lubrication, localized vaginal infections, Bartholin cysts, cystitis, retroverted uterus, uterine prolapse, endometriosis, pelvic tumors, excessive penile thrusting, and vaginismus or involuntary muscle spasms. With subsequent sexual encounter, there is the cyclical effect of anticipatory pain, inadequate arousal, and deficient lubrication. One therapeutic approach is using systemic versus local estrogen therapy. This has little effect on libido or sexual dysfunction. The management of vulvovaginal atrophy includes moisturizers, lubricants, and local or topical estrogen therapy. The American College of Obstetricians and Gynecologists do not recommend systemic progestins when low-dose estrogen therapy is administered [52]. Monitoring while on estrogen therapy is important. Providers should watch out for signs of vaginal bleeding and endometrial hyperplasia. For women with severe vulvovaginal atrophy and painful intercourse, topical lidocaine is recommended before the sex act. In one randomized study, the combination of silicone-based lubricant mixed with 4% aqueous lidocaine to the vaginal vestibule, 3 minutes prior to intercourse, resulted in better sexual function than the lubricant alone. Moreover, male partners did not experience any penile numbness from exposure to lidocaine [53].

The most prevalent sexual dysfunction in women across all ages is a lack of sexual desire [54]. Major risk factors for its development include poor health status, depression, medications, dissatisfaction with partner relationships, and history of abuse. DSM V requires that the woman experiences personal distress. The major implications affect quality of life, sense of well-being, and interpersonal relationships [55]. This is further supported by a large national survey of more than 2000 US women that revealed statistically significant decrements for health status to include mental health among women with hypoactive sexual desire [56]. Furthermore, a 2009 study showed that women with low sexual desire experience more health burdens to include more medical problems, fatigue, depression, cognitive issues, back pain, and overall poorer quality of life [57]. The approach to its management includes a combination of pharmacologic and psychological interventions. Currently, there are no FDA-approved medications for the treatment of low sexual desire in women. Conjugated estrogen and ospemifene are FDA approved for the treatment of dyspareunia which can contribute to low or absent desire [54]. Testosterone is widely prescribed off-label for postmenopausal women with decreased desire. There is evidence that it substantially improves sexual well-being, sexual desire, pleasure, arousal, and frequency of orgasm with a marked reduction in personal distress [58]. Potential adverse effects are virilization, acne, hirsutism, deepening of the voice, and androgenic alopecia. The most common formulation is 1% transdermal cream. Oral formulations are not recommended due to liver and lipid adverse effects. There is also some data pertaining to the use of bupropion as effective for low sexual desire. However, the data exists for premenopausal women [59]. As far as psychotherapeutic management is considered, cognitive behavioral therapy, sex therapy, and mindfulness training have proven some worth [60–62].

Sexually Transmitted Infections (STIs)

This section focuses on the epidemiology, prevention, diagnosis, and management of sexually transmitted infections in older patients. Sexually transmitted infections are discussed in detail in Chap. 7.

Epidemiology

Infection rates related to sexual activity have shown an upward trend for Americans older than 45 years of age. There was a twenty percent (20%) rise of overall prevalence rate for STIs in this age group from 2015 to 2016 [63]. The most common STIs included chlamydia, gonorrhea, and syphilis. The STI rates are especially high in states where there are many retirees such as Florida, Arizona, and California [64].

Background

Older adults who continue to engage in sexual activity are at risk for developing sexually transmitted infections (STIs). This risk may be the result of immunosenescence (age-related weakening of the immune system affecting humoral and cellular immunity) along with anatomic and physiological changes in aging [65]. This supports the concept that older adults have a different susceptibility than their younger cohort [66]. For older adult patients who experience urogenital atrophy after menopause, the thinning of the vaginal walls renders them at risk for tearing during sex, thereby increasing the rate of STIs to include HIV. Menopausal symptoms such as pelvic pain, postmenopausal bleeding, and deep dyspareunia could also mimic STIs, thereby rendering a challenging diagnosis at the outset [67]. Additionally, lower progesterone levels raise the risk of STIs among older cisgender women. Among older cisgender men, normal sexual changes with aging that include reduced testosterone levels that affect testicular size, sperm viability and mobility, and increased time for erection may inversely increase the risk for an older adult patient with erectile dysfunction and taking medication [68]. Older adult patients with erectile dysfunction may not properly use condoms resulting in ineffective means of engaging in safe sexual practices. Furthermore, with the advent of medications to manage erectile dysfunction, older adult patients might engage in riskier sex acts to include intercourse with multiple sexual partners, commercial sex workers, and use of illicit drugs or alcohol while engaging in sex. Milrod and Monto in 2016 looked at older men between the ages of 60 to 84 who employed commercial sex workers. About 50% of them had engaged in at least one sexual activity with a sex worker [69]. There is a tendency to forego use of condoms for both older adult women and men due to the preconceived notion that they may not be at risk and/or no longer at risk for pregnancy. This is supported by the studies of Amin and Schick [13, 70]. Using Medicare claims data in 2009, widowhood increased the risk of STIs among men but not among women [71].

Confidentiality, Reporting, and Consent

The disclosure of pertinent information relevant to sexual health is protected in the medical system through the Health Insurance Portability and Accountability Act (HIPAA) of 1996. This provides protection for individual identifiable health data known as protected health information. However, this has to be carefully balanced with reportable health data to the public health authorities for the purpose of controlling or preventing disease, injury, or disability including but not limited to public health surveillance, investigation, and intervention [72]. Healthcare providers are mandated to follow this rule, and any breach is subject to disciplinary action, civil, and criminal penalties [73]. A patient may choose to disclose protected health information and be shared with other entities provided there is informed authorization [74].

Per the CDC, the accurate and timely reporting of STDs is integral to public health efforts to assess morbidity trends, allocate limited resources, and assist local health authorities in partner notification and treatment. STD/HIV and acquired immunodeficiency syndrome (AIDS) cases should be reported in accordance with state and local statutory requirements. Syphilis (including congenital syphilis), gonorrhea, chlamydia, chancroid, HIV infection, and AIDS are reportable diseases in every state. Because the requirements for reporting other STDs differ by state, clinicians should be familiar with the reporting requirements applicable within their jurisdictions [28].

Reporting can be provider or laboratory-based or both. Clinicians who are unsure of state and local reporting requirements should seek advice from state or local health department STD programs. STDs and HIV reports are kept strictly confidential. In most jurisdictions, such reports are protected by statute or regulation. Before conducting a follow-up of a positive STD test result, public health professionals should consult the patient's healthcare provider if possible to verify the diagnosis and determine the treatments being received.

Counseling and Education

After obtaining the sexual history from patients, all healthcare providers should encourage risk reduction by providing prevention counseling. Prevention counseling is most effective if provided in a nonjudgmental and empathetic manner appropriate to the patient's culture, language, gender identity, gender expression, sexual orientation, chronologic age, and developmental level. The Centers for Disease Control and Prevention (CDC) recommends that prevention counseling for STD/HIV should be offered to all sexually active adolescents and to all adults who have received an STD diagnosis, have had an STD in the past year, or have multiple sexual partners [28]. The USPSTF found adequate evidence that intensive behavioral counseling interventions reduce the likelihood of STIs in sexually active adolescents and in adults who are at increased risk. The USPSTF determined that this benefit is of moderate magnitude. The USPSTF also found adequate evidence that intensive interventions reduce risky sexual behaviors and increase the likelihood of condom use and other protective sexual practices [75]. Intensive behavioral counseling may be delivered in primary care settings or other sectors of the healthcare system [76].

Idso described four areas for safe sex education for newly single older adult patients. These areas include sex education, STIs, safe sex practices, and communication with partner(s) to wear a condom [77]. Older adults should be educated on the age-related sexual physiology changes such as delayed erection and vaginal dryness; types of sexual transmitted infections and their symptomatology, prevention, and management; safe sexual practices including good hygiene and proper use of condoms; ED medications and vaginal lubrication enhancers; and open communication with partner(s) about safe sexual practices. Furthermore, information on self-pleasure activities such as masturbation and other non-penetrative sexual activities that serve as expressions of intimacy should be explored and discussed [77].

Screening for STIs

The CDC recommends screening for STIs in the general population. The USPSTF recommends screening for STIs starting at age 15 years to 65 years of age [28]. The decision on when to stop screening has been variable given that older adults do engage in sexual activity. The USPSTF recommends that routine screening could be stopped for women approaching menopause or at age 55 years [78]. It does not recommend screening for men who are not at increased risk. Meyers et al. in 2008 showed that there is no strong evidence to discontinue screening as individuals at any age are at risk for STI for as long as sexually active [78]. Moreover the USPSTF found inadequate evidence to make recommendations on the optimal intervals for repeat STI screening [79]. The USPSTF suggests instead that a reasonable approach is to screen patients whose sexual history reveals new or risk factors since the last negative test result [80].

Treatment of STIs

The cornerstone of STI pharmacologic management is the use of antimicrobial agents targeted to specific STIs. The details of these therapies are discussed in Chap. 10.

Insurance Coverage

Per Medicare guidelines, Part B covers screening for typical STIs (gonorrhea, syphilis, chlamydia, hepatitis B) once every 12 months for older adults. It also covers up to two individual 20–30 minute, face-to-face, high-intensity behavioral counseling sessions annually for sexually active adults at high risk for STIs [81].

HIV Prevention and Management

As of 2017, the number of adult patients affected by HIV worldwide is 35.1 million [82]. There are about 1.6 million with newly diagnosed HIV for this year. The literature is clear on the rising trend of HIV infection among individuals 50 years and above. In the United States, an estimated 428,724 individuals 50 years and above are living with HIV [83]. This group is most certainly comprised of older adults living with chronic HIV infection over the years, and another part is the rising incidence of new HIV diagnoses [84]. Sexual contact is still the most common mode of HIV transmission [83]. The risk factors for older adults developing HIV infection are the same as their younger cohort. There is a lack of knowledge of HIV prevention as well as the presence of multiple sexual partners as a consequence of being single again and dating and the perceived notion that barrier contraception is no longer necessary as pregnancy is unexpected [83]. This then creates a false sense of security foregoing safe sexual practices among older adults [85]. Injection drug use also remains a significant factor for HIV transmission in this population [86]. Furthermore, older adults are more likely than their younger counterparts to be diagnosed late of their HIV infection in part related to patients' beliefs that their risk is low, lack of interest in getting tested, and the healthcare providers' lack of proactive evaluation for sexually active patients [87].

Given the misperceptions and how underrepresented older adults with HIV infection in educational campaigns, it is important to expand targeted HIV prevention education for those at risk especially the sexually active older adults. A comprehensive sexual history and screening for high-risk sexual behavior should be done at every office visit. Counseling to include but not limited to use of condoms and risk factor or lifestyle modification such as alcohol use, illicit drug use, weight loss, and smoking is an integral educational strategy to mitigate these gaps in care. This should include the patient and the partner(s). Having timely immunizations and regular follow-up with the primary care providers are helpful preventive measures for HIV infection. Vaccinations for influenza, hepatitis A, hepatitis B, and pneumococcal vaccines should be included in the care of the HIV-infected older adult [84]. Although pre-exposure prophylaxis with daily TDF (tenofovir disoproxil fumarate) plus emtricitabine (Truvada) for adherent high-risk younger patients, the balance between risks and benefits of this intervention need to be considered among older adult patients who are already experiencing other medical problems and taking multiple medications [88].

With the advent of antiretroviral therapy (ART), people are now living with chronic HIV infection successfully. Recent clinical trials have now demonstrated that treatment of asymptomatic HIV-infected persons regardless of CD4+ cell count or viral load reduces overall morbidity and mortality [89]. As a result the older adult population living with HIV have to face a variety of new challenges including accelerated aging and higher comorbid medical illnesses. They develop geriatric syndromes and frailty earlier than uninfected people [90]. Multiple medical problems that have been implicated include coronary artery disease, stroke, osteoporosis, diabetes mellitus, renal disease, neurological complications, and malignancies such as Kaposi's sarcoma and lymphoma [90].

Immunization Recommendations

In February 2018, the Advisory Committee on Immunization Practices (ACIP) provided recommended immunization schedules for all adults aged 19 years and older. This was approved by Centers for Disease Control and Prevention (CDC), the

American College of Physicians (ACP), the American Academy of Family Physicians (AAFP), the American College of Obstetricians and Gynecologists (ACOG), and the American College of Nurse-Midwives. The schedule is published in its entirety with the *Annals of Internal Medicine* [91]. The specific recommended immunizations [91] for older adults aged 50 years and above are as follows:

1. Annual influenza vaccine.
2. One dose of Tetanus, diphtheria, pertussis (Tdap) and then tetanus diphtheria (Td) booster every 10 years.
3. Two doses of varicella vaccine (VAR), 4–8 weeks apart.
4. Two doses of zoster vaccine live (ZVL), 2–6 months apart regardless of past episode of zoster infection or receipt of live zoster vaccine.
5. Pneumococcal vaccination (PCV 13 and PPSV23) for immunocompetent adults 65 years and above: PCV 13 followed by PPSV23 at least 1 year apart; if PPSV23 were given before and no immunization for PCV 13, then PCV 13 should be given at least a year after administration of PPSV23.
6. Two to three doses of hepatitis A vaccine (HepA), at least 6 months apart.
7. Three doses of hepatitis B vaccine (HepB), at least 4 weeks apart.
8. Two doses of meningococcal vaccine, (MenACWY) at least 8 weeks apart.
9. One or three doses of Haemophilus influenzae B vaccine (HiB) if meeting criteria, e.g., anatomical or functional asplenia and hematopoietic stem cell transplant; doses are administered at least 4 weeks apart.

Cancer Prevention

In light of limited data on outcomes of screening older adults for cancer, it is important to know that the decision to screen older adults requires balancing the risks and benefits of doing the screening procedures to include its complications and impact on the overall health of the individual [92]. For clinicians, following the guidelines as recommended by USPSTF is a good place to start. It is equally vital to factor in patient preferences and risk factors in the decision-making. Generally, older adults may be categorized as maximizers who prefer more testing and minimizers who opt to follow more conservative guidelines [92]. Decision aids specific to particular screening modalities can be used to help elicit patient preferences. Examples include the Lee Schonberg index (available at www.eprognosis.org) that estimates whether adults have >50% risk of mortality within 10 years [93].

Cervical cancer is a significant cause of morbidity and mortality among women. Based on the 2018 cancer statistics data, the 5-year survival is 66.2% for all patients diagnosed with cervical cancer [94]. It is caused by a sexually transmitted infection with the human papilloma virus (HPV) [95]. The American College of Physicians (ACP) recommends that physicians stop screening after the age of 65 years for average-risk women who are immunocompromised with no prior history of high-grade, precancerous cervical lesions or cervical cancer, and no in-utero exposure to diethylstilbestrol (DES) and assuming that the patient has had three consecutive negative results on cytology or two consecutive negative results on cytology plus human papillomavirus testing within the previous 10 years and the most recent test performed within 5 years. Furthermore, if there is no more uterus and cervix result-ing from prior surgery, then cancer screening is not recommended [96]. Clinicians should consider screening >65 years old if they have never been screened before since they are at high risk for cervical cancer with the added recommendation to do an internal pelvic examination on a patient with a history of hysterectomy to clarify the anatomy if it is not clear whether or not the patient has a cervix. The widespread implementation of screening using the Pap smear has decreased the number of cases diagnosed and mortality over the last 40 years.

Anal cancer is biologically similar to cervical cancer in its relationship to HPV. Similar to cervical cancer, it is preceded by high-grade squamous intraepithe-lial lesion (HSIL). The incidence of this disease has been increasing in the general population by about 2% per year in both men and women for the last few decades [97]. By far the highest risk of anal cancer is among HIV-positive men who have sex with men followed by HIV-positive men and women who have sex with women [98, 99]. Other populations who also have considerable risk include HIV-negative men who have sex with men, women with a history of cervical or vulvar cancer, and immunosuppressed individuals who are immunosuppressed other than with HIV such as solid organ transplant patients [100]. The most specific test to identify HSIL is direct visualization with 5% acetic acid using high-resolution anoscopy (HRA). However, this is too expensive coupled with a paucity of trained clinicians. Anal cytology using anal Pap smears has limited sensitivity for detection [101]. Despite these challenges, screening for anal HSIL is recommended by some experts around the United States [102].

The occurrence of prostate cancer may be linked to sexual activity. The underly-ing pathogenesis include the following pathways: association of increased sexual activity to higher androgenic activity; increased exposure to sexually transmitted infections (STIs); and reduced ejaculation frequency leading to retention of carcino-genic secretions [103]. Sexual activity consists of multiple interrelated dimensions such as the number of sexual partners, sexual orientation, genders of sexual part-ners, ejaculation frequency, and age at first intercourse [104]. There is data to sug-gest that a history of prostatitis triggered by sexually transmitted infections increases the risk of prostate cancer [105]. More specifically, a history of gonorrhea and HPV increased the odds of developing prostate cancer [106]. Based on these studies, a potential mechanism for the role of recurring exposure to microbial agents in the etiology of prostate cancer may include the production of inflammatory cytokine mediators and genotoxic reactive oxygen radicals that increase cell proliferation and promote tumorigenesis [107]. The most widely known screening test for pros-tate cancer is the measurement of serum prostate-specific antigen (PSA) level. The evidence for benefit must be balanced with potential harms since the test itself is non-specific [108]. The psychological distress and physical harms associated with the uncertainty of a positive test and biopsy are well documented in the literature. Moreover, most men diagnosed with prostate cancer via PSA screening do not have an overall survival benefit [109]. In one study, there was no difference in prostate cancer mortality among men who received watchful waiting versus those who underwent radical prostatectomy [110]. Some known immediate risks after surgical removal of the prostate include cardiovascular events, thromboembolism, erectile dysfunction, and incontinence that can affect overall function and quality of life [111]. Currently, the USPSTF does not recommend screening PSA level for prostate cancer for men older than 70 years old. For men aged 55 to 69, the decision to undergo periodic prostate screening should be an individual one. Full informed consent discussion to include risks and benefits balanced with goals and preferences for care as they relate to risk factors (family history, comorbid conditions) should be carried out [112].

Sexual Abuse

Sexual abuse as a form of elder abuse is still sparsely represented in the medical literature. Part of this issue may be due to inaccurate categorization of sexual abuse as a form of physical abuse [113]. Moreover the concept of ageism poses a barrier in seriously taking sexual abuse of older adults. Many healthcare professionals avoid asking older adult patients about sexual abuse and refuse to believe them if this issue is raised [114]. The National Center on Elder Abuse defines sexual abuse as non-consenting sexual conduct of any kind [113]. It is the least acknowledged and underreported type of elder mistreatment. Sexual contact with any person incapable of giving consent is also considered sexual abuse. The scope of sexual abuse includes but is not limited to unwanted touching and all types of sexual assault or battery (e.g., rape, sodomy, coerced nudity, and sexually explicit photographing) [115]. Older institutionalized adults are especially vulnerable to sexual abuse by virtue of their chronic illnesses, cognitive and behavioral states, and functional dependence [116–118]. A 2015 systematic review by Malmedal et al. showed that sexual abuse in the nursing homes are committed against both men and women [119]. Perpetrators are mostly cisgender men. Staff and other residents have been implicated. It was also found that women also abuse other residents in the nursing homes. There is inadequate handling of these cases in this care setting. Therefore, there is a need for knowledge and further research on this topic as well as the need to develop guidelines and policies in reporting and managing this overlooked issue in the nursing homes. An even more vulnerable population affected by sexual abuse are the older adults with cognitive impairment. These individuals may experience accelerated dementia as a result of trauma. This worsening of cognitive deficits could represent increased stress from a disrupted environment and a subsequent chronic allostatic load [120, 121]. People with dementia may be physically frail and unable to resist sexual advances and may not be able to report abuse when it occurs. Thus sexual abuse takes place when an individual initiates a sexual relationship with a demented person without the latter's informed consent [122].

Though the majority of sexual abuse cases happen in the nursing facilities, it can also happen in other venues of care such as home, medical wards, and other facilities [123, 124]. The perpetrators could be a spouse, caregiver, strangers, staff, and other residents. In a study by Cannell et al., there was a prevalence rate of 0.9% of community-dwelling older adults who have reported sexual abuse. This roughly translated to more than 90,000 older adults across 18 states [125].

Sexual Health Considerations in Older Sexual and Gender Minority Patients (SGMs)

Sexual and reproductive health for transgender and gender nonbinary patients is presented in detail in Part 3 of this book. This section focuses on sexual and reproductive health issues of particular importance to older lesbian, gay, bisexual, transgender/gender nonbinary, and queer patients.

Throughout a lifetime of discrimination, prejudice, oppression, victimization, and prosecution, sexual and gender minority communities have been significantly impacted in various aspects of life including health care. Witten identified a link between discrimination and the biopsychosocial dimensions affecting these communities [126]. Historically there has been a negative relationship between healthcare providers and the LGBTQ patients. Previous studies have pointed out that disclosing information on sexual orientation and gender identity (SOGI) might lead to more discrimination and mistrust towards healthcare providers [127]. As a result, there is consequential delay and maybe even avoidance in seeking medical care for fear of mistreatment and disrespect thereby propagating the cycle of oppression. A 2010 survey by Lambda Legal highlighted the variability in the types of health services LGBTQ people receive [128]. It is obvious that the barriers to health care are even much more prevalent to individuals who identify as transgender and gender non-binary as opposed to gays and lesbians. For instance, about 70% of transgender respondents (sample 5000) reported having had at least one of the following experiences: being refused needed medical care, not being touched by medical providers, subjected to harsh verbal language, rough physical care, and being blamed for their health status. The *minority stress model* plays an important role in understanding the lived experiences of the LGBTQ patient [129] (see Fig. 4.1). This pertains to chronically high levels of psychological and emotional stress faced by members of a stigmatized group. Examples of triggers include poor social support, low socioeconomic status, and interpersonal prejudice and discrimination [130]. Fig. 4.1 illustrates the intersectionality of multiple identities that describe or define an individual. An older adult female who identifies as African American and lesbian may be subjected to the stress of being discriminated against based on these identities while living in a heteronormative society. Two operational theories are worth thinking about. Aldwin and Gilmer attempted to relate the *life course theory* with how older adults age over time. It essentially presupposes that a series of transitions and choice points are influenced both by the immediate social context and the larger sociohistorical period as well as gender and social roles [131]. *Goal-oriented theories* regard adulthood and late-life development as a balance between gains and losses, pursuit of goals, and the development and maintenance of self [130, 131].

**INTERSECTIONAL
IDENTITIES**

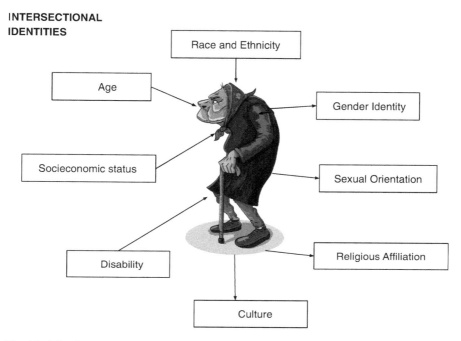

Fig. 4.1 Minority stress model and intersectionality (Javier NM original creation)

In general, the healthcare needs of the older LGBTQ adults mirror that of their cisgender heterosexual counterparts. However, there are unique aspects in this population that need more attention. It is essential to provide standardized nonjudgmental care for this population carefully considering some barriers to healthcare provision and access. Furthermore, LGBTQ individuals are subject to discrimination and prejudice in related areas of education and employment thereby affecting their ability to obtain health insurance necessary for both physical and mental health services [132]. In interfacing with the older LGBTQ patients for the first time, it is important to bear in mind that individuals may be in various stages of transition. Therefore, "no one size fits all" in terms of how they may present or express themselves. It is helpful to begin the clinical encounter with allowing the patient to take the lead in terms of disclosure of gender identity and sexual orientation. Address them using their preferred names (if not legally changed yet) and proper pronouns. Use open-ended questions such as this script: "I would like to ask personal and sensitive questions pertaining to your sexual health. I am fully committed to learning about you in every aspect of your health. I ask all my patients these questions. Whatever is shared will be kept confidential unless you authorize me to share with other providers. If you feel uncomfortable at any point, we can defer for another time. Let me ask you about your gender identity, relationship status, sexual orientation, sexual practices among other things." It is also helpful to standardize eliciting this information through intake forms that will allow options for disclosure and non-disclosure respecting patients' privacy. To enhance the experience of the patient in a clinical care setting, materials that pertain to the LGBTQ population in general may signify the institutions' welcoming spirit and universal message of acceptance and commitment to serve this population. During history taking, it is advisable to allow the patient to share their health concerns that may or may not be related to their sexual orientation, gender identity, and gender expression. In an emergency department (ED) study, patients actually preferred providers ask them questions about their SOGI. The EQUALITY study by Haider highlighted this point. In a sample of over 1500 patients and 400 ED providers, only 10% of patients reported refusal to have SOGI elicited. More than 2/3 of the providers assumed that patients will refuse disclosure of SOGI [133]. In a similar study by Maragh-Bass looking at transgender patients, close to 90% felt that gender identity was more important to disclose than sexual orientation. Both males and females who identified as transgender reported that as long as there was medical relevance, they were both willing to disclose SOGI nonetheless [134]. Another effective strategy in eliciting SOGI during history taking is asking this open-ended question: "What would you like me to know about you so I can provide holistic and efficient care?" This is the dignity question adapted from Harvey Max Chochinov [135]. For the physical examination, one compassionate strategy to keep in mind is explaining to the patient why a specific organ system or body part needs to be examined. Additionally, for anatomical parts pertaining to their genitalia, one might consider allowing the patient to name the parts they see fit. TGNB males and females might refer to their vaginas and neovaginas as "front door." The anorectal region is considered a sexual organ and is referred to as "back door" by both genders. A summary of these strategies is shown in Table 4.2.

Sexuality and intimacy are intrinsically important components on the full breadth of human experience. This is carried through during aging and regardless of gender identity and sexual orientation. Sexual health is an important personal goal for many individuals even at the point of facing a life-limiting illness. Patients with palliative care needs face unique challenges trying to balance sexual health needs and desire for sexual expression with other underlying medical illnesses and disease progression. The aging LGBTQ patient will have the same needs as the general population. Sex and sexuality are closely linked to societal role, self-esteem, pleasure, mood, and other components that affect quality of life [136]. As one ages, the chances of having and developing multiple medical problems increase. The individual will also have to contend with taking numerous medications and complications from multiple diseases that will further affect the sexual drive of the patient. Natural hormonal changes as a consequence of aging as well as diseases such as hypertension, diabetes, peripheral vascular disease, cancer, urogynecologic problems, kidney disease on hemodialysis, and rheumatologic conditions are just some of the medical conditions that can have an overall impact on the sexual health of the patient. The anatomic and physiologic changes that come with these problems will have a bearing on the perception of body image and sexual function in various capacities [137,

Table 4.2 Culturally competent, inclusive, and affirmative strategies (Javier NM original creation)

Provider level (doctors, nurses, physician assistants, nurse practitioners, social workers, medical assistants	Staff level (clerks, administrators, front-desk personnel, custodians, etc.	Institutional level
Education and in-service training	In-service training	Creation of policies to foster respect in the workplace such as anti-discrimination, visitation, etc.
Proper greeting towards patients; use of preferred names and pronouns; use of gender-neutral language	Proper greeting towards patients; use of preferred names and pronouns; use of gender-neutral language	Operationalize forms to be transgender inclusive of SOGI
Allow patients to share their story during history taking; ask open-ended questions Avoid assumptions and misconceptions; avoid inappropriate "outing" of patients and caregivers	As first point of contact with patients, ensure proper body language	Creation of a welcoming environment using flyers, brochures pertaining to LGBTQ community
Be careful not to "out" patients who have a different mindset compared to younger patients	Avoid misconceptions and pre-judgments towards patients and their caregivers	Provision of gender-neutral bathrooms
Allow patients to name body parts during physical exam	Zero tolerance towards discrimination against transgender patients by others; calling out people and advocating for this vulnerable population if prejudice were to happen	Zero tolerance for gender identity and sexual orientation discrimination
Ensure appropriate privacy in the exam room	Ensure proper record keeping with appropriate identifiers in the electronic medical records	Resources for transgender support within the medical system and outside communities whether online or on print
Provide appropriate resources for mental health, support groups, others…	Feedback opportunities on how well staff are treating patients	Provision of available medical and mental health services and resources within the institution
Offer to involve partner, significant other, spouse, "roommate" in the clinical encounter if patient so chooses	Continuing education for all providers	
Open feedback opportunities on how staff will treat patients		
Continuing education for all providers		

138]. Consequent mental health concerns such as depression, anxiety, grief, and stress could lead to more dysphoria for TGNB patients. Complicating these issues will be changes to the relationship status of partners and/or caregiving ability towards patients. Relationship factors may include partner silence, emotional distance, and even actual abuse (verbal, physical, emotional) [139]. It is therefore imperative for the healthcare professional not to overlook these issues as these may well affect the overall well-being of patients. Furthermore, clinicians may be able to give specific suggestions to older adult LGBTQ patients and their partners on ways to facilitate sexual intimacy such as referral to appropriate sex therapists and other counselors. The details pertaining to sexual function and enhancement for TGNB patients who have undergone gender-affirming surgeries are beyond the scope of this chapter. One would need the expertise of plastic surgeons, urologists, sex therapists, and gynecologists in providing appropriate sexual health care. An introduction is presented in Part 3 of this book. When patients' diseases advance, sexual health is one dimension that should be considered in providing high-quality geriatric and palliative care for as long as this continues to be of importance to the patient and partner. Lawton and colleagues reviewed recommendations for best practice and techniques to enhance communication between patients and providers, engage patients and their loved ones in this process, and include considerations of sexual orientation in sexual health care [140]. In a supporting study by Stausmire, the approach to communication should be open and nonjudgmental and that selected language should be appropriate to any sexual dynamic including gay and straight relationships [141]. Clinicians can help limit barriers by maintaining a compassionate, open-minded, and affirming approach with all patients at all times and ensuring confidentiality, privacy, and high degree of professionalism in various areas of health care.

Sexual Health in Other Care Settings (Long-Term Care, Alternate Living Facilities)

There is an estimated two million Americans who live in long-term care facilities such as nursing homes and assisted living facilities [142]. The majority of residents in the nursing homes are aged 65 years and older. There is evidence to show that these nursing home residents, both with and without cognitive impairment, ascribe at least a moderate importance to sexuality in their lives. The range of sexual activities which include kissing, hugging, holding hands, fondling, sexual intercourse, masturbation, and pornography have been cited [143, 144]. Despite the prevalence of sexual interest and desire among long-term care residents, there continues to be fear and discomfort by the staff in addressing this issue [145, 146]. Moreover, there is data to support that staff members often gossip about residents' sexuality thereby causing more emotional distress for the resident [146]. Reactions from family members and caregivers of these residents are split in half. Some feel embarrassed, angry, and humiliated by their relatives' sexuality [146]. A 2017 systematic review of sexual expression in the nursing homes showed that sexuality in the older adult must be supported. Positive predictors of attitudes by staff towards sexuality include age, level of education, and years of experience, whereas barriers to address include a lack of privacy and staff discomfort [147].

Sexual Consent Capacity

Compared to medical decision-making capacity, there is a paucity of information on the guidelines to assess capacity to consent to sexual activity [148]. The clinician must acquire a knowledge of the nature of sexual activity and the relationship of the participants. This approach is clearly distinctive from medical decision-making capacity whereby the clinician defines the nature of the proposed intervention. To date, there are no universal or standard guidelines for determining an older adult's sexual consent capacity. Organizations such as the American Psychological Association (APA) and the American Bar Association (ABA) have made recommendations [149] as follows:

1. Set up an inter-professional team comprised of psychologists, physicians, social workers, rehabilitation therapists, nurses, nursing assistants, clergy, legal guardians, family members, and ombudspersons. They can provide expert collateral information.
2. Conduct a cognitive screening and testing. Neuropsychological tools such as the Montreal Cognitive Assessment (MoCA) and Mini-Mental State Exam (MMSE) are examples of screening tests.
3. Proceed with a semi-structured interview designed to assess knowledge, reasoning, and voluntariness.
4. Acknowledge team input and collaboration especially when residents have cognitive impairment.

Situations involving cognitively impaired residents make the process more challenging. The primary ethical issue lies in balancing autonomy and privacy with the institutions' duty to protect their residents from harm [150]. It is important to note that in spite of concurrent cognitive impairments, older adults show varying levels of sexual activity and should not be precluded from sexual expression and intimacy [144]. Depending on the organic nature of the cognitive disorder such as Parkinson's disease and frontal lobe dementia, residents may manifest with disinhibition, hypersexuality, and executive dysfunction making the situation even more complicated. Lichtenberg and Strzepek [150] described an approach to the assessment of sexual consent capacity among demented residents in a nursing home, namely:

1. Awareness of with whom they are having a sexual contact and what that person's relationship is to them

2. Ability to articulate the type(s) of intimate sexual activity with which they are comfortable
3. Consistency of behavior with respect to their previously expressed beliefs and preferences
4. Ability to decline unwanted sexual activity
5. Ability to articulate what their reaction will be if the sexual activity ends

A salient feature of sexual consent capacity is that it must be determined in the moment and not ahead of time. Therefore, this functions as a continuum. One reason that explains this very nature is that decisions about participation in sexual activity are often made alone, in the spur of the moment, and without the input of other professionals. The decisions are often private and fluid as relationships change significantly over time [149].

The utility of a nuanced approach to sexual consent capacity assessments represents the first step in becoming more progressive in the nursing home setting. The American Medical Directors Association in 2013 reported that less than one quarter of nursing homes have a formal sexual consent policy in place [151]. There is therefore a call to action to further advance the steps in creating change in including sexual health as an important domain of human existence and standard medical care. The following table shows specific actionable plans that institutions such as nursing homes can take to ensure readiness for accommodating intimate sexual activity in the long-term care [152] (Table 4.3).

Table 4.3 Action steps for accommodating intimate sexual activity in long-term care [4, 5]

Preparation
Determine statutes and case law on sexual consent for your state.
Draft guidelines for your institution's management of resident sexual activity.
Establish resources to support resident sexual activity:
resident sexuality consultation team (analogous to palliative or wound care, infection control)
"intimacy room" for residents who do not have private rooms, appropriate signage
educational materials for staff, families
aids (e.g., lubricants)
Hold staff training sessions.
Management
Consult resident sexuality consultant.
Conduct sexual consent capacity assessment.
Construct individualized plan detailing approaches to maintain safety and privacy.
Hold staff support meetings.
Problem-solving resources
Ethics committee consultation
State Long-term Care Ombudsman's Office

Metzger [152]

Conclusion

Adults remain sexually active until their later years. Only a few report discussing sexual health with a physician after age 50. There is a growing body of evidence that older adults across the life course have sexual needs similar to their younger cohorts. However, despite the evidence, there persists a misconception that people become asexual as they get older and that they lose their interest in sex and their capacity for sexual behavior. Consequentially, medical providers do not address sexual health as proactively as they do other aspects of clinical care. Hence sexual health surveillance continues to be underemphasized in routine care. Healthcare professional knowledge about sexuality in the older adult should improve patient education, counseling, and the ability to recognize the spectrum of health-related and potentially treatable sexual problems. Providers can follow screening guidelines from the CDC and USPSTF as part of the standard medical care when addressing sexual health. It is also important to be mindful that sexuality and aging are relevant among patients who also reside in other care settings such as rehabilitation and long-term care units.

Bibliography

1. Facts for Features: Older Americans Month: May 2016. United States Census Bureau 2016.
2. Sexual health. World Health Organization.
3. Dominguez LJ, Barbagallo M. Ageing and sexuality. Eur Geriatr Med. 2016;7(6):512–8.
4. Wada M, Hurd Clarke L, Rozanova J. Constructions of sexuality in later life: analyses of Canadian magazine and newspaper portrayals of online dating. J Aging Stud. 2015;32:40–9.
5. DeLamater J. Sexual expression in later life: a review and synthesis. J Sex Res. 2012;49(2–3):125–41.
6. Brennan-Ing M, Seidel L, Ansell P, et al. Addressing sexual health in geriatrics education. Gerontol Geriatr Educ. 2018;39(2):249–63.
7. Taylor A, Gosney MA. Sexuality in older age: essential considerations for healthcare professionals. Age Ageing. 2011;40(5):538–43.
8. Helgason ÁR, Adolfsson J, Dickman P, et al. Sexual desire, erection, orgasm and ejaculatory functions and their importance to elderly Swedish men: a population-based study. Age Ageing. 1996;25(4):285–91.
9. Buono MD, Urciuoli O, Leo DD. Quality of life and longevity: a study of centenarians. Age Ageing. 1998;27(2):207–16.
10. Gott M, Hinchliff S. How important is sex in later life? The views of older people. Soc Sci Med. 2003;56(8):1617–28.
11. Lindau ST, Schumm LP, Laumann EO, Levinson W, O'Muircheartaigh CA, Waite LJ. A study of sexuality and health among older adults in the United States. N Engl J Med. 2007;357(8):762–74.

12. Lindau ST, Gavrilova N. Sex, health, and years of sexually active life gained due to good health: evidence from two US population based cross sectional surveys of ageing. BMJ. 2010;340(mar09 2):c810.
13. Schick V, Herbenick D, Reece M, et al. Sexual behaviors, condom use, and sexual health of Americans over 50: implications for sexual health promotion for older adults. J Sex Med. 2010;7:315–29.
14. Trompeter SE, Bettencourt R, Barrett-Connor E. Sexual activity and satisfaction in healthy community-dwelling older women. Am J Med. 2012;125(1):37–43.e31.
15. Freak-Poli R, Kirkman M, De Castro LG, Direk N, Franco OH, Tiemeier H. Sexual activity and physical tenderness in older adults: cross-sectional prevalence and associated characteristics. J Sex Med. 2017;14(7):918–27.
16. Gott M, Hinchliff S, Galena E. General practitioner attitudes to discussing sexual health issues with older people. Soc Sci Med. 2004;58(11):2093–103.
17. Nusbaum MRH, Hamilton CD. The proactive sexual health history. Am Fam Physician. 2002;66(9):1705–12.
18. Sack S, Drabant B, Perrin E. Communicating about sexuality: an initiative across the Core clerkships. Acad Med. 2002;77(11):1159–60.
19. Bouman WP. Sexuality in later life. In T. Dening & A. Thomas (Eds.), Oxford textbook of old age psychiatry. Oxford University Press: 2013; pp. 703–23. https://doi.org/10.1093/med/9780199644957.003.005. last accessed March 22, 2022.
20. Bancroft J. Human sexuality and its problems. 3rd ed. New York, NY: Churchill Livingstone; 2009.
21. Caplan RM. HIPAA: health insurance portability and accountability act of 1996. Dent Assist. 2003;72(2):6–8.
22. Hunter I, Haining Ede G, Whiddett R. Increased electronic information sharing by sexual health services: confidentiality and consent. Health Informatics J. 2014;20(1):3–12.
23. Risen CB. A guide to taking a sexual history. Psychiatr Clin N Am. 1995;18(1):39–53.
24. Tomlinson J. ABC of sexual health: taking a sexual history. BMJ. 1998;317(7172):1573–6.
25. Kingsberg SA. Taking a sexual history. Obstet Gynecol Clin N Am. 2006;33(4):535–47.
26. Granville L, Pregler J. Women's sexual health and aging. J Am Geriatr Soc. 2018;66(3):595–601.
27. Ports KA, Barnack-Tavlaris JL, Syme ML, Perera RA, Lafata JE. Sexual health discussions with older adult patients during periodic health exams. J Sex Med. 2014;11(4):901–8.
28. STD Treatment Guidelines: Clinical Prevention Guideline. Centers for Disease Control and Prevention. 2015. https://www.ncsddc.org/resource/2015-cdc-std-treatment-guidelines--summary-chart/. last accessed March 22, 2022.
29. Lindau ST, Laumann EO, Levinson W, Waite LJ. Synthesis of scientific disciplines in pursuit of health: the interactive biopsychosocial model. Perspect Biol Med. 2003;46(3):S74–86.
30. Meston CM. Aging and sexuality. West J Med. 1997;167(4):285–90.
31. DeLamater J, Moorman SM. Sexual behavior in later life. J Aging Health. 2007;19(6):921–45.
32. Corona G, Lee DM, Forti G, et al. Age-related changes in general and sexual health in middle-aged and older men: results from the European Male Ageing Study (EMAS). J Sex Med. 2010;7(4):1362–80.
33. Quek KF, Sallam AA, Ng CH, Chua CB. Prevalence of sexual problems and its association with social, psychological and physical factors among men in a Malaysian population: a cross-sectional study. J Sex Med. 2008;5(1):70–6.
34. Appa AA, Creasman J, Brown JS, et al. The impact of multimorbidity on sexual function in middle-aged and older women: beyond the single disease perspective. J Sex Med. 2014;11(11):2744–55.
35. Karavitakis M, Komninos C, Theodorakis PN, et al. Evaluation of sexual function in hypertensive men receiving treatment: a review of current guidelines recommendation. J Sex Med. 2011;8(9):2405–14.
36. Bhuvaneswar CG, Baldessarini RJ, Harsh VL, Alpert JE. Adverse endocrine and metabolic effects of psychotropic drugs: selective clinical review. CNS Drugs. 2009;23(12):1003–21.

37. Gutierrez MA, Mushtaq R, Stimmel G. Chapter 8 Sexual dysfunction in women with epilepsy. Int Rev Neurobiol. 2008;83:157–67.
38. Morgentaler A. A 66-year-old man with sexual dysfunction. JAMA. 2004;291(24):2994.
39. Wagle KC, Carrejo MH, Tan RS. The implications of increasing age on erectile dysfunction. Am J Mens Health. 2012;6(4):273–9.
40. Albaugh JA. Addressing and managing erectile dysfunction after prostatectomy for prostate cancer. Urol Nurs. 2010;30(3):167–77.
41. Lizza E, Rosen R. Definition and classification of erectile dysfunction: report of the nomenclature Committee of the International Society of Impotence Research. Int J Impot Res. 1999;11(3):141–3.
42. Corona G, Rastrelli G, Maseroli E, Forti G, Maggi M. Sexual function of the ageing male. Best Pract Res Clin Endocrinol Metab. 2013;27(4):581–601.
43. Bacon CG, Mittleman MA, Kawachi I, Giovannucci E, Glasser DB, Rimm EB. A prospective study of risk factors for erectile dysfunction. J Urol. 2006;176(1):217–21.
44. Francis ME, Kusek JW, Nyberg LM, Eggers PW. The contribution of common medical conditions and drug exposures to erectile dysfunction in adult males. J Urol. 2007;178(2):591–6.
45. Heidelbaugh JJ. Management of erectile dysfunction. Am Fam Physician. 2010;81(3):305–12.
46. Avis NE, Zhao X, Johannes CB, Ory M, Brockwell S, Greendale GA. Correlates of sexual function among multi-ethnic middle-aged women: results from the Study of Women??s Health Across the Nation (SWAN). Menopause. 2005;12(4):385–98.
47. Nusbaum MRH, Helton MR, Ray N. The changing nature of women's sexual health concerns through the midlife years. Maturitas. 2004;49(4):283–91.
48. Nappi RE, Cucinella L. Advances in pharmacotherapy for treating female sexual dysfunction. Expert Opin Pharmacother. 2015;16(6):875–87.
49. Huang AJ, Luft J, Grady D, Kuppermann M. The day-to-day impact of urogenital aging: perspectives from racially/ethnically diverse women. J Gen Intern Med. 2010;25(1):45–51.
50. Maciel M, Laganà L. Older Women's sexual desire problems: biopsychosocial factors impacting them and barriers to their clinical assessment. Biomed Res Int. 2014;2014:1–9.
51. Medina-Walpole A, Pacala JT, Potter JF. Chapter 56: Sexuality. In: Geriatrics review syllabus: a core curriculum in geriatric medicine. 9th ed. New York: American Geriatrics Society; 2016.
52. Practice Bulletin No. 141: management of menopausal symptoms. Obstet Gynecol 2014;123(1):202–216.
53. Goetsch MF, Lim JY, Caughey AB. A practical solution for dyspareunia in breast cancer survivors: a randomized controlled trial. J Clin Oncol. 2015;33(30):3394–400.
54. Kingsberg SA, Woodard T. Female sexual dysfunction: focus on low desire. Obstet Gynecol. 2015;125(2):477–86.
55. Kingsberg SA, Rezaee RL. Hypoactive sexual desire in women. Menopause. 2013;20(12):1284–300.
56. Leiblum SR, Koochaki PE, Rodenberg CA, Barton IP, Rosen RC. Hypoactive sexual desire disorder in postmenopausal women: US results from the Women??s International Study of Health and Sexuality (WISHeS). Menopause. 2006;13(1):46–56.
57. Biddle AK, West SL, D'Aloisio AA, Wheeler SB, Borisov NN, Thorp J. Hypoactive sexual desire disorder in postmenopausal women: quality of life and health burden. Value Health. 2009;12(5):763–72.
58. Snabes MC, Simes SM. COMMENTARY: approved hormonal treatments for HSDD: an unmet medical need. J Sex Med. 2009;6(7):1846–9.
59. Safarinejad MR, Hosseini SY, Asgari MA, Dadkhah F, Taghva A. A randomized, double-blind, placebo-controlled study of the efficacy and safety of bupropion for treating hypoactive sexual desire disorder in ovulating women: BUPROPION IN HYPOACTIVE SEXUAL DESIRE DISORDER. BJU Int. 2010;106(6):832–9.

60. Trudel G, Marchand A, Ravart M, Aubin S, Turgeon L, Fortier P. The effect of a cognitive-behavioral group treatment program on hypoactive sexual desire in women. Sex Relatsh Ther. 2001;16(2):145–64.
61. Hawton K, Catalan J, Martin P, Fagg J. Long-term outcome of sex therapy. Behav Res Ther. 1986;24(6):665–75.
62. Brotto LA, Basson R, Luria M. A mindfulness-based group psychoeducational intervention targeting sexual arousal disorder in women. J Sex Med. 2008;5(7):1646–59.
63. Sexually Transmitted Disease Surveillance. Ctr Dis Control Prev. 2016:2017;23-164.
64. Jameson M. Seniors' sex lives are up and so are STDs around the country. https://www.orlandosentinel.com/health/os-xpm-2011-05-16-os-seniors-stds-national-20110516-story.html. last accessed March 22, 2022.
65. Pera A, Campos C, López N, et al. Immunosenescence: implications for response to infection and vaccination in older people. Maturitas. 2015;82(1):50–5.
66. Poynten IM, Grulich AE, Templeton DJ. Sexually transmitted infections in older populations. Curr Opin Infect Dis. 2013;26(1):80–5.
67. Minkin MJ. Sexually transmitted infections and the aging female: placing risks in perspective. Maturitas. 2010;67(2):114–6.
68. Johnson BK. Sexually transmitted infections and older adults. J Gerontol Nurs. 2013;39(11):53–60.
69. Milrod C, Monto M. Condom use, sexual risk, and self-reported STI in a sample of older male clients of heterosexual prostitution in the United States. Am J Mens Health. 2016;10(4):296–305.
70. Amin I. Social capital and sexual risk-taking behaviors among older adults in the United States. J Appl Gerontol. 2016;35(9):982–99.
71. Smith KP, Christakis NA. Association between widowhood and risk of diagnosis with a sexually transmitted infection in older adults. Am J Public Health. 2009;99(11):2055–62.
72. HIPAA Privacy Rule and Public Health. Guidance from CDC and US Department of Health and Human Services. https://www.cdc.gov/mmwr/preview/mmwrhtml/m2e411a1.htm. last accessed March 22, 2022.
73. HIPAA violations & enforcement. American Medical Association. https://www.ama-assn.org/practice-management/hipaa/hipaa-violations-enforcement. last accessed March 22, 2022.
74. The HIPAA Privacy Rule: How may covered entities use and disclose health information. Privacy Rights Clearinghouse 2014. https://privacyrights.org/consumer-guides/hipaa-privacy-rule-patients-rights. last accessed March 22, 2022.
75. Final Recommendation Statement: Sexually Transmitted Infections: Behavioral Counseling. US Preventive Services Task Force. 2014. https://www.uspreventiveservicestaskforce.org/uspstf/recommendation/sexually-transmitted-infections-behavioral-counseling--september-2014. last accessed March 22, 2022.
76. Lee KC, Ngo-Metzger Q, Wolff T, Chowdhury J, LeFevre ML, Meyers DS. Sexually transmitted infections: recommendations from the U.S. Preventive Services Task Force. Am Fam Physician. 2016;94(11):907–15.
77. Idso C. Sexually transmitted infection prevention in newly single older women: a forgotten health promotion need. J Nurse Pract. 2009;5(6):440–6.
78. Meyers DS, Wolff T, Gregory K, et al. USPSTF recommendations for STI screening. Am Fam Physician. 2008;77(6):819–24.
79. LeFevre ML. Screening for Hepatitis B virus infection in nonpregnant adolescents and adults: U.S. Preventive Services Task Force Recommendation Statement. Ann Intern Med. 2014;161(1):58.
80. LeFevre ML. Screening for Chlamydia and Gonorrhea: U.S. Preventive Services Task Force Recommendation Statement. Ann Intern Med. 2014;161(12):902.
81. Sexually transmitted infections screenings & counseling. Medicare. https://www.medicare.gov/coverage/sexually-transmitted-infection-screenings-counseling. last accessed March 22, 2022.

82. UNAIDS Data 2018. UNAIDS 2018. https://www.unaids.org/sites/default/files/media_asset/unaids-data-2018_en.pdf. last accessed March 22, 2022.
83. HIV among people aged 50 and over. Centers for Disease Control and Prevention. https://www.cdc.gov/hiv/group/age/olderamericans/index.html#:~:text=In%202018%2C%20over%20half%20(51,2018%20were%20in%20this%20group. last accessed March 22, 2022.
84. Sangarlangkarn A, Appelbaum JS. Caring for older adults with the human immunodeficiency virus. J Am Geriatr Soc. 2016;64(11):2322–9.
85. Pilowsky D, Wu L-T. Sexual risk behaviors and HIV risk among Americans aged 50 years or older: a review. Subst Abuse Rehabil. 2015;6:51.
86. Skalski LM, Sikkema KJ, Heckman TG, Meade CS. Coping styles and illicit drug use in older adults with HIV/AIDS. Psychol Addict Behav. 2013;27(4):1050–8.
87. Tillman JL, Mark HD. HIV and STI testing in older adults: an integrative review. J Clin Nurs. 2015;24(15–16):2074–95.
88. Grant RM, Lama JR, Anderson PL, et al. Preexposure chemoprophylaxis for HIV prevention in men who have sex with men. N Engl J Med. 2010;363(27):2587–99.
89. Scott J, Goetz MB. Human immunodeficiency virus/acquired immunodeficiency syndrome in older adults. Clin Geriatr Med. 2016;32(3):571–83.
90. Wing EJ. HIV and aging. Int J Infect Dis. 2016;53:61–8.
91. Kim DK, Riley LE, Hunter P. On behalf of the advisory committee on immunization P. recommended immunization schedule for adults aged 19 years or older, United States, 2018. Ann Intern Med. 2018;168(3):210–20.
92. Kotwal AA, Schonberg MA. Cancer screening in the elderly: a review of breast, colorectal, lung, and prostate cancer screening. Cancer J. 2017;23(4):246–53.
93. Lee S, Smith A, Widera E, Yourman L, Schonberg M, Ahalt C. Lee Schonberg Index. ePrognosis. https://eprognosis.ucsf.edu/. last accessed March 22, 2022.
94. Cancer Stat Facts: Cervical Cancer. National Cancer Institute.
95. Helmerhorst TJM, Meijer CJLM. Cervical cancer should be considered as a rare complication of oncogenic HPV infection rather than a STD. Int J Gynecol Cancer. 2002;12(3):235–6.
96. Sawaya GF, Kulasingam S, Denberg TD, Qaseem A, for the Clinical Guidelines Committee of the American College of P. Cervical cancer screening in average-risk women: best practice advice from the clinical guidelines committee of the American College of Physicians. Ann Intern Med. 2015;162(12):851.
97. Palefsky JM. Screening to prevent anal cancer: current thinking and future directions: Clinician's corner. Cancer Cytopathol. 2015;123(9):509–10.
98. Silverberg MJ, Lau B, Justice AC, et al. Risk of anal cancer in HIV-infected and HIV-uninfected individuals in North America. Clin Infect Dis. 2012;54(7):1026–34.
99. Welbeck M. Anal pap screening for HIV-infected men who have sex with men: practice improvement. J Assoc Nurses AIDS Care. 2016;27(1):89–97.
100. Stier EA, Chigurupati NL, Fung L. Prophylactic HPV vaccination and anal cancer. Hum Vaccin Immunother. 2016;12(6):1348–51.
101. Palefsky JM, Holly EA, Hogeboom CJ, Berry JM, Jay N, Darragh TM. Anal cytology as a screening tool for anal squamous intraepithelial lesions. J Acquir Immune Defic Syndr Hum Retrovirol. 1997;14(5):415–22.
102. Kaplan JE, Benson C, Holmes KK, Brooks JT, Pau A, Masur H. Guidelines for prevention and treatment of opportunistic infections in HIV-infected adults and adolescents: Recommendations from CDC, the National Institutes of Health, and the HIV Medicine Association of the Infectious Diseases Society of America. Ctr Dis Control Prev; 2009. 2009:1-207.
103. Kotb AF, Beltagy A, Ismail AM, Hashad MM. Sexual activity and the risk of prostate cancer: review article. Arch Ital Urol Androl. 2015;87(3):214.
104. Spence AR, Rousseau M-C, Parent M-É. Sexual partners, sexually transmitted infections, and prostate cancer risk. Cancer Epidemiol. 2014;38(6):700–7.

105. Dennis LK, Coughlin JA, McKinnon BC, et al. Sexually transmitted infections and prostate cancer among men in the U.S. Military. Cancer Epidemiol Biomark Prev. 2009;18(10):2665–71.
106. Vázquez-Salas RA, Torres-Sánchez L, López-Carrillo L, et al. History of gonorrhea and prostate cancer in a population-based case–control study in Mexico. Cancer Epidemiol. 2016;40:95–101.
107. Demaria S, Pikarsky E, Karin M, et al. Cancer and inflammation: promise for biologic therapy. J Immunother. 2010;33(4):335–51.
108. Hayes JH, Barry MJ. Screening for prostate cancer with the prostate-specific antigen test: a review of current evidence. JAMA. 2014;311(11):1143–9.
109. Wingfield SA, Heflin MT. Cancer screening in older adults. Clin Geriatr Med. 2016;32(1):17–33.
110. Wilt TJ, Brawer MK, Jones KM, et al. Radical prostatectomy versus observation for localized prostate cancer. N Engl J Med. 2012;367(3):203–13.
111. Soung MC. Screening for cancer: when to stop? Med Clin N Am. 2015;99(2):249–62.
112. Final Recommendation Statement: Prostate Cancer: Screening. US Preventive Services Task Force. 2018. https://www.uspreventiveservicestaskforce.org/uspstf/recommendation/prostate-cancer-screening. last accessed March 22, 2022.
113. Teaster PB, Roberto KA. Chapter 7 sexual abuse of older women living in nursing homes. J Gerontol Soc Work. 2004;40(4):105–19.
114. Connolly M-T, Breckman R, Callahan J, Lachs M, Ramsey-Klawsnik H, Solomon J. The sexual revolution's last frontier: how silence about sex undermines health, Well-being, and safety in old age. Generations. 2012;36(3):43–52.
115. Sexual Violence in Later Life. National Sexual Violence Resource Center. 2010. https://www.nsvrc.org/sites/default/files/publication_SVlaterlife_FS.pdf. last accessed March 22, 2022.
116. Gibbs LM, Mosqueda L. Confronting elder mistreatment in long-term care. Ann Longterm Care. 2004;12(4):30–5.
117. Gorbien MJ, Eisenstein AR. Elder abuse and neglect: an overview. Clin Geriatr Med. 2005;21(2):279–92.
118. Hansberry MR, Chen E, Gorbien MJ. Dementia and Elder Abuse. Clin Geriatr Med. 2005;21(2):315–32.
119. Malmedal W, Iversen MH, Kilvik A. Sexual abuse of older nursing home residents: a literature review. Nurs Res Pract. 2015;2015:1–7.
120. McEwen BS. Sex, stress and the hippocampus: allostasis, allostatic load and the aging process. Neurobiol Aging. 2002;23(5):921–39.
121. Wicklund M, Petersen RC. Emerging biomarkers in cognition. Clin Geriatr Med. 2013;29(4):809–28.
122. Haddad PM, Benbow SM. Sexual problems associated with dementia: part 1. Problems and their consequences. Int J Geriatr Psychiatry. 1993;8(7):547–51.
123. Morgenbesser LI, Burgess AW, Boersma RR, Myruski E. Media surveillance of elder sexual abuse cases. J Forensic Nurs. 2006;2(3):121–6.
124. Roberto KA, Teaster PB, Nikzad KA. Sexual abuse of vulnerable young and old men. J Interpers Violence. 2007;22(8):1009–23.
125. Cannell MB, Manini T, Spence-Almaguer E, Maldonado-Molina M, Andresen EM. U.S. population estimates and correlates of sexual abuse of community-dwelling older adults. J Elder Abuse Negl. 2014;26(4):398–413.
126. Witten TM. End of life, chronic illness, and trans-identities. J Soc Work End Life Palliat Care. 2014;10(1):34–58.
127. Grant JM, Mottet LA, Tanis J. Injustice at every turn: a report of the National Transgender Discrimination Survey. National Center for Transgender Equality 2011. https://www.thetaskforce.org/wp-content/uploads/2019/07/ntds_full.pdf. last accessed March 22, 2022.
128. When Health Care Isn't Caring: Lambda Legal's Survey on Discrimination Against LGBT People and People Living with HIV. Lambda Legal. 2010.
129. Carroll L. Therapeutic issues with transgender elders. Psychiatr Clin N Am. 2017;40(1):127–40.

130. Van Wagenen A, Driskell J, Bradford J. "I'm still raring to go": successful aging among lesbian, gay, bisexual, and transgender older adults. J Aging Stud. 2013;27(1):1–14.
131. Aldwin CM, Gilmer DF. Health, illness, and optimal aging: biological and psychosocial perspectives. 2nd ed. New York, NY: Springer Publishing Co; 2013.
132. Puckett JA, Cleary P, Rossman K, Mustanski B, Newcomb ME. Barriers to gender-affirming care for transgender and gender nonconforming individuals. Sex Res Soc Policy. 2018;15(1):48–59.
133. Haider AH, Schneider EB, Kodadek LM, et al. Emergency department query for patient-centered approaches to sexual orientation and gender identity: The EQUALITY Study. JAMA Intern Med. 2017;177(6):819–28.
134. Maragh-Bass AC, Torain M, Adler R, et al. Is it okay to ask: transgender patient perspectives on sexual orientation and gender identity collection in healthcare. Acad Emerg Med. 2017;24(6):655–67.
135. Chochinov HM, McClement S, Hack T, Thompson G, Dufault B, Harlos M. Eliciting personhood within clinical practice: effects on patients, families, and health care providers. J Pain Symptom Manage. 2015;49(6):974–980.e972.
136. Shell JA. Sexual issues in the palliative care population. Semin Oncol Nurs. 2008;24(2):131–4.
137. Bober SL, Recklitis CJ, Bakan J, Garber JE, Patenaude AF. Addressing sexual dysfunction after risk-reducing salpingo-oophorectomy: effects of a brief, psychosexual intervention. J Sex Med. 2015;12(1):189–97.
138. Chung E, Brock G. Sexual rehabilitation and cancer survivorship: a state of art review of current literature and management strategies in male sexual dysfunction among prostate cancer survivors. J Sex Med. 2013;10:102–11.
139. Griebling TL. Sexuality and aging: a focus on lesbian, gay, bisexual, and transgender (LGBT) needs in palliative and end of life care. Curr Opin Support Palliat Care. 2016;10(1):95–101.
140. Lawton A, White J, Fromme EK. End-of-life and advance care planning considerations for lesbian, gay, bisexual, and transgender patients #275. J Palliat Med. 2014;17(1):106–8.
141. Stausmire JM. Sexuality at the end of life. Am J Hosp Palliat Care. 2004;21(1):33–9.
142. Harris-Kojetin L, Sengupta M, Park-Lee E, Valverde R. Long-Term Care Services in the United States: 2013 Overview. Vital Health Stat 3. 2013;37:1–107.
143. Mahieu L, Gastmans C. Older residents' perspectives on aged sexuality in institutionalized elderly care: a systematic literature review. Int J Nurs Stud. 2015;52(12):1891–905.
144. Roelofs TSM, Luijkx KG, Embregts PJCM. Intimacy and sexuality of nursing home residents with dementia: a systematic review. Int Psychogeriatr. 2015;27(3):367–84.
145. Archibald C. Sexuality and dementia in residential care--whose responsibility? Sex Relatsh Ther. 2002;17(3):301–9.
146. Doll GM. Sexuality in nursing homes: practice and policy. J Gerontol Nurs. 2013;39(7):30–7.
147. Aguilar RA. Sexual expression of nursing home residents: systematic review of the literature: sexual expression in nursing homes. J Nurs Scholarsh. 2017;49(5):470–7.
148. Griffith R, Tengnah C. Assessing capacity to consent to sexual relations: a guide for nurses. Br J Community Nurs. 2013;18(4):198–201.
149. Hillman J. Sexual consent capacity: ethical issues and challenges in long-term care. Clin Gerontol. 2017;40(1):43–50.
150. Lichtenberg PA, Strzepek DM. Assessments of institutionalized dementia Patients' competencies to participate in intimate relationships. The Gerontologist. 1990;30(1):117–20.
151. Elder care sex survey finds caregivers seeking more training. Bloomberg. 2013. https://www.bloomberg.com/graphics/infographics/elder-care-sex-survey-results.html. last accessed March 22, 2022.
152. Metzger E. Ethics and intimate sexual activity in long-term care. AMA J Ethics. 2017;19(7):640–8.
153. Sexually Transmitted Diseases Treatment Guidelines CDC. (2015). https://www.cdc.gov/mmwr/preview/mmwrhtml/rr6403a1.htm. Last accessed 18 Aug 2018

Part II
Special Considerations

Chapter 5
Contraception and Family Planning

Mollie Jacobs and Zoe I. Rodriguez

Contents

Most patients in the United States need contraceptive care at some point in their lives so they can plan the size and timing of their families. Primary care clinicians can provide a wide range of family planning and contraceptive services to help ensure that all patients have access to such care regardless of their gender identity, sexual practices, or medical conditions. The provision of readily accessible family planning, preconception, and contraceptive counseling offers the primary care clinician an opportunity to support patients as they consider pregnancy intent and

M. Jacobs (✉)
Department of Family Medicine, University of Colorado, Aurora, CO, USA
e-mail: mollie.jacobs@cuanschutz.edu

Z. I. Rodriguez
Department of Obstetrics, Gynecology and Reproductive Science,
Icahn School of Medicine at Mount Sinai, New York, NY, USA
e-mail: zoe.rodriguez@mountsinai.org

© Springer Nature Switzerland AG 2022
J. Truglio et al. (eds.), *Sexual and Reproductive Health*,
https://doi.org/10.1007/978-3-030-94632-6_5

timing. One Key Question, a recent practice developed in Oregon, calls on providers to screen for pregnancy intent for all patients of reproductive age by asking, "Would you like to become pregnant in the next year?" [2]. By initiating such a conversation with all patients, primary care clinicians can reduce unsafe medication prescriptions and increase the likelihood that patients will use contraception [3]. Further, by providing all patients of childbearing age preconception care services, primary care clinicians can affect not only health status prior to and during conception but also pregnancy and delivery outcomes [22].

The health considerations, indications, and contraindications for contraception discussed in this chapter apply to patients regardless of their sexual orientation or gender identity. Individuals may or may not be using contraception to avoid pregnancy depending on with whom they are partnering. Thus, it is important for primary care clinicians to elicit a patient's goals for family planning or initiating a contraceptive method and provide counseling and assistance to achieve the patient's goals. The approach to an effective and inclusive sexual history in various age groups is discussed in Part 1 of this book. This chapter will focus on the various contraception and family planning options.

Lastly, many patients use contraception for its noncontraceptive indications. For example, nearly all hormonal contraceptive methods suppress menstrual symptoms. This can benefit patients suffering from dysmenorrhea, menorrhagia, and overall discomfort during menstruation. Additionally, nearly all hormonal contraceptive methods can suppress ovulation, which can help address premenstrual syndrome symptoms (PMS) such as breast tenderness, mood swings, fatigue, etc. Some hormonal contraceptives also may help treat acne, hair loss, and hirsutism. This chapter however will focus on the contraceptive use of these medications.

Contraceptive Options

There is a wide range of contraceptive options. By providing comprehensive counseling, clinicians can help a patient choose the most appropriate, effective, safe, and tolerable contraceptive method. Contraceptive options include (a) abstinence; (b) coitus interruptus (withdrawal); (c) natural family planning (timed intercourse to avoid intercourse during ovulation); (d) barrier methods, including male and female condoms and diaphragms; (e) spermicidal agents and sponges; (f) combined hormonal contraceptives (the pill, patch, and vaginal ring); (g) progesterone-only pills; (h) the medroxyprogesterone acetate injection; (i) the progesterone-only contraceptive implant; (j) the levonorgestrel IUD; (k) the copper IUD; (l) emergency contraception; and (m) tubal ligation. The overall efficacy of each option is described in Table 5.1.

Natural family planning methods include carefully timed intercourse to avoid ovulation and coitus interruptus or withdrawal. Patients can track their ovulation by assuming they ovulate somewhere between day 10–20 of their cycle or with ovulation predictor kits or temperature tracking and avoid intercourse when they are most

Table 5.1 Efficacy comparing typical and perfect use of contraceptive methods

Natural family planning and barrier methods		
Method	% with an unintended pregnancy after 1 year of typical use	% with an unintended pregnancy after 1 year of perfect use
No method	85	85
Fertility awareness methods	24	N/A
Spermicides	28	18
Withdrawal	22	4
Female condom	21	5
Male condom	18	2
Diaphragm	12	6
Combined hormonal contraceptive pill and progesterone only contraceptive pill	9	0.3
Patch	9	0.3
Ring	9	0.3
Depo-Provera	6	0.2
Copper IUD	0.8	0.6
Levonorgestrel IUD	0.2	0.2
Subdermal etonogestrel implant	0.05	0.05
Female sterilization	0.5	0.5
Male sterilization	0.15	0.10
Trussell [25]		
How to Choose a Pill		
Absolute contraindications to estrogen		
<21 days postpartum		
>age 35 and smokes >15 cigarettes per day		
Migraine with aura		
Multiple cardiovascular risk factors		
Most patients with a history of DVT/PE or thrombogenic mutations		
Active breast cancer		
Stage 2 hypertension		
History of myocardial infarction or stroke		
Severe liver disease		
Relative contraindications to estrogen		
21–42 days postpartum with other venous thromboembolism risk factors		
>age 35 and smokes <15 cigarettes per day		
>35 and migraine without aura		
Hypertension		
Breast cancer with 5 years cancer-free		
Diabetes with nephropathy or > 20 years of disease		
Some medications, particularly anticonvulsants and antimicrobials		
High risk of using the method improperly or inconsistently [12]		

fertile. When tracking temperature, clinicians should counsel patients to take their temperature right when they wake up in the morning and write it down. They then need to make a chart. The chart will show a normal temperature starting on day 1 of the menstrual cycle, followed by an imperceptible dip on the day of ovulation and then a perceptible degree or two of rise for the subsequent days until they menstruate again. Patients should avoid intercourse on the day of the temperature decrease and the few days surrounding. However, since a temperature decrease is often imperceptible, this method cannot be used in real time but rather to predict when future ovulation may occur.

Barrier methods include male and female condoms and diaphragms. The first two methods are readily available in drugstores. Diaphragms may be more difficult to find depending on geographic location. Clinicians should perform diaphragm fittings in the office with kits that provide diaphragms of various sizes, and they should then order the most appropriate size for their patients.

Combined Hormonal Contraception

Combined hormonal contraceptives (CHCs) contain both estrogen and progesterone and include the pill, the patch, and the vaginal ring. The estrogen usually used is ethinyl estradiol, with release rates varying from steady release of 0.12mcg/day to daily oral doses of 10–50mcg/day. CHCs also each contain a synthetic progesterone, which varies in type and dose. Patients must take the pill daily, put the patch on the skin once weekly, or insert the vaginal ring once monthly. Traditionally, CHCs are self-administered for 21 days, followed by 7 days of placebo pills, or a pill, patch, or ring-free week, when a patient generally can expect to menstruate. Alternatively, patients can choose to use any of these methods continuously, without intervening placebo pills, or the contraceptive-free week to avoid their periods. Menstruation avoidance through continuous or extended (greater than 28 days) administration of CHCs long has been used to treat endometriosis, dysmenorrhea, and menstruation-associated symptoms. A 2014 Cochrane systematic review concluded that extended-cycle CHCs are as effective as traditionally dosed CHCs and may increase patient satisfaction given the suppression of menstruation-associated symptoms [15].

Contraindications to Estrogen

Given its thrombogenic properties, estrogen-use may be limited in medically complex patients. The tables below lists some common absolute and relative contraindications, which must be considered when prescribing hormonal contraceptives. This is discussed in more detail for particular populations in Chap. 9 on Congenital Heart Disease and Chap. 10 on Patients with Cancer and Survivors.

How to Choose a Pill

Absent a contraindication to estrogen, choosing an appropriate pill with a patient depends largely on its side-effect profile. Progesterone can cause three broad categories of side effects: (1) Some progesterones cause progestational side effects, including increased appetite, moodiness, decreased libido, leg vein dilation, and breast tenderness; (2) other progesterones with an androgenic profile may cause acne, increased libido, oily skin, or a deteriorated lipid profile; and (3) some progesterones themselves, or when used in higher doses, can cause endometrial side effects, which generally consist of decreased menstrual bleeding. Also, estrogen alone can cause nausea, melasma, migraines, and breast tenderness and can increase a patient's risk for blood clots.

With the above side effects in mind, a clinician should begin by checking for CHC contraindications. The clinician should then review options with the patient and inquire whether they have taken a CHC in the past, whether they were satisfied, and what they did or did not like about it. For patients without specific issues, a clinician should start a middle-of-the-road, 25–30mcg ethinyl estradiol and with a medium progestational and androgenic progesterone. Table 5.2 associates common progesterone types and dosages with their common characteristics.

Clinicians should counsel patients to use a backup contraceptive method for the first 7 days of any hormonal contraceptive method. Patients should also expect a few months of irregular spotting prior to menstrual regulation.

Progesterone-Only Contraception

For patients with a contraindication to estrogen, there are two, short-acting, progesterone-only methods available. First, the progesterone-only pill, which contains norethindrone 35mcg, can be self-administered in the same fashion as a

Table 5.2 Common progesterone formulations and associated characteristics

Pill composition	Pill characterisic
Norgestimate 25mcg-ethinyl estradiol 35mcg	Inexpensive
Levonorgestrel 15mcg-ethinyl estradiol 25mcg	Middle-of-the-road
Levonorgestrel 10mcg-ethinyl estradiol 20mcg	Low-dose
Drospirenone 30mcg-ethinyl estradiol 20mcg or norgestimate 25mcg-ethinyl estradiol 35mcg	Low androgen
Norethindrone acetate 10mcg-ethinyl estradiol 20mcg	High androgen
Norgestimate 25mcg-ethinyl estradiol 35mcg or levonorgestrel 10mcg-ethinyl estradiol 20mcg	Low progestational
Norethindrone 100mcg-eteinyl Estradiol 35mcg	High endometrial suppression (decreased breakthrough bleeding)
Any pill with 50mcg of ethinyl estradiol	High estrogen

combined hormonal contraceptive pill. The progesterone-only pill has a similar fail-ure rate to that of the combined hormonal contraceptive pill of 0.3% with perfect use and 9% with typical use [20].

The second short-acting progesterone-only option is the contraceptive injection, medroxyprogesterone acetate (Depo-Provera or Depo). This injection contains medroxyprogesterone acetate and can be injected intramuscularly by a healthcare practitioner or subcutaneously by a patient or caregiver in their home once every 3 months [24]. Depo use can cause weight gain and has been associated with lower bone mineral density after prolonged use; however, this effect appears to be revers-ible after discontinuation or a drug holiday [5].

Long-Acting Reversible Contraceptive Options

Long-acting reversible contraceptive (LARC) methods have few contraindications and, according to the American Congress of Obstetricians and Gynecologists, "should be offered routinely as safe and effective contraceptive options for most women" [11].

As of 2017, two types of LARC methods are available in the United States, the intrauterine device (IUD) and the etonogestrel single-rod subdermal implant (Nexplanon). Five IUDs are currently on the market in the United States—one copper-containing IUD and four devices that release levonorgestrel. In the past decade, LARC use has increased from 2.4% in 2002 to 11.6% in 2012 according to the National Survey of Family Growth [16]. This increase LARC in use has been credited with an historic decrease in unintended pregnancy rates [19].

A sentinel prospective cohort study, the "Contraceptive CHOICE" research proj-ect, offered 9256 women aged 14–45 a free contraceptive method of their choice. Seventy-five percent of these women chose LARC, and the study identified a sig-nificant reduction in unintended pregnancy rates among them [18].

Standard-dose levonorgestrel IUDs have been shown to provide effective con-traception for up to 7 years; however, most of them are FDA-approved only for 5 years in the United States. These IUDs also may reduce or eliminate menstrual flow. Low-dose levonorgestrel IUDs can be used effectively for up to 3 years. The copper-containing IUD is FDA approved for 10 years of use but likely can be effec-tive for 12 [28]. The copper-IUD may increase menstrual flow, although can be a good option for women who are interested in highly effective, nonhormonal con-traception. The etonogestrel subdermal implant has been FDA approved for 3 years of use; however, there is increasing evidence that it can be effective for up to 5 years [1].

Primary care clinicians can insert both IUDs and subdermal implants during a routine office visit if adequately trained to do so. The few absolute contraindications to IUDs include uterine anomalies, active endometrial or cervical cancer, active breast cancer (levonorgestrel IUDs and implants only), and some clotting disorders (levonorgestrel IUDs and implants only). IUDs do not increase the risk of sexually transmitted infection [13]. The risk of infective endocarditis in select patients is discussed in Chap. 9, Congenital Heart Disease.

Emergency Contraception

Four types of emergency or postcoital contraception are currently available in the United States: (1) combined hormonal pills, which contain estrogen and progesterone; (2) levonorgestrel-only pills, commonly known as Plan B; (3) a progestin antagonist known as Ella, which contains ulipristal acetate; and (4) the copper IUD. In addition, the levonorgestrel IUD is under study to confirm its likely postcoital contraceptive efficacy [26]. Patients should use postcoital contraception as soon as possible after intercourse and, at a maximum, 120 hours after unprotected intercourse. Generally speaking, estrogen-containing emergency contraception can be safely used in patients in whom ongoing CHC would be contraindicated.

The efficacy of emergency contraception is very difficult to quantify given difficulties in controlling for the time at which a patient takes it during their cycle as well as the amount of days post-intercourse a patient takes it. Estimates of efficacy range from 52% to 100% for levonorgestrel, 56–89% for combined hormonal contraceptives, and 62–85% for ulipristal acetate. The copper IUD is highly effective. More than 7000 insertions for postcoital contraception have been reported in the literature since 1976 with only 10 known failures [26].

The hormonal emergency contraception methods delay or impair ovulation and thus prevent pregnancy. The copper-IUD prevents implantation. Of the three hormonal emergency contraceptive pills, ulipristal is the most effective. Unlike its levonorgestrel-containing counterpart, its use is unaffected by body mass index [26]. Emergency contraceptive pills should be available over the counter without a prescription. However, a recent study of ulipristal acetate, the most effective of these available pills, found that despite high-quality evidence for the increased efficacy of ulipristal over levonorgestrel emergency contraception, its availability in a sample of major US cities remains limited [23]. Another recent study in Colorado found significant barriers for women in obtaining legal, over-the-counter, levonorgestrel emergency contraception [9].

Common side effects of hormonal emergency contraception include nausea, vomiting, breast tenderness, breakthrough bleeding, headache, dizziness, and fatigue. Side effects usually do not last more than a few days after treatment. Since ulipristal acetate antagonizes progesterone, practitioners should counsel patients starting or continuing a progesterone-only birth control method to use a backup method of contraception for 14 days after using ulipristal.

Tubal Ligation

Permanent sterilization remains an effective option for many women. This can be achieved via various operative methods.

According to a 2014 study, the expected pregnancy rates per 1000 women at 1 year are 57 for Essure insertion (since removed from the market) and between 3 and 7 for various techniques of operative tubal ligation. At 10 years, pregnancy rates per 1000 women increase to 96 for Essure insertion and between 24 and 30 for operative tubal ligation [17].

Rare operative complications can result from tubal ligation such as damage to the bowel, bladder, uterus, or major blood vessels; adverse reaction to anesthesia; improper healing or wound infection; and prolonged, undifferentiated pelvic pain.

Contraceptive Options for Men or Patients with Male Sex Organs

Contraceptive options for men have long-included barrier methods, such as condoms and permanent sterilization, also known as vasectomy. Vasectomy is a safe, minimally invasive procedure performed by urologists and many family doctors, which blocks the vas deferens and thus inhibits sperm from traveling outside the body. Vasectomy is highly effective, with a 0.1% chance of unintended pregnancy after a year of perfect use [25], and should be considered irreversible. However, some practitioners may offer vasectomy reversal procedures with varying degrees of success. Of note, following vasectomy, a couple must use backup contraception for a number of weeks until a semen sample reveals the absence of sperm in order to avoid conception with residual downstream sperm.

Hormonal contraception for men has also been synthesized. A recent study demonstrated near complete reversible suppression of spermatogenesis through the administration of an intramuscular formulation of progesterone and testosterone every 8 weeks to male subjects. However, the study was terminated due to increased frequency of reportedly intolerable side effects, including acne and severe depression [4]. Research in this area is continuing.

Initiation of Contraception

If a patient has not had unprotected intercourse since their last menstrual period, contraception may be initiated safely at any time. Some patients prefer to start the birth control pill, patch, or ring on a Sunday or Monday in order to remember to start a new pill package or change their patch or ring on the first day of the week. Patients may also prefer to start a pill, patch, or ring on the first day of their menstrual cycle in order to keep it as regular as possible. However, if a patient is likely to have unprotected intercourse prior to their next period, clinicians should always offer to start immediately. It is important that clinicians counsel patients that they may experience irregular spotting for the first several months when changing or starting birth control. Additionally, all hormonal methods require that a patient use a backup method for 1 week upon initiation of a new method.

Initiating any method of contraception can become complicated if a patient has had unprotected intercourse since their last menstrual period (LMP) and if the LMP was more than 7 days prior. Under these circumstances, a urine pregnancy test may not yet be positive, and clinicians may not be able to rule out pregnancy definitively prior to method initiation. Clinicians can offer patients several options to address these issues. A clinician can counsel a patient on the risk of early pregnancy not yet evident on a pregnancy test and can initiate a contraceptive method, assuming the patient has been informed and understands the risk, or a clinician can offer to wait until the first day of the patient's next menstrual period to initiate a contraceptive method. If the patient chooses the former option, she should take a pregnancy test at home 2 weeks later and be offered option counseling if her test result is positive [12].

Option Counseling and Unintended Pregnancy

In 2011, nearly half (45% or 2.8 million) of the 6.1 million pregnancies in the United States were unintended [16]. Patients who become pregnant, whether intentionally or not, should have ready access to all of their options. Pregnancy options include continuation of the pregnancy and parenting, continuation of the pregnancy followed by adoption, and abortion. There are two types of abortion. Medication abortion can safely be administered up to 10 weeks after conception, and surgical abortion can safely be offered and administered up to the gestational age permitted in the state in which the abortion will occur. Primary care providers should counsel patients on their pregnancy options in a nonjudgmental manner and connect them with the resources they desire in a timely fashion. Of note, crisis pregnancy centers are not appropriate referrals for pregnancy options counseling as they provide judgmental counseling and services from a staunchly antiabortion prospective [21].

Contraception and Family Planning for Special Populations

Clinicians should offer to all patients counselling about all available contraceptive and pregnancy options. The following are some special considerations clinicians may take into account for specific populations.

Transgender and Gender Nonbinary Patients

As described in the introduction to this chapter, all aspects of contraception and family planning discussed in this chapter pertain to patients regardless of their gender identity. The need for and utility of various forms of contraception depend on the sex organs that are present and the sexual behaviors of the patient. Of note, depending on their sexual activity and sexual partners, patients on testosterone should be counseled that testosterone does not provide adequate contraception.

The reproductive desires of transgender patients have not been well studied, but data suggest that 50% of the patients would like to have biological children of their own [14, 27]. The primary care clinician as part of the sexual history should ask all trans and nonbinary patients what their parenting goals are. With improved assisted reproductive technology and greater access to fertility preservation procedures, more and more patients are opting to preserve their capacity for birthing or parenting biologic children. The hormone prescribing clinician should make themselves familiar with these options as gender-affirming hormones can have lasting or permanent effects on natal gonads that may render the patient sterile. The impact of various gender-affirming hormonal and surgical treatments on fertility is discussed in more detail in Part 3 of this book. Additionally, many of the surgical procedures that are available to transgender patients do impart permanent sterility.

Referral for a consultation by a reproductive endocrinologist prior to the initiation of gender affirming hormones is a crucial step in helping transgender and gender nonbinary patients achieve their parenting goals. The consultant will clearly and explicitly describe the fertility options available to the patient which may include oocyte or sperm cryopreservation.

Individuals with Intellectual Disabilities

Please see Chap. 11 for additional details on sexual and reproductive health in individuals with intellectual disabilities. Briefly, individuals with intellectual disabilities should receive standard contraceptive and family planning counseling. Such counseling should be offered directly to the patient unless that individual is unable to participate in such a conversation. Caregivers also may be involved in these conversations as needed, but, absent legal decision-making authority, should not be relied upon to make decisions for the patient.

Some individuals with intellectual disabilities desire contraceptive initiation to assist with menstrual hygiene. This is an appropriate use of many forms of contraception; however, providers should not assume that patients with intellectual disabilities are not sexually active.

Adolescents

Barring additional medical indications or contraindications, adolescents may be offered all contraceptive options, including long-acting reversible contraceptive options. Contraceptive counseling for teens may be influenced, however by the fact that the teen population experiences a higher incidence of sexually transmitted infections (STIs). According to the CDC, young people aged 15–24 years experience half of all new STIs, and 1 in 4 sexually active adolescent females has an STI [8]. While this increased prevalence does not affect a teen's candidacy for any particular birth control method, it should inform a clinician's counseling and encourage him or her to stress that non-barrier contraceptive methods do not protect against STIs. Additionally, intrauterine devices should not be placed during an active chlamydia or gonorrhea infection. Such infections should be treated prior to IUD insertion. If a patient does not know if she has an STI, she can be screened for gonorrhea and chlamydia at the time of insertion, and if positive, she can receive treatment followed by a test of cure without removing her IUD.

Such increase in STI prevalence among adolescents should not dissuade clinicians from offering LARCs to patients in this group, as LARCs remain a highly effective option. For example, in 2008, Colorado received funding for the Colorado Family Planning Initiative. This program provided no- or low-cost LARCs to low-income women statewide, including teens. According to the program's executive summary, by the middle of 2015, the initiative provided LARCs to more than 36,000 women. "Between 2009 and 2014, birth and abortion rates both declined by nearly 50 percent among teens aged 15–19 and by 20 percent among young women aged 20–24" [10].

Preconception Counseling

Many patients seek advice from their primary care clinician prior to planning a pregnancy. Primary care clinicians should counsel patients on basic fertility management such as ways to track ovulation, when to have intercourse in order to achieve pregnancy, and basic health considerations regarding preconception. Providers should counsel patients to stop smoking, avoid excess alcohol, and avoid illicit drugs and should review patients' medications for any possible contraindications in pregnancy. The CDC recommends folic acid supplementation starting at least 1 month prior to conception. Thus, when a couple is actively trying to conceive, providers should recommend starting a prenatal vitamin with folic acid [6, 7].

Patients should be counseled that once they stop their contraception method, they immediately become at risk for pregnancy, even though conception sometimes takes up to 1 year to occur. For patients who desire pregnancy, intercourse ideally should be timed around ovulation, which can be tracked by simply assuming it happens between day 10 and 20 of a woman's cycle or by more technical methods such as ovulation predictor kits or temperature tracking.

Infertility and Assisted Reproduction

Specialty referral for evaluation of infertility or assisted reproduction is reasonable for patients under the age of 35 who have been trying to conceive for 1 year and for those over the age of 35 who have been trying for 6 months. Same-sex couples and uncoupled individuals may also seek and should be readily referred for assisted reproductive technologies to conceive children.

The CDC estimates that about 12% of women in the United States suffer from infertility [6, 7]. Infertility can be caused by male factors such as decreased or impaired sperm production or function. It also can be caused by female factors such as impaired ovulation, fallopian tube dysfunction or distortion, unusual uterine anatomy, endometriosis, and, in many cases, indeterminate causes.

Primary care clinicians can initiate an infertility work-up by ordering a semen analysis in male patients and, if comfortable, a small laboratory evaluation in female patients including a TSH, prolactin, FSH, estradiol, and anti-mullerian hormone.

Assisted reproduction has become more effective in recent decades. Primary care clinicians can refer patients to reproductive endocrinologists where they can obtain ovulation inducing drugs, intrauterine insemination procedures, and in vitro fertilization procedures. Specialized urologists can provide counselling and treatment to men who struggle with infertility.

Conclusion

Primary care clinicians can help their patients achieve their overall health and personal goals by fostering a trusting relationship and ensuring that all patients have access to the necessary family planning and contraceptive services.

References

1. Ali M, Akin A, Bahamondes L, Brache V, Habib N, Landoulsi S, Hubacher D. Extended use up to 5 years of the etonogestrel-releasing subdermal contraceptive implant: comparison to levonorgestrel-releasing subdermal implant. Hum Reprod. 2016;31(11):2491–8. https://doi.org/10.1093/humrep/dew222.
2. Allen D, Hunter MS, Wood S, Beeson T. One key question: first things first reproductive health. Matern Child Health J. 2017;21(3):387–92. https://doi.org/10.1007/s10995-017-2283-2.

3. American Academy of Pediatrics/American College of Obstetricians and Gynecologists. Guidelines for perinatal care. 5th ed. Elk Grove Village, IL: American Academy of Pediatricians; 2012.
4. Behre H, Zitzmann M, Anderson R, Handelsman D, Lestari S, McLachlan R, Meriggiola C, Misro M, Noe G, Wu F, Festin M, Habib N, Vogelsong K, Callahan M, Linton K, Colvard D. Efficacy and Safety of an Injectable Combination Hormonal Contraceptive for Men. J Clin Endocrinol Metab. 2016;101(12):4779–88. https://doi.org/10.1210/jc.2016-2141.
5. Bigrigg A, Evans M, Gbolade B, Newton J, Pollard L, Szarewski A, Thomas C, Walling M. Depo Provera: position paper on clinical use, effectiveness and side effects. Br J Fam Plann. 1999;25(2):69–76.
6. Center for Disease Control and Prevention (CDC). *Infertility FAQs*. 2017a. Retrieved from https://www.cdc.gov/reproductivehealth/infertility/index.htm.
7. Center for Disease Control and Prevention (CDC). Planning for pregnancy. 2017b. Retrieved from https://www.cdc.gov/preconception/planning.html.
8. Center for Disease Control and Prevention (CDC). *STDs in adolescents and young adults*. 2016. Retrieved from https://www.cdc.gov/std/stats15/adolescents.htm.
9. Chau V, Stamm C, Borgelt L, Gafney M, Moore A, Blumhagen R, Rupp L, Topp D, Gilroy C. Barriers to single-dose levonorgestrel-only emergency contraception access in retail pharmacies. Womens Health Issues. 2017;27(5):518–22.
10. Colorado Department of Public Health and Environment (CDPHE), Taking the Unintended Out of Pregnancy: Colorado's Success with Long-Acting Reversible Contraception, January 2017. Retrieved from https://www.colorado.gov/pacific/sites/default/files/PSD_TitleX3_CFPI-Report.pdf.
11. Committee on Practice Bulletins—Gynecology, Epsey E, Hofler L. Long-acting reversible contraception: Implants and intrauterine devices. ACOG Practice Bulletin Number 186, November, 2017. https://www.acog.org/Resources-And-Publications/Practice-Bulletins/Committee-on-Practice-Bulletins-Gynecology/Long-Acting-Reversible-Contraception-Implants-and-Intrauterine-Devices.
12. Curtis KM, Jatlaoui TC, Tepper NK, et al. U.S. selected practice recommendations for contraceptive use, 2016. MMWR Recomm Rep. 2016;65(RR-4):1–66. https://doi.org/10.15585/mmwr.rr6504a1.
13. Curtis K, Tepper N, Jatlaoui T, Berry-Bibee E, Horton L, Zapata L, Simmons K, Pagano P, Jamieson D, Whiteman M. US medical eligibility criteria for contraceptive use, 2016. Morb Mortal Wkly Rep. 2016;65(3):1–104.
14. DeSutter P, et al. The desire to have children and the preservation of fertility in transsexual women: a survey. Int J Transgenderism. 2002;6:215–21.
15. Edelman A, Micks E, Gallo MF, Jensen JT, Grimes DA. Continuous or extended cycle vs. cyclic use of combined hormonal contraceptives for contraception. Cochrane Database Syst Rev. 2014;29(7):CD004695. https://doi.org/10.1002/14651858.CD004695.pub3.
16. Finer LB, Zolna MR. Declines in unintended pregnancy rates in the United States 2008-2011. N Engl J Med. 2016;374:843–52. Retrieved from http://nejm.org/doi/full/10.1056/NEJMsa1506575.
17. Gariepy A, Creinin M, Smith K, Xu X. Probability of pregnancy after sterilization: a comparison of hysteroscopy versus laparoscopic sterilization. Contraception. 2014;90(2):174–81.
18. Harper CC, Rocca CH, Thompson KM, Morfesis J, Goodman S, Darney PD, et al. Reductions in pregnancy rates in the USA with long-acting reversible contraception: a cluster randomized trial. Lancet. 2015;386:562–8.
19. Peipert JF, Madden T, Allsworth JE, Secura GM. Preventing unintended pregnancies by providing no-cost contraception. Obstet Gynecol. 2012;120:1291–7.
20. Phelps R, Murphy P, Godfrey E, et al. A quick reference guide for clinicians: choosing a birth control method. Association of Reproductive Health Professionals. September, 2011. http://www.arhp.org/Publications-and-Resources/Quick-Reference-Guide-for-Clinicians/choosing/failure-rates-table.

21. Rosen J. The public health risks of crisis pregnancy centers. Perspect Sex Reprod Health. 2012;44:201–5.
22. Schwarz EB, Parisi S, Fischer G, et al. Effect of a "contraceptive vital sign" in primary care: a randomized controlled trial. Contraception. 2010;82:183–216.
23. Shigesato M, Elia J, Tschann M, Bullock H, Hurwitz E, Wu Y, Salcedo J. Pharmacy access to ulipristal acetate in major cities throughout the United States. Contraception. 2017;pii:s0010-7824(17):30497–3. https://doi.org/10.1016/j.contraception.2017.10.009.
24. Simon MA, Shlman LP. Subcutaneous versus intramuscular depot medroxyprogesterone acetate: a comparative review. Women's Health (Lond). 2006;2(2):191–7. https://doi.org/10.2217/17455057.2.2.191.
25. Trussell J. Contraceptive failure in the United States. Contraception. 2011;83(5):397–404.
26. Trussell, J, Raymond, E, Cleland, K. Emergency contraception: a last chance to prevent unintended pregnancy. Office of Population Research, Princeton University. Princeton, NJ: 2017.
27. Wierckx K, et al. Reproductive wish in transexual men. Hum Reprod. 2012;27:483–7.
28. Wu J, Pickle S. Extended use of the intrauterine device: a literature review and recommendations for clinical practice. Contraception. 2014;89(6):495–503.

Chapter 6
Sexually Transmitted Infections

John Koeppe

Contents

Introduction

Sexually transmitted infections (STIs) are common infections, especially in adolescents and young adults. Primary care clinicians play an important role in the diagnosis and treatment of STIs, with approximately 22–33% of these infections diagnosed in primary care settings [1]. Depending upon proposed cuts to federally funded family planning clinics, [2] the role of the primary care clinicians could become even more important in the coming years. Thus, having a basic understanding of prevention, screening, diagnoses, and treatment of STIs is important for all primary care clinicians to have.

J. Koeppe (✉)
Department of General Internal Medicine, University of Colorado at Denver and Health Sciences Center, Denver, CO, USA
e-mail: John.Koeppe@cuanschutz.edu

© Springer Nature Switzerland AG 2022
J. Truglio et al. (eds.), *Sexual and Reproductive Health*,
https://doi.org/10.1007/978-3-030-94632-6_6

145

This chapter will review the prevention, diagnosis, and treatment of STIs in non-pregnant, immunocompetent adults. An approach to the prevention, diagnosis, and treatment of STIs in adolescent patients can be found in Chap. 2. The prevention and diagnosis of HIV will be discussed, including the role or pre-exposure prophylaxis for HIV; however, the treatment of HIV and prevention of vertical transmission will not. The chapter is divided into three main sections: common STIs in the United States; uncommon STIs in the United States; and an emerging STI—*Mycoplasma genitalium*.

Prevention

Effective counseling on prevention of STIs is dependent on obtaining an accurate sexual history with particular attention to sexual practices. Inclusive approaches to sexual history are presented in Part 1 of this book.

Condoms offer effective prevention from STIs, especially infections transmitted by genital secretions such as gonorrhea, chlamydia, trichomonas, and HIV. The true efficacy of condoms is not known due to the reliance on observational studies with self-reported condom use. Condoms are less effective for the prevention of infections such as herpes simplex virus (HSV) and the human papillomavirus (HPV) due to the transmission being largely through skin-to-skin contact for these infections [3].

Other forms of barrier protection are often overlooked, especially when discussing sexual practices with women who have sex with women (WSW). Female condoms [4], dental dams [5], gloves during digital genital stimulation, and covers/condoms with sex toys [6] can all help prevent STI transmission.

The use of medications for prevention, where appropriate, is discussed under each disease heading.

Common Sexually Transmitted Infections in the United States

Chlamydia and Gonorrhea

Epidemiology Chlamydia is the most common reportable infection in the United States, and rates of new chlamydia infections have been increasing since at least 2000 with young women being the most commonly affected population. Although increased testing is likely part of the explanation, most experts also feel there has been an increase in actual infections. The case rate in 2016 in the United States among females was 657.3 per 100,000, and among men, it was 330.5 per 100,000 [1].

Rates of gonorrhea have also been increasing since 2009, with the greatest increases being seen in men. Similar to chlamydia, the increased rates of gonorrhea may in part be explained by increased testing, but most experts feel there has been an increase in the actual number of infections. The case rate in 2016 in the United States among men was 170.7 per 100,000 and 121.0 per 100,000 among women [1].

Clinical Presentation Chlamydia infection is most often asymptomatic with between 84.8% and 92.9% of women reporting no symptoms and between 94.1% and 98.2% of men reporting no symptoms in one large study. For gonorrhea between 84.2% and 88.5% of women and between 86.4% and 92.6% of men reported no symptoms in the same study [7]. Cervical and urethral discharge is the most common symptom in women and men, respectively. Discharge and pain can be present rectally and orally when infections are present at these sites. Systemic manifestations including disseminated infection, septic arthritis (gonorrhea), perihepatitis, and conjunctivitis (chlamydia) are also seen but are beyond the scope of this chapter.

Screening and Testing The United States Preventive Services Task Force (USPSTF), the Centers for Disease Control (CDC), the American Academy of Family Physicians (AAFP), and the Canadian Health Agency all recommend screening sexually active women under the age of 25 and women over the age of 25 with any risk factors [8]. Neither the USPSTF nor the AAFP recommend screening in men; however, the CDC recommends screening men who are at risk, and the Canadian Health Agency recommend screening men under the age of 25 [8, 9]. Questions about sexual activity should be included as part of routine care, and men with any concerns or at high risk should be offered routine screening.

Testing is done using nucleic acid amplification tests (NAATs). In women a vaginal swab is preferred, and first catch urine is considered an acceptable alternative. In men a first catch urine is the preferred test [10].

Extragenital testing should also be offered to any persons reporting receptive oral or anal intercourse. In one study of men who have sex with men (MSM) and women who reported a history of receptive anal intercourse (RAI), over 75% of infections were found only extragenitally in men, and over 15% were found only extragenitally in women [11]. A study of self-identified gay and bisexual men looking urinary samples and anal swabs found gonorrhea and chlamydia threefold more often rectally than in urine samples [12]. Extragenital testing is done using the same NAAT swabs but is not validated in all labs and thus may not yet be available in some labs.

Treatment Treatment of chlamydia and gonorrhea in adults with genitourinary, oral, or rectal infections has recently been updated [13] and is shown in Tables 6.1 and 6.2.

Follow-Up Test-of-cure follow-up testing is not recommended for either gonorrhea or chlamydia that is treated with recommended regimens. Most follow-up testing that is positive is felt to be new infections. Additionally tests done within the first few weeks after treatment may be false positives due to the extreme sensitivity of NAAT testing.

Table 6.1 Treatment of genitourinary, oral, and rectal chlamydia infections (Ref. [10])

Recommended regimens
Non-Pregnant Adults: Doxycycline 100 mg orally twice a day for 7 days
Pregnant Adults: Azithromycin 1 gram orally as a single dose
Alternative regimens
Erythromycin base 500 mg orally four times a day for 7 days
OR
Erythromycin succinate 800 mg orally four times a day for 7 days
OR
Levofloxacin 500 mg orally once daily for 7 days
OR
Ofloxacin 300 mg twice a day for 7 days

Table 6.2 Treatment for genitourinary, oral, and rectal gonorrhea infections (Ref. [10])

Recommended regimen
Ceftriaxone 500 mg IM in a single dose
Alternative regimen
Cefixime 800 mg orally as a single dose
PLUS
Azithromycin 1 gram orally as a single dose

Treatment of Sex Partners Both chlamydia and gonorrhea are reportable conditions, and the laboratories that do the testing should notify their respective State Health Departments. Sexual partners in the last 60 days and the last potential exposure if the last sexual encounter was more than 60 days ago should be referred for counseling, testing, and treatment. Persons should abstain from sex for at least 7 days after receiving treatment. If there are concerns about sexual partners getting in for testing and treatment, expedited partner therapy (EPT) can be given in most states (for a list of states where EPT is legal, go to https://www.cdc.gov/STI/ept/legal/default.htm). EPT involves either prescribing for the partner or providing the patient with a prescription for the partner (doxycycline 100 mg orally twice daily for 7 days for chlamydia and cefixime 800 mg as a single dose for gonorrhea) [13]. The CDC does not recommend the routine use of EPT for MSM due to a higher risk of other STIs such as HIV that may be missed with EPT [14]. However, each patient should be assessed individually, and there are situations where EPT can be appropriate for MSM.

Trichomonas

Epidemiology It is estimated that there are over a one million new infections caused by *Trichomonas vaginalis* in the United States annually [15] with self-identified heterosexual Black women being the most heavily affected population. Of note, any such observations regarding racial inequities should be interpreted as a manifestation of social and structural forces, not biological differences between races, and the application of these data individualized to each patient or community.

Clinical Presentation Seventy to eighty-five percent of persons may be asymptomatic. Women may present with vaginal discharge that may be malodorous and have associated vulvar irritation. Men may present with urethritis, epididymitis, or prostatitis [14]. Infection may last for years, and it is estimated that prevalence may be 3 – 4fold greater than the incidence of disease [14, 15].

Screening and Testing NAAT is considered is the preferred method of detecting trichomonas. In women vaginal swabs and urine testing are considered equally sensitive (95.3–100%) and specific (95.2–100%, Ref. 14). Recently NAAT has also been found to have a sensitivity 97.2% and a specificity of 99.9% in male urine samples [16]. Wet mount microscopy can be a rapid way to diagnose trichomonas and is available in many clinics but suffers from poor sensitivity (51–65%) compared to NAAT [14].

Treatment Treatment is with metronidazole or tinidazole, both 2 grams orally as a single dose. Metronidazole 500 mg orally twice daily for 7 days is an alternative.

Follow-Up Follow-up test of cure is recommended by the CDC due to high rates of reinfections and emerging resistance to metronidazole (4–10%). Retesting with NAAT can be done within 2 weeks of completing therapy [14].

Treatment of Sex Partners All sex partners should be treated as well with the same regimens used for patients. Patients and their partners should abstain from sex until both have been treated and symptoms have resolved [14].

Syphilis

Epidemiology The rates of primary and secondary (P & S) syphilis (i.e., new infections) have been increasing every year since about 2000 when they were at an all-time low. In 2016 the rate among men was 15.6 per 100,000 and 1.9 per 100,000 among women. During most of this time, the increase has largely been in MSM; however, starting in 2013 rates in women also started to increase. Congenital syphilis cases tend to rise when rates in women increase, and indeed rates of congenital syphilis have increased from 8.4 per 100,000 in 2012 to 15.7 per 100,000 in 2016 [1].

Clinical Presentation Syphilis is often called the great masquerader and can present with protean manifestations. The most common presentation of primary syphilis is a clean based, painless ulcer at the infection site. For secondary syphilis a rash, often involving the palms and soles of the feet is the most common symptom. A discussion of all the manifestations of secondary and tertiary syphilis is beyond the scope of this chapter. However, anyone with unexplained symptoms and risk factors for syphilis should be tested [14]. The CDC website offers a concise discussion of the presentation of syphilis in its various stages (https://www.cdc.gov/STI/syphilis/

STIfact-syphilis-detailed.htm) along with images of its various manifestations (https://phil.cdc.gov/QuickSearch.aspx).

Screening and Testing Screening is recommended in HIV positive men and MSM with intervals as often as every 3 months for persons with multiple sexual partners [17]. It is also the opinion of the author that any person requesting STI testing should be offered syphilis screening.

In the primary care setting, testing for syphilis is generally done using serologic testing. Two sets of serologic tests are available, treponemal (TPPA, FTA-ABS) and non-treponemal tests (RPR, VRDL). Neither test alone is sufficient to diagnosis syphilis [14]. Characteristics of the tests are shown in Table 6.3. Although the reported specificity of both tests is high [17, 18], there is no gold standard to truly base this on, and false positives are more commonly reported with non-treponemal tests. Most centers today first perform a treponemal test (i.e., TPPA) and if this is positive will reflex to a non-treponemal test (i.e., RPR). Interpretation of testing is often confusing for providers without a lot of experience, and Table 6.4 offers interpretations of the most common scenarios seen in primary care.

Treatment Penicillin is the preferred treatment for all stages of syphilis. Treatments for syphilis are shown in Table 6.5 and are based on CDC guidelines [14]. According to the CDC, secondary syphilis can be treated the same as primary and early latent syphilis (infection of less than 1 year's duration); however, given the frequent uncertainty in the staging of syphilis, consideration should be made to treat with three injections of benzathine penicillin. Thus, the recommended treatment can be separated into three clinical scenarios. (1) Infection of less than 1 year should be treated with benzathine penicillin 2.4 million units one time. (2) Infection that is of unknown duration or more than 1 year's duration but does not involve the central nervous

Table 6.3 Characteristics of serologic tests for syphilis (Ref. [10, 14, 15])

	Treponemal	Non-treponemal
Test names	TPPA, FTA-AB	RPR, VDRL
Antigens tested	*Treponemal pallidum*	Cardiolipin, cholesterol, lecithin
Remains positive after treatment	Yes	Not usually. Should decline and hopefully become undetectable with therapy
Can be used to follow response to therapy	No	Yes, titer should drop with therapy. A fourfold or greater drop is considered an appropriate response
Sensitivity		
Primary	84–88%	78–86%
Secondary	100%	100%
Latent	97–100%	96–98%
Late	94–96%	71–73%
Specificity	96–97%	98% False positive seen in autoimmune diseases, HIV, pregnancy, intravenous drug abuse

Table 6.4 Interpretation of syphilis tests

Clinical scenario	Treponemal test (TPPA, FTA-AB)	Non-treponemal test (RPR, VDRL)	Interpretation
Asymptomatic screening	Positive	Negative	In most cases, this represents previously treated syphilis. However, this scenario could be seen in late disease, and confirmation of prior treatment is essential
Asymptomatic screening	Positive	Positive with a titer of 1:2 or greater	In most cases this means active disease and treatment are indicated. However, this could also be seen in someone with prior disease that has been treated. If a fourfold drop in the titer is documented from pre-treatment levels, this may indicate an appropriate response to therapy and not active disease
Symptomatic testing	Positive	Positive with a titer of 1:2 or greater	This indicates active disease. Unless documentation of a fourfold drop in titer with prior treatment and a good alternative for patients symptoms is available, treatment is indicated
Symptomatic testing or asymptomatic screening	Negative	Positive with a titer or 1:2 or greater	This usually indicates a false positive non-treponemal test. This scenario is less common today due to most laboratories doing the treponemal assay first and only doing the non-treponemal test if that is positive

Table 6.5 Treatment of syphilis (Ref. [10])

Clinical scenario	Treatment
Primary syphilis or disease of less than 1 year's duration (i.e., prior screening test done less than a year ago was negative)	Benzathine penicillin G 2.4 million units IM in a single dose ALTERNATIVES Doxycycline 100 mg orally twice daily x 14 days OR Ceftriaxone 1–2 grams IM or IV for 10–14 days
Disease duration unknown or greater than 1 year, but not neurosyphilis	Benzathine penicillin G 2.4 million units IM × 3 doses, each a week apart ALTERNATIVE Doxycycline 100 mg orally twice daily × 28 days
Neurosyphilis	Aqueous crystalline penicillin 3–4 million units every 4 hours or 18–24 million units as a continuous drip for 10–14 days. ALTERNATIVES Procaine penicillin G 2.4 million units IM daily for 10–14 days PLUS Probenecid 500 mg orally four times daily for the same duration OR Ceftriaxone 2 grams IM or IV daily for 10–14 days

system (CNS) should be treated with three injections, each a week apart of benzathine penicillin 2.4 million units each. (3) Neurosyphilis should be treated with IV penicillin 3–four million units every 4 hours and usually requires hospital admission to at least begin therapy (Table 6.5).

Follow-Up All persons with syphilis require close follow-up to assess response to therapy. The non-treponemal (RPR or VDRL) titer should be followed, with a response to therapy considered a fourfold or greater drop in the titer (i.e., 1:16 drops to 1:4), although ideally these titers become undetectable. In some patients these titers will not drop, and in those cases they should be evaluated for possible undertreated syphilis, and consideration should be given to getting a lumbar puncture (LP) if not done as part of the initial work-up. However, in many cases these patients are what's known as serofast. The serofast state is when the titers do not drop despite appropriate therapy and represent the imperfection of antibody-based tests [14].

Treatment of Sex Partners Syphilis is only considered transmittable during the primary and secondary stages. Persons who have had sexual contact with the patient in the last 90 days during either of these stages should be tested and then treated presumptively for syphilis. Persons who have had a sexual exposure with the patient within the first year of infection should be tested, and consideration should be given to presumptive treatment. Long-term sexual partners should be tested and treated based on the results of testing [14].

Genital Herpes Simplex Virus (HSV)

Epidemiology Approximately 50 million Americans are infected with HSV-2, the most common cause of genital ulcers in the United States. Although HSV-1 is more commonly associated with oral mucosal ulcers, it can also cause genital ulcers [14].

Clinical Presentation HSV usually presents as painful blistering ulcer on an erythematous base. Infection is generally self-limited in the absence of immune compromising conditions. HSV is a lifelong infection and can recur throughout a person's life, although many patients may only have one episode in their life.

Screening and Testing Routine screening for HSV is not recommended. Testing in patients with symptoms is done with either viral culture or more commonly polymerase chain reaction (PCR) of active lesions [14].

Treatment Acyclovir, valacyclovir, and famciclovir can all be used to treat herpes infections. Various dosing regimens can be used; common ones are shown in Table 6.6. For outbreaks treatment is most likely to be beneficial if started within the first 24 hours of lesion appearance and will shorten the duration of illness by 1–2 days. For persons with HIV or who may be immunecompromised, higher dos-

Table 6.6 Treatment for genitourinary herpes simplex infections. Other dosing regimens are available (Ref. [10])

Drug (duration of therapy)	Primary infection (7–10 days)	Recurrent infection (5 days)	Chronic suppressive therapy (indefinite)
Acyclovir	400 mg thrice a day	400 mg thrice a day	400 mg twice a day
Valacyclovir	1 gram twice a day	1 gram daily	1 gram daily
Famciclovir	250 mg thrice a day	125 mg twice a day	250 mg twice a day

ages and longer treatment durations should be considered [14]. Daily suppressive therapy can be given for patients with recurrent infections. The decision of when it is appropriate to do this relies on patient preference and shared decision-making. Factors such as how bothersome they find the outbreaks, the likelihood of transmission to a partner, and their feelings about daily medication should all be considered.

Follow-Up Follow-up is not required for HSV although patients should be told to contact their provider if symptoms fail to improve.

Treatment of Sex Partners Treatment of sex partners is not required. Suppressive therapy for persons who are concerned about transmitting the virus to a partner can be given. Serologic testing of the partner to see if they have already been infected is reasonable in this setting.

Human Papillomavirus (HPV)

Epidemiology Human papillomavirus is the most common STI in the United States [15], and most sexually active persons will become infected at least once in their lifetime [14].

Clinical Presentation Most of these infections are asymptomatic and clear on their own, but persistent infection can lead to genital warts and cancer depending upon the serotype present. Most cervical, vulvar, vaginal, penile, anal and oropharyngeal cancers are caused by HPV [14]. There are more than 200 serotypes of HPV that can infect humans with 12 serotypes that are associated with human cancers (16,1 8,31,33,35,39,45,51,52,56,58,59) (Ref. 19).

Screening and Testing It is well agreed that screening for cervical cancer with cervical cytology decreases the incidence and mortality from cervical cancer [20]. Since the initiation of pap smear screening of women, mortality from cervical cancer has dropped almost fivefold [20]. Cervical cancer screening for average risk patients is covered in more detail in Part 1 of this book. Screening for other forms of HPV-related cancer is more controversial. The HIV Medical Association recommends anal pap smears for HIV-positive MSM, women with a history or receptive anal intercourse or abnormal pap smears, and anyone with genital warts [21]. There are currently no guidelines that recommend anal cancer screening in HIV-negative individuals who have receptive anal intercourse. Despite this, many providers feel anal paps should be offered to any individuals at risk for HPV-related anal cancer. Anal paps can be done by inserting a moistened polyester fiber swab into the anal canal and turning several times and then sending the swab for cytology. No other extragenital screening for HPV and or its manifestations is currently recommended.

Treatment and Prevention There is no available therapy to treat the HPV. When abnormalities are noted on cervical cytology, women should generally be referred for colposcopy. Patients with abnormal cytology on anal pap smears should generally be referred for high resolution anoscopy (HRA) which is analogous to colposcopy of the rectum. HRA is not available at all centers, further complicating the question of screening for anal cancer.

There are three licensed vaccines to prevent HPV, but currently only the nine-valent vaccine is available in the United States. The vaccine appears to be greater than 96.0% effective in preventing HPV-related infection from the strains included in the vaccine. The nine valent offers protection against serotypes 16, 18 (which cause the majority of HPV-related cancers), 31, 33, 45, 52, and 58 (together these 7 strains cause 75% or more of HPV-related cancers). It also offers protection against serotypes 6 and 11 that are responsible for 90% of genital warts [22]. The vaccine can be given as a two shot series for girls and boys between the ages 9 and 14. For persons ages 15–26, it is recommended as a three-shot series [23].

Human Immunodeficiency Virus (HIV)

This section will focus on screening and testing for HIV, along with prevention through pre-exposure prophylaxis (PrEP). The treatment of HIV and the use of anti-retrovirals to prevent vertical transmission of HIV are beyond the scope of this book.

Epidemiology There are approximately 1.1 million people over the age of 13 with HIV in the United States, with an estimated 37,600 new infections in 2014. The number of new infections has declined since 2008 when there were 45,700 new infections [24].

Screening and Testing HIV screening is recommended for all persons age 15–65 at least once. Persons younger and older than this should also be screened if risks for HIV are identified. Persons at high risk for HIV, such persons reporting unprotected vaginal or anal intercourse with more than one partner, persons who use injection drugs, and persons who report sex with HIV-positive partners or exchanging sex for money or drugs, should be screened annually or more often depending upon provider judgement of risks [25]. Most laboratories now use a fourth or fifth generation assay for HIV that combines both antibody detection as well as detection of the HIV p24 antigen. Such infection can usually be detected 11–14 days after infection [26]. If there is concern that an infection may be more recent than 14 days, HIV quantitative PCR testing can be ordered. If all of this is negative and concern remains high, testing should be repeated in 4 weeks.

Pre-exposure Prophylaxis (PrEP) PrEP consists of taking one tablet of the fixed-dose formulation Truvada (tenofovir disoproxil fumarate and emtricitabine) daily to prevent HIV. Truvada has been a part of many HIV treatment regimens since its approval in 2004. Eight randomized control trials have been performed evaluating the efficacy of PrEP [27–34]. In the five trials with the highest-risk patients, the number of persons that would need to be treated for a year to prevent one case of HIV (NNT) was between 12.8 and 52.6 [27, 28, 30, 33, 34]. Most cases in which persons on PrEP have acquired HIV are thought to be due to poor adherence to the study medication. However, recently a case of transmission despite good adherence and absence of drug resistance mutations has been documented [35], highlighting the continued importance of condoms and limiting the numbers sexual partners.

In the PrEP trials, the following side effects were more common in patients given Truvada: nausea and/or vomiting [27, 29–31, 33], an elevation in creatinine [32, 33], and grade 1 or 2 ALT elevation [31]. None of these differences were noted in all studies, and discontinuation of Truvada due to toxicity was rare. Only one study assessed the effect on bone mineral density, and this study did show a greater decrease in patients on Truvada [30].

Target Population PrEP should be considered for HIV negative men and women who are sexually active and may have sex with someone who is or may be HIV-positive, as well as persons who use intravenous drugs and may share their drug paraphernalia. The epidemiology of HIV suggests MSM are at the greatest risk. However, before PrEP is prescribed, a detailed sexual history should be obtained. A man who only engages in oral sex is unlikely to benefit from PrEP, whereas a man who has receptive and/or insertive anal intercourse without condoms, with multiple different partners, clearly could. Individuals with opposite sex partners may also benefit from PrEP if they are having sex with HIV-positive persons or persons of unknown HIV status. Because many variables play into a person's risk of contracting HIV, an online risk calculator has been developed [36] that may helpful in some situations when either the patient or the provider are unsure about starting PrEP (https://prephere. org/). Further, unless contraindications exist, PrEP should generally be considered for any patient who requests it, regardless of the sexual practices that individual is comfortable sharing with the clinician. The CDC estimates the number of people in the United States who could qualify for PrEP to be about 1.2 million [37].

Monitoring Recommended laboratory testing and monitoring for PrEP is shown in Table 6.7. Hepatitis B testing should be included as part of baseline testing. The

Table 6.7 Laboratory testing for pre-exposure prophylaxis (PrEP) with Truvada

Test	Baseline	Every 3–6 months
HIV Ag/Ab	Yes	Yes
HIV pcr	If concern for acute infection within the last 14 days. See text	If concern for acute infection within the last 14 days. See text
Renal function	Yes	Yes
Hepatitis B sAg, sAb	Yes	Depends on results of baseline testing[a]
Gonorrhea and chlamydia testing[b]	Yes	Offer

[a]See text
[b]Consider extragenital testing if patient report any history of receptive anal intercourse or receptive oral sex

reason for this is that both medications in Truvada have activity against hepatitis B. If a person has active hepatitis B, the Truvada will suppress its replication but not cure the infection. If the Truvada is stopped after a prolonged period of time, there can be recurrence similar to acute hepatitis B. Any person who is not immune to hepatitis B at baseline should be vaccinated. Patients should be seen every 3–6 months, and testing for HIV and renal function should be repeated. Providers should have a very low threshold for testing for other STIs at these follow-up visits Guidelines have recently been updated to recommend HIV pcr testing along with HIV Ag/Ab testing at each visit [38].

On-demand PrEP For individuals who are sexually active on an intermittent basis and can reliably predict when they will be sexually active, on-demand PrEP may be an option. On-demand PrEP has been evaluated in a randomized control trial and was found to be efficacious, with a number need to treat (NNT) of 17.6. In this study patients took two Truvada tablets with food 2–24 hours before sex, a third tablet 24 hours after the first tablets, and a forth tablet 24 hours later [34]. On-demand PrEP has an A1a recommendation (highest recommendation) from the International Antiviral Society—USA Panel (IAS-USA) and should be considered an option for persons who are intermittently sexually active [39].

Newer Options for PrEP Descovy (Tenofovir alafenamide and emtricitabine) has recently been approved for PrEP [40]. Descovy is very similar to Truvada but has a better safety profile with regard to kidney function and bone density [41]. Descovy has not been studied for on-demand PrEP. Cabotegravir is a long-acting antiretroviral that can be injected every 2 months and was approved in December 2021. Cabotegravir has been shown to be more effective in preventing HIV among MSM, transgender women and heterosexual women than Truvada [42, 43]. Traditional PrEP with Truvada failed to show benefit in heterosexual women [29, 30], thus the dramatic benefits of Cabotegravir are very exciting [43].

Rare Sexually Transmitted Infections in the United States

Chancroid

Epidemiology Chancroid is caused by *Haemophilus ducreyi* and is rare in the United States. Prevalence has declined in both the United States and the world; however, due the difficulty in culturing this organism, it's true prevalence may be underreported [1, 14].

Clinical Presentation The presence of a painful genital ulcer and tender, suppurative inguinal lymphadenopathy should raise suspicion for Chancroid.

Diagnosis Culturing of *H. ducreyi* requires special media that may not be available in all labs. A clinical diagnosis of chancroid can be made if the above clinical scenario is met and the patient tests negative for both syphilis and HSV.

Treatment Treatment for chancroid is shown in Table 6.8. All sex partners of the patient should be examined, and anyone with symptoms OR who has had sex with the patient within 10 days of symptom onset should be treated [14].

Lymphogranuloma Venereum (LGV)

Epidemiology Lymphogranuloma venereum is caused by *Chlamydia trachomatis*, serovars L1, L2, or L3. This has previously been thought to be rare disease in developed countries, but more recent studies suggest it may be more common than previously thought, especially in persons who have receptive anal intercourse [39].

Clinical Presentation Typical presentations include tender, usually unilateral, inguinal lymphadenopathy. A self-limited genital ulcer may also be present at the site of inoculation [14]. Patients who have anal receptive sex may present with proctitis and proctocolitis that can resemble inflammatory bowel disease [14, 39].

Table 6.8 Treatment for chancroid, *Haemophilus ducreyi* (Ref. [10])

Azithromycin 500 mg orally × 1
OR
Ceftriaxone 250 mg IM × 1
OR
Ciprofloxacin 500 mg orally twice a day for 3 days
OR
Erythromycin base 500 mg orally thrice a day for 7 days

Diagnosis NAAT do not distinguish between LGV-chlamydia and non-LGV-chlamydia and will be positive in both settings. Tests to distinguish between the two types of chlamydial infections have been developed but are not commercially available outside or research settings. The diagnosis of LGV is made based on proper epidemiology and clinical findings along with a positive chlamydia NAAT and the exclusion of other possible etiologies [14, 39].

Treatment Treatment of LGV is with either doxycycline 100 mg orally twice daily or erythromycin base 500 mg orally four times daily. Both should be given for 21 days. Anyone who has had sex with the patient within 60 days of symptoms onset should be examined and tested for chlamydial infection. Presumptive therapy of a sex partner, in the absence of disease manifestations, is with antichlamydial therapy (i.e., Azithromycin 1 gram orally × 1).

Granuloma Inguinale (Donovanosis)

Epidemiology Granuloma inguinale is caused by *Klebsiella granulomatis* and is rare in the United States but is endemic in some tropical and developing areas such as India, Papua New Guinea, the Caribbean, Central Australia, and Southern Africa [14].

Clinical Presentation Granuloma inguinale is characterized by painless, slowly progressive, highly vascular ulcers on the genitals and in the perineum. Lymphadenopathy is typical absent although subcutaneous granulomas may be present. Lesions can spread to involve intra-abdominal organs, bone, and the mouth. Ulcers may become superinfected [14].

Diagnosis The diagnosis is made by visualization of "Donovan bodies" on biopsy specimens. The organism is difficult to culture, and no FDA-approved molecular tests exist [14].

Treatment Treatment for granuloma inguinale is shown in Table 6.9, but data clearly demonstrating the superiority of one regimen over another are lacking [14].

Sexually Transmitted Disease Uncertainty

Mycoplasma Genitalium

Mycoplasma genitalium may be the cause of 20–25% of cases nongonococcal/non-chlamydia urethritis and perhaps as high as 30% of persistent urethritis cases [10]. Several factors make the development of clear guidelines on the diagnosis and management of this organism difficult. First is the lack of a FDA-approved test to diagnose this infection [14, 44], although non-FDA-approved tests are available in some

Table 6.9 Treatment of granuloma inguinale (donovanosis) (Ref. [10])

Recommended regimen
Azithromycin 1 gram weekly for 3 weeks and until all lesions have resolved
OR
Azithromycin 500 mg daily for 3 weeks and until all lesions have resolved
Alternative regimens
Doxycycline 100 mg twice daily for 3 weeks and until all lesions have resolved
OR
Ciprofloxacin 750 mg twice daily for 3 weeks and until all lesions have resolved
OR
Erythromycin base 500 mg four times daily for 3 weeks and until all lesions have resolved
OR
Trimethoprim/sulfamethoxazole DS (160/800) twice daily for 3 weeks and until all lesions have resolved

centers [44]. Second is the lack of a clear correlation between this infection and adverse health outcomes—although associations exist. The difficulty of isolating this organism has made studying its epidemiology difficult. Third, there is a rising rate of antibiotic resistance among isolates, but currently there is no commercially available test for resistance [44]. Currently, the CDC recommends 1 gram azithromycin one time for nongonococcal urethritis that may be due to *Mycoplasma genitalium*. If this treatment if ineffective, then a 5-day course of azithromycin (500 mg on day 1, followed by 250 mg daily for 4 days) may be more effective. If this is ineffective, then moxifloxacin 400 mg daily for 7–14 days is recommended [14, 44]. Because resistance in this organism has arisen so quickly, some authors now recommend combination therapy, although this is not part of a guideline currently [44]. Sexual partners should be tested (if available) and treated like the source patient [14, 44].

Conclusion

Sexually transmitted infections are common and contribute to significant morbidity. Up to a third of infections are diagnosed in a primary care setting [1], and primary care clinicians play a critical role in the prevention, diagnosis, and treatment. Depending upon what changes are made to healthcare coverage and funding, the role of the primary care provider is likely to only become more critical in the future.

References

1. Centers for Disease Control and Prevention. Sexually transmitted disease surveillance 2016. https://www.cdc.gov/STI/stats16/default.htm. Downloaded 3 Jan 2018.
2. Davis, JH. Trump signs law taking aim at planned parenthood funding. NY Times, April 13, 2017. https://www.nytimes.com/2017/04/13/us/politics/planned-parenthood-trump.html. Last accessed 3 Jan 2018.

3. Condoms and STIs: Fact Sheet for Public Health Personnel. https://www.cdc.gov/condomef-fectiveness/docs/Condoms_and_STIS.pdf. Last accessed 8 Jan 2018.
4. Female Condom Use. https://www.cdc.gov/condomeffectiveness/Female-condom-use.html . Last accessed 5 Sept 2018.
5. Dental Dam Use. https://www.cdc.gov/condomeffectiveness/Dental-dam-use.html. Last accessed 5 Sept 2018.
6. Rowen TS, Breyer BN, Lin TC, Li CS, Robertson PA, Shindel AW. Use of barrier protection for sexual activity among women who have sex with women. Int J Gynaecol Obstet. 2013;120(1):42–5.
7. Detels R, Green AM, Klausner JD, Katzenstein D, Gaydos C, Handsfield H, et al. The incidence and correlates of symptomatic and asymptomatic chlamydia trachomatous and Neisseria gonorrhoeae infections in selected populations in five countries. Sex Transm Dis. 2011;38(6):503–9.
8. LeFevre ML, USPSTF. Screening for chlamydia and gonorrhea: U.S. preventive services task force recommendation statement. Ann Intern Med. 2014;161(12):902–10.
9. Lee KC, Ngo-Metzger Q, Wolff T, Chowdhury J, Lefevre ML, Meyers DS. Sexually transmitted infections: recommendations of the U.S. preventive services task force. Amer Fam Phy. 2016;94(11):907–15.
10. Papp JR, Schachter J, Gaydos C, Van Der Pol C. Recommendations for the laboratory-based detection of chlamydia trachomatous and Neisseria gonorrhea. MMWR. 2014;63(0):1–19.
11. Danby CS, Cosentino LA, Rabe LK, Priest CL, Damare KC, Macio IS, Meyn LA, et al. Patterns of Extragenital chlamydia and gonorrhea in women and men who have sex with men reporting a history of receptive anal intercourse. Sex Transm Dis. 2016;43(2):105–9.
12. Grov D, Cain D, Rendia J, Ventuneac A, Parsons JT. Characteristics associated with urethral and rectal gonorrhea and chlamydia diagnoses in a U.S. National Sample of gay and bisexual men: results from the one thousand strong panel. Sex Transm Dis. 2016;43(3):165–17.
13. St. Cyr S, Barbee L, Workowski KA, Bachmann LH, Pham C, Schlanger K, et al. Update to CDC's Treatment Guidelines for Gonoccoccal Infection 2020. MMWR. 2020;69(50):1911–6.
14. Workowski KA, Bolan GA. Sexually transmitted diseases treatment guidelines, 2015. MMWR. 2015;64(3):1–137.
15. Satterwhite CL, Torrone E, Meites E, Dunne DF, Mahajan R, Banez Ocfemia MC, et al. Sexually transmitted infections among US women and men: prevalence and incidence estimates, 2008. Sex Transm Dis. 2013;40(3):187–93.
16. Schwebke JR, Gaydos CA, Davis T, Marrazzo J, Furgerson D, Taylor SN, et al. Clinical evaluation of the Cepheid Xpert TV assay for detection of trichomonas vaginalis with prospectively collected female and male specimens. J Clin Microbiol. 2017;56(2):e01091–17.
17. Cantor AG, Pappas M, Daegas M, Nelson HD. Screening for Syphilis: Updated Evidence Report and Systematic Review for the US Preventive Services Task Force. JAMA. 2016;315(21):2328–37.
18. Larsen SA, Steiner BM, Rudolph AH. Laboratory diagnosis and interpretation of tests for syphilis. Clin Microbiol Rev. 1995;8(1):1–21.
19. Araldi RP, Sant Ana TA, Modolo DG, de Melo TC, Spadacci-Morena DD, de Cassia SR, et al. The human papillomavirus related cancer biology: an overview. Biomed Pharmocother. 2018;106:1537–56.
20. Saslow D, Solomon D, Lawson HW, Killackey M, Kulasingam S, Cain J, et al. American Cancer Society, American Society of Colposcopy and Cervical Pathology screening guidelines for the prevention and early detection of cervical cancer. CA Cancer J Clin. 2012;62(3):147–72.
21. Aberg JA, Gallant JE, Ghanem KG, Emmanuel P, Zingman BS, Horberg MA. Primary care guidelines for the care of persons infected with HIV: 2013 update by the HIV Medical Association of the Infectious Diseases Society of America. Clin Infect Dis. 2014;58(1):1–10.

22. Petrosky E, Bocchini JA, Hariri S, Chesson H, Curtis R, Saraiya M. Use of the 9-valent human papillomavirus (HPV) vaccine: updated HPV vaccination recommendations of the advisory committee on immunization practices. MMWR. 2015;64(11):300–4.
23. Meites E, Kempe A, Markowitz LE. Use of a 2-dose schedule for human papillomavirus vaccination—updated recommendations of the advisory committee on immunization practices. MMWR. 2016;65(49):1405–8.
24. CDC HIV Statistics. https://www.cdc.gov/hiv/basics/statistics.html. Last accessed 01/23/18.
25. Moyer VA, USPSTF. Screening for HIV: a United States preventive services task force recommendation statement. Ann Intern Med. 2013;159:51–60.
26. Alexander TS. Human immunodeficiency virus diagnostic testing: 30 years of evolution. Clin Vaccine Immunol. 2016;23(4):249–53.
27. Grant RM, Lama JR, Anderson PL, McMahan V, Liu AY, Vargas L, et al. Preexposure chemophrphylaxis for HIV prevention in men who have sex with men. NEJM. 2010;363(27):2587–99.
28. Baeten JM, Donnell D, Ndase P, Mugo NR, Campbell JD, Wangisi J, et al. Antiretroviral prophylaxis for HIV prevention in heterosexual men and women. NEJM. 2012;367(5):399–410.
29. Damme LV, Corneli A, Ahmed K, Agot K, Lombaard J, Kapiga S. Preexposure prophylaxis for HIV infection among African women. NEJM. 2012;367(5):411–22.
30. Thigpen MC, Kebaabetswe PM, Paxton LA, Smith DK, Rose CE, Segolodi TM, et al. Antiretroviral preexposure prophylaxis for heterosexual HIV transmission in Botswana. NEJM. 2012;367(5):423–34.
31. Choopanya K, Martin M, Suntharasamai P, Sangkum U, Mock PA, Leethochawalit M, et al. Anitretroviral prophylaxis for HIV infection in injection drug users in Bangkok, Thailand (the Bangkok Tenofovir study):a randomized, double-blind, placebo-controlled phase 3 trial. Lancet. 2013;381:2083–90.
32. Marrazzo JM, Ramjee G, Richardson BA, Gomez K, Mgodi N, Nair G, et al. Tenofovir-based preexposure prophylaxis for HIV infection among African women. NEJM. 2015;372(6):509–18.
33. Molina JM, Capitant C, Spire B, Pialoux G, Cotte L, Charreau I, et al. On-demand preespsure prophylaxis in men at high risk of HIV-1 infection. NEJM. 2015;373(23):2237–46.
34. McCormack S, Dunn DT, Desai M, Dolling DI, Gafos M, Gilson R, et al. Pre-exposure prophylaxis to prevent the acquistion of HIV-1 infection (PROUD): effectiveness results from the pilot phase of a pragmatic open-label randomised trial. Lancet. 2016;387:53–60.
35. Hoornenborg E, Prins M, Achterbergh RCA, Lr W, Cornelissen S, Jurriaans N, et al. Acquisition of Wild-Type HIV-1 infection in a patient on pre-exposure prophylaxis with high intracellular concentrations of Tenofovir diphosphate: a case report. Lancet HIV. 2017;4(11):e522–8.
36. Beymer MR, Weiss RE, Sugar CA, Bourque LB, Gee GC, Morisky DE, et al. Are Centers for Disease Control and Prevention Guidelines for preexposure prophylaxis specific enough? formulation of a personalized HIV Risk score for pre-exposure prophylaxis initiation. Sexually Transmitted Diseases. 2017;44(1):49–57.
37. Smith DK, Van Handel M, Wolitski RJ, Stryker JE, Hall HI, Prejean J, et al. Vital signs: estimated percentages and numbers of adults with indications for preexposure prophylaxis to prevent HIV acquisition—United States, 2015. MMWR. 2015;64(46):1291–5.
38. https://www.cdc.gov/hiv/pdf/risk/prep/cdc-hiv-prep-guidelines-2021.pdf
39. Saag MS, Benson CA, Gandhi RT, Hoy JF, Landovitz RJ, Mugavero MJ, et al. Antiretroviral drugs for treatment and prevention of HIV infection in adults 2018 recommendations of the international antiviral society–USA Panel. JAMA. 2018;320(4):379–96.Stoner BP, Cohen SE. Lymphogranuloma venereum 2015: clinical presentation, diagnosis and treatment. Clin Infect Dis 2015:61(Suppl 8):S865-S873.
40. https://www.fda.gov/news-events/press-announcements/fda-approves-second-drug-prevent-hiv-infection-part-ongoing-efforts-end-hiv-epidemic.
41. Mayer KH, Molina JM, Thompson MA, Anderson PL, Mounzer KC, De WEJJ, et al. Emtricitabine and tenofovir alafenamide vs emtricitabine and tenofiovir disoproxil fumarate

for HIV pre-exposure prophylaxis (DISCOVER): primary results from a randomized, double-blind, multicenter, active-controlled, phase 3, non-inferiority trial. Lancet. 2020;396:239–54.

42. Landovitz RJ, Donnell D, Clement ME, Hanscom B, Coelho L, et al. Cabotegravir for HIV Prevention in Cisgender Men and Transgender Women. NEJM. 2021;385(7):595–608.

43. https://www.hptn.org/news-and-events/announcements/hptn-084-study-demonstrates-superiority-of-injectable-cabotegravir-to.

44. Sethi S, Zaman K, Jain N. Mycoplasma genitalium infections: current treatment options and resistance issues. Infect Drug Resist. 2017;10:283–91.

Chapter 7
Sexual Dysfunction

Aaron Grotas and Marissa Kent

Contents

Introduction

Sexual health contributes to quality of life at all ages with many individuals placing high importance on sexuality in survey studies [1]. Sexual dysfunction in a broad sense refers to a problem which prevents an individual or an individual's partner from experiencing satisfaction from sexual activity [2]. It has been estimated that 10–52% of men and 25–63% of women experience some form of sexual

A. Grotas (✉) · M. Kent
Department of Urology, Mount Sinai, New York, NY, USA
e-mail: aaron.grotas@mountsinai.org

© Springer Nature Switzerland AG 2022
J. Truglio et al. (eds.), *Sexual and Reproductive Health*,
https://doi.org/10.1007/978-3-030-94632-6_7

dysfunction. Sexual problems can be a challenge to identify and treat as they are often correlated with other health conditions, such as cardiovascular disorders, diabetes, and mental health [3].

This chapter delves into the topic of sexuality discussing how to diagnose sexual dysfunction, what treatments are available, and how to counsel individuals. When reading this chapter and applying it as a point of reference, it is important to note that the current guidelines set by the American Urological Association (AUA) and other major associations categorize sexual dysfunction based on male or female sex. These guidelines are evidence-based and currently the best available resource for clinicians. In order to provide the best evidence-based and up-to-date information, this chapter is likewise organized according to male and female sexual dysfunction. We recommend applying these guidelines within the same gender-affirming framework described throughout this book. For transgender and gender nonbinary (TGNB) patients, these guidelines can easily be applied by focusing on the sex organs present, as opposed to the gender identity of the patient. Please refer to Part 3 of this book for individuals who have had gender-affirming surgery or who take gender-affirming medications and experience sexual dysfunction that may be specifically related to these treatments.

Male Sexual Dysfunction

Introduction

Male sexual dysfunction includes erectile dysfunction (ED), ejaculation problems, delayed or inhibited orgasm, and low libido (hypoactive sexual desire) [4]. Of these, erectile dysfunction and premature ejaculation and hypoactive sexual desire are the most common complaints and will be the focus of this section [5, 6].

Hypoactive Sexual Desire (HSD)

Hypoactive sexual desire is defined as "persistently or recurrently deficient (or absent) sexual fantasies and desire for sexual activity that causes significant distress." [7]

The National Health and Social Life Survey found 14–17% of men aged 18–44 years reported low sexual desire [8]. The true biologic basis of sexual desire is largely unknown but thought to involve an interplay between internal thoughts, neurophysiological arousal, and one's emotional state [9]. There are many psychiatric diagnoses, medical conditions, and medications which have been shown to be associated with low sexual desire. These include depression, androgen deficiency, stroke, relationship conflict, renal failure, and coronary artery disease to name a few [7].

Diagnostic Workup

Initial workup should include a thorough history making sure to include medications, medical history, urologic history, relationship history, and any potential mood disorders. Two objective ways to assess for low sexual desire include The International Index of Erectile Function's sexual desire domain [10] and The Sexual Desire Inventory [11].

Physical exam should be performed including testicular size and a digital rectal exam.

Initial laboratory testing should include thyroid-stimulating hormone, prolactin, and testosterone to test for the more common causes of HSD along with routine lab work and tests directed at any suspected diagnoses based on history and physical exam [7].

Treatment

If any underlying medical condition was found on the initial workup, these conditions should be addressed or referral made to the appropriate specialist. This includes counseling or psychiatry referral for those with suspected depression or anxiety. Individuals with suspected relationship problems should be referred for couples' therapy [7].

Currently there are no FDA-approved medications for the treatment of hypoactive sexual desire. For individuals where no cause of low desire is found, this presents a great challenge as providers are left with offering psychotherapy or off-label pharmacotherapy. Exogenous testosterone therapy has shown in some studies to improve libido in hypogonadal men [12], but in eugonadal men, there is no clinical benefit [13].

Erectile Dysfunction

Erectile dysfunction is defined as the inability to achieve or maintain an erection sufficient for satisfactory sexual performance [14].

Many epidemiological studies have demonstrated a high prevalence of ED with increasing incidence with age. The first large community-based study on the prevalence of ED was the Massachusetts Male Aging Study which found 52% of men between the ages of 40–70 had ED. [15] The incidence rate of ED, based on this study, was estimated to be 26 per 1000 men annually [16]. Another study called the Cologne study looked at men aged 30–80 years and found an age-related increase in ED with 2.3% prevalence in the younger population aged 30–39 years, which increased to 53.4% in those 70–80 years old [17].

Erectile dysfunction shares many risk factors with cardiovascular disease. This may include obesity, hypercholesterolemia, sedentary lifestyle, metabolic syndrome, diabetes, and smoking. The same holds true for men with mild ED, and therefore many consider ED a potential indicator of associated underlying cardiovascular disease [18]. Additional causes of ED include medication side effect, endocrine disorders, psychologic, trauma, or a result of prior urologic treatment such as prostatectomy or radiation therapy [19].

Diagnostic Workup

History, Physical Exam, Laboratory Testing

Any patient presenting with ED should undergo a detailed history including sexual, medical, and psychosocial histories [19]. There are validated psychometric questionnaires, such as the International Index for Erectile Function (IIEF), which may assist in identifying the sexual dysfunction and aide in monitoring progress of a given treatment [20].

Every patient should be given a physical exam which includes the genitourinary, endocrine, vascular, and neurological systems [21]. Both the European Association of Urology (EAU) and AUA recommend a digital rectal examination in any patient above the age of 40 with a prostate [19, 21]. Patients with enlarged prostate and urinary symptoms may need further workup before supplementing testosterone. In addition, patients with abnormal prostate exam may need prostate imaging or biopsy prior to testosterone therapy. This may be of importance when considering the use of testosterone in the management of sexual dysfunctions.

Laboratory tests should be individualized based on the patient's risk factors with the goal being to identify comorbid conditions that may predispose the patient to ED and that may contraindicate certain therapies [19, 21]. It is recommended by the EUA that individuals should have glucose-lipid profile and total testosterone along with routine laboratory tests [21].

Referral and Cardiac Considerations

Prior to initiating treatment for ED, individuals should be risk stratified based on their cardiovascular risk to determine if it is safe to initiate treatment or engage in sexual activity. The Princeton Consensus conferences on sexual dysfunction and cardiac risk created a risk stratification (see Table 7.1 below) which categorizes individuals into low, intermediate, or high risk. Individuals with low risk do not require additional cardiac testing prior to initiating ED treatment. Those with high risk should be referred to a cardiologist prior to initiating treatment. Individuals in intermediate risk category is at the discretion of the provider [21].

Table 7.1 Cardiac risk stratification based on Princeton Consensus

Low risk	
	Asymptomatic with < 3 risk factors for CAD
	Mild, stable angina
	Uncomplicated previous MI
	NYHA Class 1 or 2 LVD/CHF
	Post-successful coronary revascularization
	Controlled HTN
	Mild valvular disease
Intermediate risk	
	≥3 Risk factor for CAD
	Moderate, stable angina
	Recent MI (>2, <6 weeks)
	NYHA Class 3 LVD/CHF
	Noncardiac sequelae of atherosclerotic disease
High risk	
	High-risk arrhythmias
	Unstable or refractory angina
	Recent MI (>2 weeks)
	NYHA class 4 LVD/CHF
	Hypertrophic obstructive and other cardiomyopathies
	Uncontrolled HTN
	Moderate to severe valvular disease

CAD coronary artery disease, *CHF* congestive heart failure, *LVD* left ventricular dysfunction, *MI* myocardial infarction, *NYHA* New York Heart Association, *HTN* hypertension

First-Line Treatment

Lifestyle Modifications and Modifying Risk Factors

Lifestyle changes and risk factor modification may occur before or concurrent with initiating first-line treatment for ED. If any identifiable cause of ED was found during evaluation, it should be treated. Concomitant medical comorbidities should be optimized, including hypertension, diabetes, or endocrine conditions [21]. It is generally recommended that individuals make lifestyle modifications to improve their cardiovascular health such as avoidance of smoking, maintaining an ideal body weight, and regular exercise but high-quality research is lacking as to exactly how much lifestyle modification improves erectile function [19].

Table 7.2 PDE-5 inhibitors for erectile dysfunction

Drug	Dose	Starting dose	Timing	Side effects[a]
Sildenafil	25 mg, 50 mg, 100 mg	50 mg	Effective after 30–60 min after administration last 4–6 hrs	Facial flushing, nasal congestion, headache, and dyspepsia, visual effects
Tadalafil	2.5 mg, 5 mg daily or 5 mg, 10 mg, 20 mg on demand	10 mg on demand or 2.5 mg daily	Effective after 30 min from administration and lasts up to 36 hours	Facial flushing, nasal congestion, headache, and dyspepsia, back pain
Vardenafil	2.5 mg, 5 mg, 10 mg, 20 mg on demand	10 mg	Effective after 30 min from administration, lasts ~4–6 hours	Facial flushing, nasal congestion, headache, and dyspepsia, visual effects, QT prolongation

[a]Side effects listed are not all inclusive and providers should refer to product labeling

Pharmacotherapy

Standard first-line therapy for ED is the administration of an oral phosphodiesterase type 5 (PDE5) inhibitor, unless otherwise contraindicated. The three FDA-approved PDE5 inhibitors for treatment of ED are sildenafil, tadalafil, and vardenafil (see Table 7.2). There is insufficient data to support the use of one agent over the other [19]. Of note, none of these medications initiate an erection on their own and require sexual stimulation to initiate an erection [21].

PDE5 inhibitors are contraindicated in the following patients [21]:

- Recent myocardial infarction, stroke, or life-threatening arrhythmia within the last 6 months
- Resting hypotension (<90/50 mmHg) or hypertension (>170/100 mmHg)
- Unstable angina, angina with sexual intercourse, or class 4 congestive heart failure
- Patients taking any form of nitrates

Patients who do not have initial success with the use of PDE5 inhibitors should have their drug dose titrated and be counseled to ensure proper use of the drug, including timing and frequency of drug dosing and adequate sexual stimulation. If one fails a trial of one PDE5 inhibitor, another drug in the class may be tried, but there is no good evidence to suggest the other drug will be more successful [19].

Second-Line Therapy

All patients who fail first-line therapy with PDE5 inhibitors should be counseled on alternative treatment options including intraurethral suppositories, intracavernous drug injection, vacuum constriction devices, and as a third-line therapy, penile prostheses. It is recommended that first time administration of both intraurethral suppositories and intracavernous drug injection be performed by a healthcare provider due to safety concerns [19]. If the provider does not feel comfortable administering either of these therapies in the office, the patient should be referred to a specialist at this time.

Vacuum Constriction Devices

Vacuum constriction devices (VCD) work by providing passive engorgement of the corpora cavernosa; then once an adequate erection is achieved, a ring is placed at the base of the penis to retain the blood within the corpora [21]. Patients do not need a prescription to purchase a VCD but should be advised to buy one with a vacuum limiter to avoid injury to the penis [19]. Common side effects include inability to ejaculate, pain, bruising, petechiae, and numbness. The ring should be removed within 30 min of finishing sexual activity [21].

Intraurethral Suppositories

Alprostadil is a synthetic vasodilator identical to PGE1. It is administered 125–1000 µg in a medicated pellet which is given as a transurethral suppository. Hypotension occurs in 3% of patients after the first dose, and therefore the first dose should be administered under the supervision of a healthcare provider [19]. Side effects include but are not limited to pain, dizziness, urethral bleeding, urinary tract infections, penile fibrosis, and priapism [21].

Intracavernous Drug Injection

Alprostadil, papaverine, and phentolamine are the most commonly used drugs for intracavernous injection. Alprostadil and papaverine are sold as monotherapy and are available from most pharmacies. Combination formulas, bimix and trimix, are common alternatives which are only available at compounding pharmacies. Intracavernous drug therapy is considered the most effective nonsurgical treatment for ED but has the highest rate of priapism. First time administration should be performed under the supervision of a healthcare provider, and individuals who are prescribed this medication should be counseled on priapism and need for urgent treatment should this happen [19].

Third-Line Therapy

Individuals who fail first- and second-line therapy who have not been referred to a specialist should be referred at this time to discuss the potential for a penile prosthesis.

Penile Prosthesis

There are two main types of penile prosthesis, a malleable or noninflatable and an inflatable. The inflatable prothesis comes in a two-piece or three-piece version. Those with an inflatable penile prothesis consider it closer to a normal flaccidity and erection over the malleable version. Possible complications include but are not limited to infection, erosion, nerve damage, penile shortening, mechanical failure, and diminished efficacy of other treatments if the device is subsequently removed [19].

Experimental Therapies

Shock Wave Therapy

Low-intensity extracorporeal shock wave therapy has been examined for the use in ED in a randomized, double-blind, sham-controlled study. It has demonstrated positive short-term clinical and physiological effect on erectile function in patients who respond to PDE5 inhibitors, and preliminary data shows improvement in penile hemodynamics and endothelial function [21].

Premature Ejaculation

There is no universally accepted definition of premature ejaculation (PE). For purposes of this book, the definition by the AUA will be used.

Premature ejaculation is "ejaculation that occurs sooner than desired, either before or shortly after penetration, causing distress to either one or both partners." [22]

Premature ejaculation has been estimated to have a prevalence rate of 31% according to the National Health and Social Life Survey study which looked at men aged 18–59 [23]. It is typically subdivided into acquired PE or lifelong. Lifelong PE is differentiated from acquired in that it starts when a patient first becomes sexually active. The pathophysiology and etiology of PE are unknown. There is weak evidence that it may be associated with anxiety, penile hypersensitivity, or 5-HT receptor dysfunction [24].

Diagnostic Workup

History, Physical Exam, Laboratory Testing

The diagnosis of premature ejaculation can be made based on sexual history alone. All patients presenting with complaints of PE should undergo a detailed medical and sexual history to ensure no other concomitant problem exists. If the patient has

ED, it should be treated prior to undergoing treatment for PE; see section above on Erectile Dysfunction [22].

A physical exam may be performed as part of the initial evaluation for PE to look for other medical conditions. Neurologic deficits or evidence of hypogonadism like testicular atrophy are two examples of physical exam findings that may contribute to PE.

Laboratory testing for routine PE is not indicated unless history or physical exam reveals something which warrants further investigation [22].

Treatment

Behavioral Modification and Psychosexual Counseling

Individuals who have mild bother from PE should be offered education and referral for psychosexual counseling. For those with acquired PE, behavioral techniques may be offered as first line to patients who are uncomfortable with pharmacologic management, but the long-term outcomes using these techniques are unknown. The two most well-known techniques are the "stop-start" and "squeeze" technique. Both are typically conducted in a cycle of three before proceeding to orgasm [21].

Stop-start technique: The patient's penis is stimulated by his partner until he feels the urge to ejaculate at which time he instructs his partner to stop until the urge passes.

Squeeze technique: The patient's penis is stimulated by his partner until he feels the urge to ejaculate then the partner squeezes the glans until the urge passes.

Pharmacotherapy

Currently there are no medical therapies approved by the US Food and Drug Administration (FDA) for the specific indication of PE. The risks and benefits of initiating therapy should be discussed with each patient. Table 7.3 presents medications and dosing for various pharmacotherapies based on the recommendations from the American Urological Association [22].

Female Sexual Dysfunction

Epidemiology

Female sexual dysfunction (FSD) is a complex issue involving both physical and psychological components. In the National Health and Social Life Survey, 43% of women reported some degree of sexual difficulty [23]. For many years FSD was not clearly defined and as a result led to very few advances in the field. Most clinicians

Table 7.3 Pharmacotherapy for premature ejaculation as recommended by the American Urological Association

Drug class	Drug	Dose	Timing	Side effects[a]
Nonselective serotonin reuptake inhibitor	Clomipramine	25-50 mg day Or 25 mg prn	Daily or 4–24 hrs prn prior to intercourse	Dizziness, drowsiness, dry mouth, constipation, stomach upset, flushing, sweating, blurry vision, memory, and concentration problems
Selective serotonin reuptake inhibitor	Fluoxetine Paroxetine Sertraline	5–20 mg day 10–40 mg or 20 mg prn 25–200 mg or 50 mg prn	Daily or 4–24 hrs prn prior to intercourse	Hives, inability to sit, restlessness, joint or muscle pain, above side effects in lesser degree
Topical therapy	Lidocaine/ prilocaine cream2.5%/2.5%	1 gram of cream to glans and shaft cover with condom	20–30 min prior to intercourse	Prolonged application which may lead to loss of erection or numbness to the partner.

[a]Not a complete list of side effects; in addition all of these drugs may make sexual experience worse rather than better

use the definition of FSD as put forth by the Diagnostic and Statistical Manual of Mental Disorders in the fourth edition [25] and more recently revised in the fifth edition [26]. The three recognized disorders include:

- *Female sexual interest/arousal disorder*
- *Genitopelvic pain/penetration disorder*
- *Female orgasmic disorder*

To be considered a dysfunction, the sexual problem must be present for more than seventy-five percent of the time for greater than 6 months. Additionally, the problem must produce significant distress and cannot be explained by another condition [26].

Diagnostic Workup

History, Physical Exam, Laboratory Testing

Women presenting with sexual dysfunction should undergo a detailed history including sexual, medical, and psychosocial histories. There are validated questionnaires, such as The Female Sexual Function Index (FSFI), which may assist in identifying the sexual dysfunction [27].

A complete physical exam should be performed which includes a thorough pelvic exam looking at the external, internal, and neurologic components [28].

There is no specific laboratory testing that is indicated unless history or physical exam reveals something which warrants further investigation.

Treatment

Once an initial evaluation has been completed, treatment may be initiated or a referral can be made to a sex therapist or marriage counselor [29].

Female Sexual Interest/Arousal Disorder

The mainstay of treatment consists of psychotherapy and antidepressants for patients with associated anxiety. The FDA has approved flibanserin, a serotonin receptor 1A agonist and 2A antagonist, as the first targeted treatment for women with hypoactive sexual desire disorder.

This medication may cause severe hypotension and syncope and is contraindicated in patients who take certain CYP3A4 inhibitors or who have liver impairment [28]. Transdermal testosterone has been shown to be effective for short-term therapy, but there is little evidence to support its continued use beyond 6-month duration [29].

Genitopelvic Pain/Penetration Disorder

Conjugated estrogens have been FDA approved for the treatment of dyspareunia. Vaginal atrophy or estrogen deficiency responds better to estrogen than vulvodynia or vaginismus. In postmenopausal women with dyspareunia, ospemifene is a selective estrogen receptor modulator that acts as an estrogen agonist in vaginal epithelium and is FDA approved for dyspareunia in postmenopausal women. The recommended daily dose is 60 mg [28].

In individuals with vaginismus, the most effective treatment is a combination of cognitive and behavioral psychotherapy known as systematic desensitization. The treatment consists of individuals learning muscle relaxation techniques and inserting dilators of increasing diameter into the vagina. If this is ineffective, a referral may be made for pelvic physical therapy [29].

Female Orgasmic Disorder

There is no effective therapy for individuals with unexplained primary orgasmic disorder who have never achieved orgasm through any means. If individuals have primary orgasmic disorder associated with abuse, psychotherapy and couple counseling may be helpful. Secondary orgasmic disorder usually improves with treatment of the primary dysfunction [29].

Conclusion

Sexual dysfunction is common, impacts the overall health and wellness of patients, and may be associated other physical and mental health conditions. Primary care clinicians are well positioned to address sexual dysfunction, applying current best practices to individual patients using a gender-affirming, patient-centered approach to sexual health.

References

1. Flynn KE, Li L, Bruner DW, et al. Sexual Satisfaction and the Importance of Sexual Health to Quality of Life Throughout the Life Course of U.S. Adults. J Sex Med. 2016;13(11):1642–50.
2. The Cleveland Clinic Foundation (2015, January 24.) An overview of sexual dysfunction. my.clevelandclinic.org/disorders/sexual_dysfunction/hic_an_overview_of_sexual_dysfunction.aspx
3. Heiman JR. Sexual Dysfunction: Overview of prevalence, etiological factors, and treatments. J Sex Res. 2002;39(1):73–8.
4. Parmet S. Male Sexual Dysfunction. JAMA. 2004;291(24):3076.
5. Rosenberg MT, Sadovsky R. Identification and diagnosis of premature ejaculation. Int J Clin Pract. 2007;61(6):903–8. http://www.ncbi.nlm.nih.gov/pubmed/17504352.
6. Produced by Bob Phillips, Chris Ball, Dave Sackett, Doug Badenoch, Sharon Straus, Brian Haynes, Martin Dawes since November 1998. Updated by Jeremy Howick March 2009. http://www.cebm.net/index.aspx?o=1025 [Access date February 2014].
7. Krakowsky Y, Grober ED. Hypoactive Sexual Desire in Men. In: Lipshultz L, Pastuszak A, Goldstein A, Giraldi A, Perelman M. (eds) Management of Sexual Dysfunction in Men and Women. Springer, New York, NY 2016;171–87.
8. Laumann EO, Paik A, Rosen R. Sexual dysfunction in the United States: prevalence and predictors. JAMA. 1999;281:537–44.
9. Bancroft J. Sexual desire and the brain. J Sex Marital Ther. 1988;3:11–27.
10. Rosen RC, Riley A, Wagner G, Osterloh IH, Kirkpatrick J, Mishra A. The international index of erectile function (IIEF): a multidimensional scale for assessment of erectile dysfunction. Urology. 1997;49:822–30.
11. Spector IP, Carey MP, Steinberg L. The sexual desire inventory: development, factor structure, and evidence of reliability. J Sex Marital Ther. 1996;22:175–90.
12. Isidori AM, Giannetta E, Gianfrilli D, Greco EA, Bonifacio V, Aversa A, Isidori A, Fabbri A, Lenzi A. Effects of testosterone on sexual function in men: results of a meta-analysis. Clin Endocrinol. 2005;63:381–94.
13. Morales A, Heaton JP. Hormonal erectile dysfunction. Evaluation and management. Urol Clin N Am. 2001;28:279–88.
14. Impotence. NIH Consens Statement, 10: 1, 1992
15. Feldman HA, Goldstein I, Hatzichristou DG, et al. Impotence and its medical and psychosocial correlates: results of the Massachusetts Male Aging Study. J Urol. 1994;151(1):54–61. http://www.ncbi.nlm.nih.gov/pubmed/8254833.
16. Johannes CB, Araujo AB, Feldman HA, et al. Incidence of erectile dysfunction in men 40 to 69 years old: longitudinal results from the Massachusetts Male Aging Study. J Urol. 2000;163(2):460–3. http://www.ncbi.nlm.nih.gov/pubmed/10647654.
17. Braun M, Wassmer G, Klotz T, et al. Epidemiology of erectile dysfunction: results of the 'Cologne Male Survey'. Int J Impot Res. 2000;12(6):305–11.

18. Lee JC, Bénard F, Carrier S, et al. Do men with mild erectile dysfunction have the same risk factors as the general erectile dysfunction clinical trial population? BJU Int. 2011;107(6):956–60. http://www.ncbi.nlm.nih.gov/pubmed/20950304.

19. Montague DK, Jarow JP, Broderick GA, et al. The management of erectile dysfunction: an AUA update. J Urol. 2005;174(1):230–9.

20. Rosen RC, Riley A, Wagner G, et al. The international index of erectile function (IIEF): a multidimensional scale for assessment of erectile dysfunction. Urology. 1997;49(6):822–30. http://www.ncbi.nlm.nih.gov/pubmed/9187685.

21. Hatzimouratidis K, Giuliano F, Moncada I, et al. EUA guidelines on erectile dysfunction, premature ejaculation, penile curvature and priapism. Presented at the EAU Annual Congress Munich 2016. http://uroweb.org/guideline/male-sexual-dysfunction/

22. Montague DK, Jarow JP, Broderick GA, et al. AUA guideline on the pharmacologic management of premature ejaculation. J Urol. 2004;172(1):290–4.

23. Laumann EO, Paik A, Rosen RC. Sexual dysfunction in the United States: prevalence and predictors. JAMA. 1999;281(6):537–44.

24. McMahon CG, Abdo C, Incrocci L, et al. Disorders of orgasm and ejaculation in men. J Sex Med. 2004;1(1):58–65.

25. American Psychiatric Association. Diagnostic and Statistical Manual of Mental Disorders. (4th ed, text revision). Washington, DC;1994.

26. American Psychiatric Association. Sexual Dysfunction. In: Diagnostic and Statistical Manual of Mental Disorders. (5th ed). Washington, DC;2013.

27. Rosen R, Brown C, Heiman J, Leiblum S, Meston CM, Shabsigh R, Ferguson D, D'Agostino R., Jr The Female Sexual Function Index (FSFI): A multidimensional self-report instrument for the assessment of female sexual function. J Sex Marital Ther. 2000;26:191–208.

28. Dawson ML, Shah NM, Rinko RC, et al. The evaluation and management of female sexual dysfunction. J Fam Pract. 2017;66(12):722–8.

29. Armstrong C. ACOG Guideline on Sexual Dysfunction in Women. Am Fam Physician. 2011;84(6):705–9.

Chapter 8
Pregnancy and the Peripartum Period

Srilakshmi Mitta

Contents

S. Mitta (✉)
Department of Obstetric Medicine, Brown University Medical School, Women & Infants'
Hospital, Providence, RI, USA
e-mail: Srilakshmi_mitta@brown.edu

© Springer Nature Switzerland AG 2022
J. Truglio et al. (eds.), *Sexual and Reproductive Health*,
https://doi.org/10.1007/978-3-030-94632-6_8

Introduction

Between 2011 and 2013, there was an estimated 61 million women of childbearing age (15–44 years) living in the United States [7]. Birth rates for those >35 years of age have been steadily increasing [8] as well as rates of pregnancies in patients with chronic illness [9, 10]. Given that childbearing is a common and desired occurrence in the United States, it is vital that primary care clinicians be well versed with preconception, intrapartum, and postpartum care of these patients. However given constraints on time, resources, and a trend to specialization and superspecialization of medical care, it can be difficult to keep up to date on such topics. Therefore this chapter will focus on presenting the basics of how to approach care for this population, as well as specific diseases to be aware of before, during, and after pregnancy.

Preconception Care

Preconception care and counseling are a key component in the care of patients of childbearing age and have been recommended by the CDC because there is a proven improvement in pregnancy outcomes for both parent and baby. However, despite the known benefits, preconception counseling is not consistently being done in daily practice. Barriers to providing preconception care include lack of resources, lack of provider knowledge and comfort in this area, and appropriate education and outreach done to improve education [2]. Further, bias about who can or wishes to get pregnant may cause certain groups to not get any counseling at all – such as women with chronic illness, transgender or gender nonbinary (TGNB) patients, or women who have sex with women or identify as lesbian. However, regardless of these barriers, physicians believe that preconception care and counseling are important and needed for optimal care [1]. The delaying of childbearing, increase in chronic medical illness, and improvement in reproductive techniques have only heightened this need and make preconception counseling and awareness all the more relevant to current practice. Various forms of preconception counseling exist, but the two most pertinent to primary care clinicians would be counseling in healthy patients with no known risks and counseling in patients with known chronic medical problems.

Universal Preconception Counseling

Upwards of 50% of pregnancies in the United States are unplanned making the routine screening for pregnancy possibility and pregnancy planning essential during regular preventive care visits. Much of what a preventive visit already includes such as nutrition, diet, and exercise, smoking cessation, alcohol use, illicit drug use,

Table 8.1 General points of discussion for preconception

Counseling topics	Counseling points
Nutrition	Folic acid deficiency prepregnancy is associated with increased risk of neural tube defects.
	Supplementation *before* pregnancy is most effective for prevention.
	Folic acid 400mcg daily is recommended to reduce the incidence of neural tube defects
Elevated BMI/ obesity	Extremes of weight (very low and very high BMI) can be associated with poor pregnancy outcomes.
	Obesity increases the risk for gestational diabetes, preeclampsia, and cesarean sections.
	Prepregnancy screening for diabetes, hypertension, and hyperlipidemia to better counsel and prepare for pregnancy
	Modest amounts of weight loss can impact change in pregnancy outcomes, and patient should be referred to a nutritionist and counseled about exercise.
	Bariatric surgery should also be considered prepregnancy in appropriate patients and has led to drastic improvement in pregnancy outcomes
Tobacco, alcohol, and substance use	Associated with spontaneous miscarriage, placental abruption, still births, and sudden infant death syndrome
	Tobacco cessation can reduce these outcomes.
	Nicotine replacement therapy is the safest for pregnancy.
	Alcohol abuse during pregnancy can be teratogenic to the heart, eyes, and kidneys and causes growth restriction, facial abnormalities, and neurodevelopmental delays also common
Vaccinations	Assess immune status for rubella, varicella, and hepatitis B

intimate partner violence screening, and immune/vaccine status are also the foundation for preconception care [3, 4]. These concepts should be continued and reiterated when discussing the possibility of pregnancy with patients to ensure safe and healthy outcomes for the parent and baby as detailed in Table 8.1.

Preconception Care in Patients with Chronic Illness

The approach to preconception care in patients with chronic illness would include all that was already discussed as well as condition-specific recommendations. Anticipation of condition-specific complications or management changes needed for pregnancy can be done in a timely manner before conception or in early pregnancy. Primary care clinicians are usually in a unique position of having a relationship with and knowing a patient over time, making it a safe environment for the patient to explore their reproductive options. Details for condition-specific counseling will be further discussed at the end of the chapter, as well as in select chapters in Part 2 of this book.

Pregnancy Care: The Basics

When caring for a pregnant patient, clinicians may struggle with balancing the needs of their patient versus those of the developing fetus. The choice to avoid medications or certain imaging studies is common due to concern of fetal effects, though this may not always be the correct decision. Often times caring for a pregnant patient will include the use of medications or necessitate imaging for diagnostic purposes, just as with any other patient. Being familiar with pregnancy physiology and approaching pregnant patients with the thought that maternal health is equal to fetal health will ease the decision-making process for both clinician and patient.

Pregnancy Physiology

Pregnancy is a time of significant physiologic changes, both anatomically and metabolically, that occur to accommodate the needs of the developing fetus as well as prepare for labor and delivery. Many of these changes mimic disease states; therefore, it is important to understand and differentiate what is normal for pregnancy from a true pathologic state. For example, erythrocyte sedimentation rate (ESR) is elevated in pregnancy due to changes in blood volume and increased rates of anemia, making it an unreliable marker for inflammation. Other findings of edema, new murmurs, hydronephrosis, or anemia can all be attributed the expected rise in blood volume. Table 8.2

Table 8.2 Basic physiologic changes in pregnancy

Pregnancy physiologic changes and normal values		
Cardiovascular system		
	Direction of change	*% change or normal range in pregnancy*
Blood pressure	Decreases	Drops 10–15 mmHg
Blood volume	Increases	30–50% increase
Cardiac output	Increases	40% increase
Heart rate	Increases	70–105 beats/min
Vascular resistance	Decreases	25–30% decrease
Respiratory system		
	Direction of change	*% change or normal range in pregnancy*
Tidal volume	Increases	45% increase
Respiratory rate	No change	
Peak expiratory flow	No change	
Functional residual capacity	Decreases	10–25% decrease
Arterial PCO2	Decreases	27–32 mmHg
Arterial PO2	Increases	100–105 mmHg
Renal system		

Table 8.2 (continued)

Pregnancy physiologic changes and normal values

	Direction of change	% change or normal range in pregnancy
Renal plasma flow	Increases	
Glomerular filtration rate	Increases	50% increase
Creatinine clearance	Increases	120–160 ml/min
Creatinine	Decreases	0.4–0.7 mg/dL
BUN	Decreases	8–12 mg/dL
24 hour urinary protein excretion	Increases	≤ 300 mg
Hematologic system		
	Direction of change	% change or normal range in pregnancy
Hemoglobin	Decreases	10–13 gm/dL
White blood cell count	Increases	$10–16 \times 10^9$/L
Platelets	Decreases in the third trimester	Lower limit of normal 100,000/L
Sedimentation rate	Increases	6–120 mm/hr (increases with gestation)

gives further information about common physiologic changes in pregnancy that will aid in understanding how pregnancy can affect a disease process as well as its care and management.

Drug Prescribing and Safety in Pregnancy

Prescribing

Many times the need for medication use in pregnancy can be anxiety provoking for both clinician and patient, but when approached in a logical manner, much of this worry can be alleviated. First, understanding your patient's fears, value system, and decision-making process is crucial when counseling them about any management or treatment plan. Many times a patient's past experiences, the media, social circles, pharmacist, or other doctors have caused this patient to have preconceived ideas about medication use in pregnancy which should be addressed first and taken into account when deciding to prescribe a drug or not.

Next a clinician must think about whether a medication is really necessary. For example, a self-limiting acute illness, such as an upper respiratory tract infection or headache, may not always need treatment, whereas some conditions, like asthma, will warrant pharmacologic intervention to improve maternal disease and thereby fetal wellbeing. Lastly, consideration of a medication's safety profile and whether any alternatives may exist is needed to formulate a mutually agreed upon management course.

Drug Safety in Pregnancy and Lactation

Traditionally, teratogenic effects of drugs have been noted as anatomic malformations, and the fetus is most vulnerable to these in the first trimester. However, medications may adversely affect fetal neurological and behavioral development, fetal survival, or function of specific organs even after the first trimester [12]. For most drugs, it is not known whether or when an absolutely "safe" period exists when the medication can be deemed to be without effect [13]. Similarly, drug levels and safety in breastfeeding are a balance between maternal need for treatment and benefits of breastfeeding for patient and baby.

Old and New Drug Labeling

Since 1979, the Food and Drug Administration (FDA) has regulated the labeling of drug safety and use for pregnancy and lactation. The five FDA pregnancy categories for medications include A, B, C, D, and X; however, there are several shortcomings with such classification. The categories are often seen as a grading system where the risk increases from the lowest in Category A to highest in Category X, while the safety information in the accompanying narrative is not always appreciated by prescribers. Drugs in a particular category may be perceived as carrying a similar risk. However, 65–70% of all medications are in Category C. This category includes medications with adverse animal data or no animal data at all. In addition, adverse animal data may vary in severity from decreased fetal weights to major structural malformation and fetal loss, indicating difference in expected risk. So while the FDA pregnancy risk classification was useful as a quick reference with regard to available safety data, it was confusing and inadequate when used as the only source. Similarly past labeling for safety in lactation was sparse and usually gave vague recommendation to either stop a medication if possible or to use it with caution.

Since 2015, however, due to the abovementioned problems, the FDA has made an official change to its labeling rule. The first and most significant is the elimination of the pregnancy drug categories, followed by changes in categories to include pregnancy, lactation and reproductive potential, and lastly the use of pregnancy registries [14]. The sections for pregnancy and lactation are further divided into three subsections of Risk Summary, Clinical Considerations, and Data. The Risk Summary for pregnancy will include a summary of available animal, human, and pharmacologic data and for lactation will include information about the excretion of the drug into human milk, the possible effects on the breastfed infant, and effects on maternal milk production. The Clinical Consideration for pregnancy will give details about disease associated risk and adverse reactions to mother and baby, as well as any pertinent dose adjustments and information about labor and delivery. The section Lactation the Clinical Considerations gives a more concrete guide on how to best minimize drug exposure to the breastfed infant and also how to monitor the infant for any expected adverse drug effects. Lastly the Data portion for both will give a detailed summary of what research exists on the drug during pregnancy or lactation and how the recommendations for the other two sections were obtained [15].

Imaging in Pregnancy

Assessing the need for imaging and deciding what type of imaging is appropriate and can be difficult and worrisome for the patient, family, and the provider. Even so, pregnant patients do get sick and will warrant imaging to help aid diagnosis and treatment. Again, the same principal approach used when prescribing medications, parental well-being is fetal well-being, can be applied here as well. In the case of diagnostic imaging however, there are several frequently used modalities that include both ionizing and nonionizing radiation.

Ionizing Radiation

Possible adverse fetal outcomes related to radiation exposure during pregnancy include teratogenicity, genetic damage, intrauterine death, and increased risk of malignancy in later life for the baby. The extent to which radiation exposure causes injury depends upon level of exposure as well as timing (gestational age) of exposure [34]. A highly vulnerable time of exposure includes the first trimester when organogenesis occurs, but fetal growth and neurologic development are susceptible at any time in gestation. During pregnancy, ionizing radiation doses of <10 rads have not been shown to cause congenital malformations, fetal growth restriction, or miscarriage. Given this, the National Commission on Radiation Protection advises limiting ionizing radiation exposure to <5 rads during pregnancy [33]. However, most diagnostic procedures outside of the abdomen and pelvis will lead to fetal absorbed doses of less than 0.1 rads of radiation, well below the allowed recommendations, as detailed in Table 8.3.

Table 8.3 Fetal radiation exposure for common imaging techniques

Imaging	Mean fetal radiation exposure, Rads (mGy)
Head CT	< 0.001 (< 0.01)
Chest X-ray (2 views)	< 0.001 (< 0.01)
Chest CT	0.006 (0.06)
Ventilation/perfusion scan	Ventilation portion: 0.01–0.03 (0.1–0.3) Perfusion Portion: 0.04–0.06 (0.4–0.6)
Abdominal CT	0.8 (8)
Pelvic CT	2.5 (25)
Upper or lower extremity X-ray	0.001 (0.01)
Lumbar spine CT	0.17 (1.7)

Commonly used ionizing radiation studies in pregnancy are X-rays, CT scans, and V/Q scans. These studies provide valuable data for diagnosing and treating potentially harmful diseases and conditions for patient and baby such as infections, pulmonary emboli, or pleural effusions. A provider's understanding of the risks of imaging versus the risk of misdiagnosis is critical, with the former being more difficult to become comfortable with. Table 8.3 summarizes the extent of fetal radiation exposure with certain studies and can help when counseling patients of the fetal risks.

Non-ionizing Radiation

Both ultrasound and magnetic resonance imaging (MRI) are invaluable alternatives when caring for a potentially sick pregnant patient, and imaging is needed for diagnosis. Ultrasounds are commonly performed on the obstetric side but should also be considered for initial testing when possible for non-obstetric-related pathology. MR imaging has not been shown to cause any harm to the growing fetus; however, the use of gadolinium based contrast is not endorsed since it does cross the placenta and the effects on the fetus are unknown [22]. For example, when evaluating a patient with new onset prolonged headaches, MR imaging including MR venography or MR angiography can be done without contrast to help diagnosis possible aneurysm, arteriovenous malformations, bleed, or mass.

Common Medical Problems in Pregnancy

This next portion will focus on certain commonly encountered medical problems or diseases in the context of pregnancy. The impact of the disease on pregnancy and the effect of pregnancy on the disease will be the basic approach, along with management and possible risks of which to be aware. Preconception care can range from a few years to just a few months before pregnancy, whereas the postpartum period refers specifically to the 6 weeks after delivery. The role for primary care clinicians in providing preconception, intrapartum, and postpartum care is critical since these diseases can affect a patient's future health and require long-term screening and follow-up.

Hypertension

Hypertension is one of the most commonly encountered and treated conditions in a primary care office. The CDCs National Health and Nutrition Examination Survey showed that the prevalence of hypertension among adults was 29.0% from 2011 to 2014, with 7.3% between the ages of 18–39 and continued to increase with age [11].

Recent studies and data predict that the incidence of hypertension in patients of childbearing age is likely to increase congruent with the increasing rates of obesity, hyperlipidemia, and metabolic syndrome worldwide. In addition, with many people delaying pregnancy until after the age of 35, the rates of pregnant patients with pre-existing hypertension is likely to rise. Consequently, the role of primary care clinicians in counseling and managing in these patients becomes pivotal.

Effect of Pregnancy on Hypertension

The normal vascular changes that occur in pregnancy can considerably impact a patient's blood pressure. Progesterone-mediated smooth muscle relaxation causes significant vasodilation and a lowering of blood pressure in the first half of pregnancy. Specifically arterial blood pressure decreases about 10–15 mmHg with a greater drop in diastolic pressure than that in the systolic. Blood pressure steadily decreases starting in the first trimester with its nadir at the end of the second trimester around 24 weeks of gestation. Blood pressure then starts to rise, and by the beginning of the third trimester, it returns to prepregnancy levels. Due to this initial drop in blood pressure, many times patients with known hypertension can be taken off of medications and given a "medication holiday" during pregnancy.

Effects of Hypertension on Pregnancy

Preexisting hypertension in pregnancy is associated with poor pregnancy outcomes such as intrauterine growth restriction, placental abruption, preterm delivery, and low birth weight. In addition to this, the most concerning complication that could occur is preeclampsia and the sequela associated with it. Preeclampsia is a systemic condition that occurs in 25–40% of patients with preexisting hypertension (compared to 5–7% of non-hypertensive primagravid patients), causing proteinuria and severe elevation in blood pressure [16]. The American Congress of Obstetricians and Gynecologists' (ACOG) revised diagnostic criteria for preeclampsia are detailed in Table 8.4. In addition to this, in patients who develop preeclampsia, there is an increased risk of future development of ischemic heart disease and stroke, and this should routinely be asked about to assess a patient's long-term risk [6].

Management of Hypertension in Pregnancy

Management of preexisting hypertension entails both controlling blood pressure as well as preventing and/or recognizing the development of preeclampsia. Blood pressure goals are controversial, and guidelines vary around the world. The aim of

Table 8.4 Criteria for the diagnosis of preeclampsia

Criteria for the diagnosis of preeclampsia
Systolic blood pressure ≥ 140 mmHg or diastolic blood pressure ≥ 90 mmHg on two occasions at least four hours apart after 20 weeks of gestation in a previously normotensive patient If systolic blood pressure is ≥160 mmHg or diastolic blood pressure is ≥110 mmHg, confirmation within minutes is sufficient
AND
Proteinuria ≥0.3 g in a 24 hour urine specimen or protein/creatinine ratio ≥ 0.3 (mg/mg) (30 mg/mmol) Or dipstick ≥1+ if a quantitative measurement is unavailable
OR
Platelet count <100,000/microL
Serum creatinine >1.1 mg/dL (97.2 micromol/L) or doubling of the creatinine concentration in the absence of other renal disease
Liver transaminases at least twice the upper limit of the normal concentrations for the local laboratory
Pulmonary edema
Cerebral or visual symptoms (new or persistent, blurred vision, flashing lights, or scotomata)

Adapted from Hypertension in pregnancy. Report of the American College of Obstetricians and Gynecologists' Task Force on Hypertension in Pregnancy [6]

antihypertensive therapy is to reduce the risk of severe range blood pressure (stroke, myocardial damage, and renal injury) while balancing the need for adequate fetal perfusion [23]. The extent to which the high blood pressure may be tolerated differs among societies. Both the National Institute for Health and Care Excellence(NICE) and the Society of Obstetricians and Gynaecologists of Canada (SOGC) recommend initiating therapy when blood pressure exceeds 150/100 mmHg. The American Congress of Obstetricians and Gynecologists (ACOG) is less stringent and recommend treatment only for blood pressures over 160/110 mmHg, since complications are significantly increased with blood pressure over this limit. Given all this, options for management include (1) stopping all antihypertensive medications and only restart if above blood pressure limit, (2) continuing current medications with the aim of keeping blood pressure under limit, or (3) switching patient to a pregnancy preferred antihypertensive agent if need be. Blood pressure is routinely checked at all OB visits, which are monthly in the first and second trimester and then weekly after 34 weeks of gestation. Commonly used antihypertensive medications in pregnancy and postpartum include methyldopa or labetalol, but other possible choices could be nifedipine or hydralazine as listed in Table 8.5.

Risk of Preeclampsia

The development of preeclampsia is significant in patients with preexisting hypertension and preventive measures when possible should be started. Multiple hypotheses exist regarding the etiology of preeclampsia, though no one single cause has

Table 8.5 Antihypertensive drugs in pregnancy

Stage of pregnancy	Relatively contraindicated[1]	Absolutely contraindicated	Drugs that may be used
First trimester[2]		ACE inhibitors	Methyldopa
		A-II receptor antagonists	Labetalol and beta-blockers
			Calcium channel blockers
Second trimester	Beta-blockers	ACE inhibitors	Methyldopa
	Diuretics	A-II receptor antagonists	Nifedipine
			Labetalol
Third trimester	Beta-blockers	ACE inhibitors	Methyldopa
	Diuretics	A-II receptor antagonists	Nifedipine
			Labetalol
			Doxazosin
			Prazosin
Puerperium		None	Labetalol and beta-blockers
			Nifedipine
			Diuretics
			ACE inhibitors
			A-II receptor antagonists

[1]Can be used but avoid unless necessary
[2]Avoid all drugs in the first trimester unless necessary

Table 8.6 Primary prevention of preeclampsia

Probably or definitely ineffective	May be effective for at least some patients
Weight restriction	Low-dose aspirin and other antiplatelet agents
Salt restriction	Calcium supplements Aerobic exercise
Anti-oxidant vitamins (vitamins C and E)	
Diuretics	
Antihypertensive agents	
Fish oil supplements	

been identified yet [16]. Prevention of preeclampsia has been a major area of research, and many strategies have been studied to assess efficacy (Table 8.6). However, mainly low-dose aspirin and calcium supplementation in patients with low dietary intake have been shown to be helpful for prevention [24, 25]. Possibly even more important than trying to prevent preeclampsia is the need for the clinician to recognize and diagnose preeclampsia. New-onset headache or change in headaches, vision changes, epigastric pain, and RUQ pain are common clinical manifestations, and if present, communication with the patient's obstetrician is the most important next step in order to rule out and/or manage possible preeclampsia [6].

Diabetes

Roughly 9.4% of the US population has diabetes mellitus with the prevalence doubling as rates of obesity increase. With this increase, roughly 1–2% of pregnancies are now affected by preexisting diabetes [29]. Reliable and consistent prenatal care and control, as well as appropriate preconception counseling, are essential to decreasing poor outcomes for both parent and baby.

Effect of Pregnancy on Diabetes

The effects of insulin change and fluctuate tremendously throughout pregnancy. Early on, pregnancy causes an accelerated starvation state and therefore increased ketone production. Additionally, early in pregnancy, there is an increase in insulin sensitivity causing hypoglycemia and a drop in fasting plasma glucose levels. However, by the end of the second trimester, insulin sensitivity declines (insulin resistance increases) by 50% due to increases in maternal prolactin and cortisol, as well as growth in the placenta to produce human placental lactogen and human placental growth hormone.

Microvascular complications of diabetes are also accelerated due to pregnancy. Retinopathy in type 1 diabetics is increased by 50% in pregnancy and can lead to irreversible vision changes and even vision loss in a small number of patients [29]. This is possibly thought to be due to the increase in cardiac output and an increase in production of growth factors. Nephropathy also is affected and can worsen due to the increased proteinuria seen in pregnancy along with the increased risk of preeclampsia and hypotension in diabetic patients. For most patients however renal function will improve or revert back to prepregnancy levels after delivery.

Effect of Diabetes on Pregnancy

Maternal complications in pregnancy include the above acceleration of certain underlying disease processes, as well as other pregnancy-related complications. Poor glycemic control early in pregnancy is associated with increased fetal loss and congenital anomalies. Incidence of congenital malformations such as cardiac and neural tube defects is directly associated with increasing HgbA1c levels in the first trimester, whereas hyperglycemia in later pregnancy is associated with macrosomia, complicated vaginal deliveries, and increased risk of operative delivery. Hypertensive disorders of pregnancy, especially preeclampsia, are markedly increased as well [26, 27]. Antepartum urinary tract and genital and respiratory infections also are increased when compared to nondiabetic controls.

Management of Diabetes in Pregnancy

Diabetes care in pregnancy includes preconception and intrapartum care for patients with Type I, Type II, and gestational diabetes. Primary care clinicians are most often going to be caring for these patients prepregnancy or early in pregnancy, which will be the focus in this section, with emphasis given to preconception care, counseling, and management.

Adequate glycemic control with a goal HgbA1c of <7% is recommended by the International Diabetes Federation to help improve poor pregnancy outcomes [28]. Prior to pregnancy, this can be achieved by either using oral agents or having the patient become accustomed to an insulin regimen. Insulin is still the preferred medication for treating hyperglycemia in all types of diabetes during pregnancy, since it does not cross the placenta in large amounts. NPH, rapid-acting insulin or long-acting insulin Detemir appears to be the safest and best studied of all the insulin types. Metformin and glyburide have both been shown to cross the placenta, though safety data in pregnancy thus far appears favorable [30, 32]. However, all oral agents lack long-term safety data, and this should be discussed with the patient. In addition to this, risk of preeclampsia is increased, and patients should be advised to start low dose aspirin for primary prevention [31].

Venous Thromboembolism

Population-based studies have shown an increasing incidence of venous thromboembolism (VTE) in pregnancy, which may be due in part to increasing vigilance on the part of clinicians as well as improved diagnostic techniques and standards [17, 21]. In addition to this, the postpartum period has been identified as a time of even greater risk, with one study showing that the annual incidence was 5 times higher among postpartum patients than pregnant patients [21].

Effect of Pregnancy on Venous Thromboembolism

Pregnancy and the puerperium (the 6–8 week postpartum period between childbirth and the return of the uterus to its normal size) are times of increased risk for VTE secondary to fulfilling Virchow's triad of hypercoagulability, venous stasis, and vascular injury [18]. Pregnancy is a hypercoagulable state due to an increase in procoagulants (Factor V and VIII) and a decrease in anticoagulants (protein S). Progesterone-mediated vasodilation causes increased venous stasis which is present from the first trimester onwards. Additional risk factors for peripartum VTE are essential determinants for diagnoses, treatment, and outcomes and can be found in Table 8.7.

Table 8.7 Risk factors for postpartum VTE

Risk factors for postpartum VTE
Past history of VTE
Family history of VTE
Thrombophilia
Obesity
Age > 35 years
Tobacco use
Cesarean section
Preeclampsia
Prolonged bed rest or immobility

Table 8.8 VTE treatment options for pregnancy and postpartum

VTE treatment options for pregnancy and postpartum		
Agent	Antepartum	Postpartum
LMWH	Preferred option	Preferred Can be started 12–24 hours after delivery Safe for breastfeeding
UFH	Second-line option	Can be started 12–24hours after delivery Safe for breastfeeding
Fondaparinux	Acceptable (especially if HIT develops)	Not recommended for breastfeeding
Warfarin	Avoid	Can be started the day after delivery Safe for breastfeeding
DOACs	Avoid	Avoid if breastfeeding

HIT heparin-induced thrombocytopenia, *DOAC* direct acting oral anticoagulant

While VTE is relatively rare in otherwise healthy young patients, it can be up to 10 times more common in pregnant patients of similar age. In fact, VTE has been recognized for many years as a leading cause of maternal morbidity and mortality worldwide, especially among developed and developing nations [17, 19]. A high index of suspicion for VTE should be had when assessing pregnant patients with complaints suggestive of either deep vein thrombosis or pulmonary embolism. Many symptoms of DVT or PE, such as lower extremity edema, dyspnea, and musculoskeletal complaints, are common occurrences in pregnancy and may delay the diagnosis.

Effective and safe treatment options for both therapy and prophylaxis of VTE include low molecular weight heparin (LMWH) and unfractionated heparin (UFH) which are the most utilized [20]. Other options are available, and more information regarding medications for VTE in pregnancy can be found in Table 8.8.

Effect of Venous Thromboembolism on Pregnancy

As described above, acute VTE is more common in pregnancy, and the subsequent treatment needed can affect choice of treatment and also affect labor and delivery planning. However, the focus of this section will be on preconception counseling and pregnancy management in patients who may need prophylactic anticoagulation. All pregnant patients are at increased risk of VTE; however, risk stratification of all patients should be considered and include personal history of VTE, family history of VTE, and existing diagnosis of a thrombophilia. Table 8.9 summarizes risk groups and recommended treatment options.

Table 8.9 Summary of guidelines for thromboprophylaxis in patients with previous VTE and/or thrombophilia

Summary of guidelines for thromboprophylaxis in patients with previous VTE and/or thrombophilia		
Very high risk	Previous VTE on long-term oral anticoagulant therapy	Antenatal therapeutic/high-dose LMWH Postpartum need continued anticoagulation with LMWH or switched back to oral anticoagulant
	Antithrombin III deficiency Antiphospholipid antibody syndrome	*These patients require specialist management by experts in hemostasis and pregnancy*

High risk	Any previous VTE:
	  Previous unprovoked VTE or estrogen associated VTE
	  Previous VTE + thrombophilia
	  Previous VTE + family history of VTE
	Asymptomatic high-risk thrombophilia (combined defects, homozygous FVL, homozygous PT gene mutation)
		Antenatal and 6 weeks postpartum prophylactic LMWH

Intermediate risk	Single previous provoked VTE (by a transient risk factor that is no longer present, such as surgery) without thrombophilia, family history, or other risk factors Asymptomatic protein C or S deficiency *with* a family history of VTE	Six weeks postpartum prophylactic LMWH and close antenatal surveillance for other risk factors
Low risk	Asymptomatic low-risk thrombophilia (PT gene mutation or FVL)	No anticoagulation – recommend antenatal and postpartum surveillance for other risk factors

Adapted from RCOG Green Top Guideline, [5] and ASH Guidelines 2018
Asymptomatic = no history of VTE
FVL Factor V Leiden
PT Prothrombin Gene

Medical Complications in Pregnancy and Future Health Risks

Pregnancy is an amazing time of physiologic changes that creates an extra burden to the human body but can also reveal a patient's possible predisposition for chronic disease. Pregnancy-induced syndromes such as preeclampsia or gestational diabetes can be markers for subsequent disease and aid in risk stratification and counseling for long term health. Primary care clinicians can provide a bridge between pregnancy and future health care needs, which is why pregnancy complications and outcomes must be integrated as part of routine intake and assessment. Table 8.10 highlights certain conditions that warrant further attention and counseling both before and after pregnancy.

Box 8.1

	Preconception care checklist
Hypertension	☐ Discussed safe medications in pregnancy and switched patient if needed ☐ Discussed risk of preeclampsia ☐ Advised taking baby aspirin for prevention of preeclampsia ☐ Advised increased calcium intake for prevention of preeclampsia ☐ If patient has a history of preeclampsia, counseled on the risk of recurrence and also the long-term risk of cardiovascular disease in the future ☐ Reiterated need for a healthy diet and exercise ☐ Monitor renal function and assess for proteinuria
Diabetes	☐ Discussed the importance of pregnancy planning and to achieve optimal glucose control before conceiving ☐ Ideal HgbA1c < 7% (< 6.5% if possible) ☐ Discussed the maternal and fetal complications ☐ Evaluateed for microvascular complications (nephropathy and retinopathy) ☐ Folic acid supplementation of 400mcg daily preconception ☐ Reviewed current medication regimen and made changes accordingly (stopping ACE-I and some oral hypoglycemic agents)
Venous thromboembolic disease	☐ Discussed the increased risk of VTE in pregnancy with past history of personal VTE ☐ Discussed the need for antenatal and postpartum prophylaxis ☐ Discussed medication options of LMWH or Unfractionated Heparin as well as side effects ☐ If a patient is on an oral anticoagulant, discussed timing of stopping those meds and transitioning to injectable anticoagulants

Table 8.10 Pregnancy and long-term health risks

Pregnancy complication that points to a future health risk	Future health risk	Office Checklist
1. Preeclampsia prior to 37 weeks 2. Recurrent preeclampsia or who have delivered pre-term or growth restricted infants	Cardiovascular disease (ischemic heart disease and stroke)	Smoking cessation Daily regular exercise Achieve and maintain ideal body weight Undergo cholesterol screening postpartum Yearly blood pressure measurement and the subsequent appropriate treatment
	Renal disease	Ensure that preeclampsia-related proteinuria completely resolves, and if persistent, initiate appropriate investigations Yearly blood pressure measurement and the subsequent appropriate treatment Consider yearly urinalysis
Thromboembolic disease	Recurrent thromboembolism	Consider screening patient for thrombophilia to help quantitate future risk Smoking cessation Achieve and maintain ideal body weight Avoid estrogen containing medications Consider thromboprophylaxis with any prolonged bed rest, surgery,or a subsequent pregnancy Educate patient as to signs and symptoms of acute VTE, and encourage them to seek medical attention early if any of them occur at a subsequent date
Gestational diabetes	Type 2 diabetes	Glucose tolerance test 6 weeks postpartum and a screening HgbA1c Daily regular exercise Achieve and maintain ideal body weight Consider yearly screening with HgbA1c Consider initiation of metformin if evidence of impaired glucose tolerance
Postpartum thyroiditis	Hypothyroidism	Check thyroid peroxidase antibodies (anti-TPO) to assess risk of recurrence/subsequent hypothyroidism Check TSH yearly. Check TSH prior to and/or early in the first trimester and 3–6 months after subsequent pregnancies Patients who are known to have an elevated anti-TPO should have their TSH checked at 3 and 6 months postpartum
Peripartum cardiomyopathy	Persistent or worsening cardiac dysfunction	Follow cardiac function with serial echocardiograms, and optimize congestive heart failure therapy Warn patient of risk of worsening disease with subsequent pregnancies
Postpartum depression	Recurrent depression	Screen patient for depression yearly and with any presenting complaint potentially attributable to recurrent depression

Conclusion

Primary care clinicians can have a significant positive impact on the health of anyone who is or who may become pregnant by engaging in proactive care and guidance before, during and after pregnancy.

References

1. Kukreja R, Locke RG, Hack D, Paul DA. Knowledge of preconception health care among primary care physicians in Delaware. Del Med J. 2012;84(11):349–52. PMID: 23409465.
2. Berghella V, Buchanan E, Pereira L, Baxter JK. Preconception care. Obstet Gynecol Surv. 2010;65(2):119–31. https://doi.org/10.1097/OGX.0b013e3181d0c358. PMID: 20100361.
3. Farahi N, Zolotor A. Recommendations for preconception counseling and care. Am Fam Physician. 2013;88(8):499–506. Erratum in: Am Fam Physician. 2014;89(5):316. Dosage error in article text. PMID: 24364570.
4. Dean SV, Lassi ZS, Imam AM, Bhutta ZA. Preconception care: nutritional risks and interventions. Reprod Health. 2014;11 Suppl 3(Suppl 3):S3. https://doi.org/10.1186/1742-4755-11-S3-S3. Epub 2014 Sep 26. PMID: 25415364; PMCID: PMC4196560.
5. Royal College of Obstetricians and Gynaecologists. Reducing the Risk of Venous Thromboembolism during Pregnancy and the Puerperium. Green Top Guideline No. 37a. London: RCOG; 2015
6. Hypertension in pregnancy. Report of the American College of Obstetricians and Gynecologists' Task Force on Hypertension in Pregnancy. Obstet Gynecol. 2013;122(5):1122–31. https://doi.org/10.1097/01.AOG.0000437382.03963.88. PMID: 24150027.
7. Daniels K, Daugherty J, Jones J. Current contraceptive status among women aged 15–44: United States, 2011–2013. NCHS Data Brief. 2014;(173):1–8. PMID: 25500343.
8. Martin JA, Hamilton BE, Osterman MJ, Curtin SC, Matthews TJ. Births: final data for 2013. Natl Vital Stat Rep. 2015;64(1):1–65. PMID: 25603115.
9. Kersten I, Lange AE, Haas JP, Fusch C, Lode H, Hoffmann W, Thyrian JR. Chronic diseases in pregnant women: prevalence and birth outcomes based on the SNiP-study. BMC Pregnancy Childbirth. 2014;14:75. https://doi.org/10.1186/1471-2393-14-75. PMID: 24552439; PMCID: PMC3943445.
10. Barfield WD, Warner L. Preventing chronic disease in women of reproductive age: opportunities for health promotion and preventive services. Prev Chronic Dis. 2012;9:E34. https://doi.org/10.5888/pcd9.110281. Epub 2012 Jan 12. PMID: 22239749; PMCID: PMC3310066.
11. Bateman BT, Shaw KM, Kuklina EV, Callaghan WM, Seely EW, Hernández-Díaz S. Hypertension in women of reproductive age in the United States: NHANES 1999-2008. PLoS One. 2012;7(4):e36171. https://doi.org/10.1371/journal.pone.0036171. Epub 2012 Apr 30. PMID: 22558371; PMCID: PMC3340351.
12. Sachs HC. Committee On Drugs. The transfer of drugs and therapeutics into human breast milk: an update on selected topics. Pediatrics. 2013;132(3):e796–809. https://doi.org/10.1542/peds.2013-1985. Epub 2013 Aug 26. PMID: 23979084.
13. Spencer JP, Gonzalez LS 3rd, Barnhart DJ. Medications in the breast-feeding mother. Am Fam Physician. 2001;64:119.
14. Pernia S, DeMaagd G. The new pregnancy and lactation labeling rule. P T. 2016;41(11):713–5.
15. Tillett J. Medication use during pregnancy and lactation: the new FDA drug labeling. J Perinat Neonatal Nurs. 2015;29(2):97–9. https://doi.org/10.1097/JPN.0000000000000097. PMID: 25919597.

16. Sibai B, Dekker G, Kupferminc M. Pre-eclampsia. Lancet. 2005;365(9461):785–99. https://doi.org/10.1016/S0140-6736(05)17987-2. PMID: 15733721.
17. Andersen BS, Steffensen FH, Sørensen HT, Nielsen GL, Olsen J. The cumulative incidence of venous thromboembolism during pregnancy and puerperium--an 11 year Danish population-based study of 63,300 pregnancies. Acta Obstet Gynecol Scand. 1998;77(2):170–3. PMID: 9512321.
18. Bagot CN, Arya R. Virchow and his triad: a question of attribution. Br J Haematol. 2008;143(2):180–90. https://doi.org/10.1111/j.1365-2141.2008.07323.x. Epub 2008 Sep 6. PMID: 18783400.
19. Cantwell R, Clutton-Brock T, Cooper G, Dawson A, Drife J, Garrod D, Harper A, Hulbert D, Lucas S, McClure J, Millward-Sadler H, Neilson J, Nelson-Piercy C, Norman J, O'Herlihy C, Oates M, Shakespeare J, de Swiet M, Williamson C, Beale V, Knight M, Lennox C, Miller A, Parmar D, Rogers J, Springett A. Saving Mothers' Lives: Reviewing maternal deaths to make motherhood safer: 2006-2008. The Eighth Report of the Confidential Enquiries into Maternal Deaths in the United Kingdom. BJOG. 2011;118 Suppl 1:1–203. https://doi.org/10.1111/j.1471-0528.2010.02847.x. Erratum in: BJOG. 2015;122(5):e1. Erratum in: BJOG. 2015;122(5):e1. PMID: 21356004.
20. Greer IA, Nelson-Piercy C. Low-molecular-weight heparins for thromboprophylaxis and treatment of venous thromboembolism in pregnancy: a systematic review of safety and efficacy. Blood. 2005;106:401–7.
21. Heit JA, Kobbervig CE, James AH, Petterson TM, Bailey KR, Melton LJ 3rd. Trends in the incidence of venous thromboembolism during pregnancy or postpartum: a 30-year populationbased study. Ann Intern Med. 2005;143(10):697–706. https://doi.org/10.7326/0003-4819-143-10-200511150-00006. PMID: 16287790.
22. Webb JA, Thomsen HS, Morcos SK; Members of Contrast Media Safety Committee of European Society of Urogenital Radiology (ESUR). The use of iodinated and gadolinium contrast media during pregnancy and lactation. Eur Radiol. 2005;15(6):1234–40. https://doi.org/10.1007/s00330-004-2583-y. Epub 2004 Dec 18. PMID: 15609057.
23. SMFM Publications Committee. Electronic address: pubs@smfm.org. SMFM Statement: benefit of antihypertensive therapy for mild-to-moderate chronic hypertension during pregnancy remains uncertain. Am J Obstet Gynecol. 2015;213(1):3–4. https://doi.org/10.1016/j.ajog.2015.04.013. Epub 2015 May 21. PMID: 26004324.
24. Magee LA, Pels A, Helewa M, Rey E, von Dadelszen P; Canadian Hypertensive Disorders of Pregnancy (HDP) Working Group. Diagnosis, evaluation, and management of the hypertensive disorders of pregnancy. Pregnancy Hypertens. 2014;4(2):105–45. https://doi.org/10.1016/j.preghy.2014.01.003. Epub 2014 Feb 25. PMID: 26104418.
25. National Collaborating Centre for Women's and Children's Health (UK). Hypertension in Pregnancy: The Management of Hypertensive Disorders During Pregnancy. London: RCOG Press; 2010. PMID: 22220321.
26. McCance DR. Diabetes in pregnancy. Best Pract Res Clin Obstet Gynaecol. 2015;29(5):685–99. https://doi.org/10.1016/j.bpobgyn.2015.04.009. Epub 2015 Apr 28. PMID: 26004196.
27. American Diabetes Association. (12) Management of diabetes in pregnancy. Diabetes Care. 2015;38 Suppl:S77–9. https://doi.org/10.2337/dc15-S015. PMID: 25537713.
28. American Diabetes Association. 13. Management of Diabetes in Pregnancy: Standards of Medical Care in Diabetes-2018. Diabetes Care. 2018;41(Suppl 1):S137–43. https://doi.org/10.2337/dc18-S013. PMID: 29222384.
29. Blumer I, Hadar E, Hadden DR, Jovanovič L, Mestman JH, Murad MH, Yogev Y. Diabetes and pregnancy: an endocrine society clinical practice guideline. J Clin Endocrinol Metab. 2013;98(11):4227–49. https://doi.org/10.1210/jc.2013-2465. PMID: 24194617.
30. Coustan DR. Pharmacological management of gestational diabetes: an overview. Diabetes Care. 2007;30 Suppl 2:S206–8. https://doi.org/10.2337/dc07-s217. Erratum in: Diabetes Care. 2007;30(12):3154. PMID: 17596473.

31. Balsells M, García-Patterson A, Solà I, Roqué M, Gich I, Corcoy R. Glibenclamide, metformin, and insulin for the treatment of gestational diabetes: a systematic review and metaanalysis. BMJ. 2015;350:h102. https://doi.org/10.1136/bmj.h102. PMID: 25609400; PMCID: PMC4301599.

32. Jiang YF, Chen XY, Ding T, Wang XF, Zhu ZN, Su SW. Comparative efficacy and safety of OADs in management of GDM: network meta-analysis of randomized controlled trials. J Clin Endocrinol Metab. 2015;100(5):2071–80. https://doi.org/10.1210/jc.2014-4403. Epub 2015 Mar 24. PMID: 25803270.

33. International Commission on Radiological Protection. Pregnancy and medical radiation. Ann ICRP. 2000;30(1):16–9. https://doi.org/10.1016/s0146-6453(00)00037-3. PMID: 11108925.

34. Lowe SA. Diagnostic radiography in pregnancy: risks and reality. Aust N Z J Obstet Gynaecol. 2004;44(3):191–6. https://doi.org/10.1111/j.1479-828X.2004.00212.x. PMID: 15191441.

Chapter 9
Patients with Congenital Heart Disease

Alexandra Dembar, Joseph Truglio, and Barry Love

Contents

Introduction

There are an increasing number of patients with congenital heart disease (CHD), and, thanks to advances in treatment options for complex congenital heart disease, adults with CHD now outnumber children with CHD. With this demographic shift comes an increasing need to provide sexual and reproductive health for patients with CHD. Congenital heart disease remains one of the most common causes of

A. Dembar
Gustave L Levy, Mount Sinai School of Medicine, New York, NY, USA
e-mail: alexandra.dembar@icahn.mssm.edu

J. Truglio
Departments of Internal Medicine, Pediatrics and Medical Education, Icahn School of Medicine Mount Sinai, New York, NY, USA
e-mail: joseph.truglio@mssm.edu

B. Love (✉)
Department of Pediatrics and Medicine, Icahn School of Medicine at Mount Sinai, New York, NY, USA
e-mail: barry.love@mssm.edu

© Springer Nature Switzerland AG 2022
J. Truglio et al. (eds.), *Sexual and Reproductive Health*,
https://doi.org/10.1007/978-3-030-94632-6_9

maternal morbidity and mortality in the United States [17]. Despite this risk, women with congenital heart disease are often not counseled on pregnancy-related risk or appropriate contraception. A recent study of over 500 sexually active women with congenital heart disease revealed one in five women to be using a contraindicated birth control option, 28% not using any contraception, and nearly half not having received counseling on pregnancy-related risk [20]. Furthermore, given the genetic risk for CHD in the offspring of adults with congenital heart disease (ACHD) and the impact of functional limitations on sexual activity, sexual and reproductive health should be addressed in all adults with CHD, regardless of their sexual orientation or gender identity. The role of the primary care clinician is to advocate for appropriate counseling on sexual and reproductive health and identify when patients need to be referred to subspecialists. The most common issues include puberty, contraceptive counseling, pregnancy and delivery, genetic counseling, functional limitations that impact sexual activity, management of perimenopausal symptoms, and gender-affirming therapies for transgender and gender nonbinary patients with CHD.

Puberty

As children with CHD make the physiologic transition to adulthood by way of puberty, primary care clinicians should partner with the child and child's caregivers to provide anticipatory guidance on expected development, with particular attention to potential differences based on their heart conditions. These may include delayed menarche and increased likelihood of menstrual abnormalities. Patients with genetic conditions that are associated with congenital heart disease such as coarctation of the aorta and Turner's syndrome may not undergo puberty at all in the absence of endocrine supplementation. Delayed puberty may be the first indication of underling genetic condition in some.

Patients with more complex heart anomalies or those with cyanotic defects are typically significantly older than the general population at their first menarche – the mean age at menarche for women with simple (acyanotic) heart disease was 13, whereas the mean age at menarche for the complex group was 14.5 [11, 19], compared with the mean age of 12–12.5 years in the United States. Furthermore, patients with CHD are far more likely to experience menstrual cycle irregularities, menstrual pain, severe menstrual bleeding, and amenorrhea than their healthy counterparts [19]. The most common menstrual abnormality for which women with CHD seek care is menorrhagia, both for patients with complex (cyanotic) and simple (acyanotic) disease [11]. These findings are consistent with other studies demonstrating associations between menstrual complaints and cyanosis, increased number of surgical interventions, and severity of underlying cardiac disease [6]. Finally, patients on anticoagulation therapy demonstrate close to a threefold increased risk of menorrhagia [19]. Providers should be vigilant in screening these women for menorrhagia and, subsequently, for iron deficiency anemia.

Contraception

Chapter 5 of this book provides a detailed discussion of contraception and family planning options. Here we focus on applying this approach to patients with CHD.

To aid clinicians and patients in selecting safe and effective contraception options, the World Health Organization provides guidance for the safety of contraceptive options and a classification system to determine risk of pregnancy in patients for a wide variety of underlying medical conditions. This ranges from risk class I ("no increased risk in maternal mortality and no-to-mild increased risk in maternal morbidity") to risk class IV ("extremely high risk of maternal mortality or severe morbidity").

The major concern in adults with CHD is the risk of thromboembolism. Estrogen-containing birth control increases the risk of thromboembolism, and the use of combined oral contraceptives is cautioned for patients in WHO risk class 3 and contraindicated for patients in WHO risk class 4 [18]. For patients with CHD, this generally includes patients with cyanotic lesions, pulmonary arterial hypertension, prior Fontan procedure, atrial fibrillation not on anticoagulation, Bjork-Shiley or Starr-Edwards valves, a dilated left atrium greater than 4 centimeters, prior thrombotic events, left ventricular (LV) dysfunction with LV ejection fractions at or below 30%, Kawasaki disease with coronary artery involvement, pulmonary arteriovenous malformations, or complicated valvular heart disease (with pulmonary hypertension or atrial fibrillation). The risk of thromboembolism in these conditions must be individualized in conjunction with a CHD specialist. It should be noted, however, that there are no data to suggest that a single dose of emergency contraception would increase a patient's risk for thromboembolism.

Progesterone-only forms of contraception are often the preferred alternative for patients at elevated risk for thromboembolic disease. However, the risk of fluid overload should be discussed in patients with heart failure. Furthermore, providers should be sure to do a full medication reconciliation on all CHD patients before utilizing the progesterone only "minipill" as the primary means of contraception. For example, for women with pulmonary hypertension, preventing pregnancy is of utmost importance, as being pregnant is associated with a high mortality rate. These women are often treated with the endothelin antagonist bosentan, which is an enzyme inducer that can reduce the efficacy of the progesterone-only minipill [18]. Thus, other methods of contraception should be considered in this population of patients.

Intrauterine devices (IUDs) are widely available in a variety of hormone and nonhormone-containing versions. There are concerns regarding infections with IUD use, particularly in ACHD who may be at increased risk of IE. However, studies have shown only a modestly increased risk of IE in women with ACHD using IUD, meaning that IUDs may still be the best birth control option given their superior efficacy [23]. When considering IUD placement, caution must also be exercised with women who have a Fontan circulation or pulmonary vascular disease. The insertion of the IUD is associated with a vasovagal reaction in up to 5% of women which could potentially lead to fatal cardiovascular collapse in these populations. For these women, the risk of a vasovagal response may be managed with intravenous atropine or reduced by utilizing a paracervical block or combined spinal and epidural block. For these reasons, some patents may prefer the Implanon to the IUD [18]. This same patient population may also have similar risks if undergoing surgical termination of pregnancy. For more information, see the section on termination below.

Table 9.1 provides the contraindications to the mainstays of birth control therapy (estrogen-containing birth control and IUDs), as well as recommendations for alternative options for women in whom these options are contraindicated

Pregnancy

Pregnancy and delivery are safe for most adults with congenital heart disease. All patients of childbearing age should receive counseling on any potential risks for their specific lesion, as well as genetic counseling as appropriate (see section below on genetic counseling). For adults with complex congenital heart disease at elevated risk for adverse events, clinicians should ensure that a multidisciplinary team is in place and that the most appropriate timing and setting are planned for the safest possible pregnancy and delivery. Table 9.2 presents selected common congenital heart lesions with their associated World Health Organization risk stratification. In a systematic review of the literature examining sexual and reproductive health for patients with CHD, Hargrove et al. demonstrated that in general, CHD patients have

Table 9.1 Contraception contraindications and alternative options for patients with CHD

Type of birth control	Contraindications	Other special considerations	Alternative options
Estrogen-containing birth control (including combined OCPs, vaginal ring)	Adults with: Cyanotic lesions Pulmonary arterial HTN Prior Fontan procedure Atrial fibrillation WHO risk class 4	Estrogen-containing birth control should also be used with caution in women with migraines, smokers, and women with history of VTE	Progesterone-only "minipill" Intrauterine devices (IUDs) Medroxyprogesterone acetate etonogestrel implant
IUD	Fontan circulation Pulmonary vascular disease	Modest increase in rate of infective endocarditis with IUD; should exercise clinical judgment	Use of paracervical block or combined spinal/epidural block on insertion etonogestrel implant Medroxyprogesterone acetate

a poor understanding of topics related to contraception, fertility, and risks related to pregnancy [9]. Identifying this gap in knowledge is important, as other studies have demonstrated that patients with CHD are just as likely as their healthy peers to engage in sexual activity [10].

There are a number of congenital heart conditions in which pregnancy is contra-indicated, as it poses a severe threat to the mother's health. These conditions are listed in Table 9.2 and include but are not limited to stenotic left-sided lesions (aor-tic stenosis, mitral stenosis), pulmonary artery hypertension of any cause, severe systemic ventricular dysfunction (LVEF <30%, NYHA III–IV), Marfan syndrome with aorta dilated >45 mm, and native severe coarctation [18]. For patients with pulmonary hypertension, a 50% risk of maternal death has been reported [9]. The modified WHO classification of maternal cardiovascular risk is currently the most

Table 9.2 Conditions associated with WHO risk classes [18]

WHO risk class	Conditions associated

I
No detectable increased risk of maternal mortality and no/mild increase in morbidity
	Uncomplicated, small, or mild:
	  Pulmonary stenosis
	  Patent ductus arteriosus
	  Mitral valve prolapse
	Successfully repaired simple lesions
	Atrial or ventricular ectopic beats, isolated

II *Small increased risk of maternal mortality or moderate increase in morbidity*	Unoperated atrial or ventricular septal defect Repaired Tetralogy of Fallot Most arrhythmias Mild LV impairment Hypertrophic cardiomyopathy Marfan syndrome without aortic dilatation Aorta <45 mm in aortic disease associated with bicuspid aortic valve Repaired coarctation
III *Significantly increased risk of maternal mortality or severe morbidity. Expert counseling required. If pregnancy is decided upon, intensive specialist cardiac and obstetric monitoring needed throughout pregnancy, childbirth, and the puerperium*	Mechanical valve Systemic right ventricle Fontan circulation Cyanotic heart disease (unrepaired) Other complex congenital heart disease Aortic dilatation 40–45 mm in Marfan syndrome Aortic dilatation 45–50 mm in aortic disease associated with bicuspid aortic valve
IV *Extremely high risk of maternal mortality or severe morbidity; pregnancy contraindicated. If pregnancy occurs, termination should be discussed. If pregnancy continues, care as for class III*	Pulmonary artery hypertension of any cause Severe systemic ventricular dysfunction (LVEF <30%, NYHA III–IV) Severe mitral stenosis Severe symptomatic aortic stenosis Marfan syndrome with aorta dilated >45 mm Aortic dilatation >50 mm in aortic disease associated with bicuspid aortic valve Native severe coarctation

reliable predictor of maternal cardiovascular complications. The most common maternal cardiovascular complications are arrhythmia and heart failure [1].

Providers can further characterize non-lesion-specific maternal risk by screening for the presence of the following risk factors: cyanosis (SaO2 < 90%), NYHA symptoms > functional class II, systemic ventricular ejection fraction <40%, and prior cardiovascular event (arrhythmia, pulmonary edema, stroke, or transient ischemic attack) [17]. If one of the aforementioned risk factors is present, the additional risk of an adverse cardiac event during pregnancy is 27%; however, if there are two or more risk factors present, the risk of an adverse event increases to 75% [18]. All patients with congenital heart disease who are planning pregnancy should be seen and counseled by a cardiologist with experience in congenital heart disease.

In addition to the risk of pregnancy to the mother herself, the risk of congenital heart disease in her offspring is increased. For certain conditions such as the 22q deletion most strongly associated with tetralogy of Fallot, Truncus arteriosus, and interrupted aortic arch, the risk of fetal cardiac anomalies is 50%. For left-sided cardiac conditions such as bicuspid aortic valve, aortic stenosis, and coarctation, the risk may be as high as 10%. For other cardiac conditions, the usual figure quoted is between 3 and 5%. Genetic counseling prior to conception is strongly advised for patients at highest risk.

An additional consideration for pregnancy in this patient population is medication teratogenicity. ACE Inhibitors, angiotensin II receptor blockers and warfarin are commonly used teratogenic medication in this patient population. As with all patients of childbearing age on such medications, clinicians should discuss the need for effective contraception and must be prepared to discuss alternative treatment options with patients that wish to become pregnant. See the Chap. 8 on pregnancy for more information.

Termination of Pregnancy

The approach to discussing termination in general is included in Chap. 3 Sexual and Reproductive Health for Adults Age 18–65, with the various options discussed in Chap. 5 Contraception and Family Planning. Patients with CHD may face unique challenges when choosing to terminate a pregnancy. These generally fall into three categories: the risk of bleeding due to anticoagulation, the risk of circulatory compromise during cervical dilatation, and the general perioperative risk for anesthesia.

The risk of bleeding for women on anticoagulation is highest with medication abortion. Medication abortion can typically which can be performed safely during the first 10 weeks since the patient's last menstrual period regardless of the patient's underlying cardiac lesion. However, it should not be used in women who are anticoagulated where the anticoagulation cannot safely be held for a period of time. For women who are anticoagulated or who have a bleeding diathesis, surgical management may be preferable [8].

For patients with complex congenital heart disease undergoing surgical abortions, the pre-procedure circulatory physiology should clearly be defined by an adult-congenital cardiologist in order to identify patients at high risk for circulatory compromise with cervical dilatation. This includes Fontan circulation and more commonly pulmonary arterial hypertension. These patients should be managed by a trained medical team.

Genetic Screening

An identifiable genetic or environmental cause is found in approximately 20–30% of cases of congenital heart disease [2]. Defining a genetic cause may help identify other organ systems at risk for complications, provide prognostic information, and help clarify the risk of CHD in their offspring and other family members [5]. Clinicians should also consider re-evaluating older adults with CHD periodically as new genetic tests become available and new syndromes are recognized. In addition to considering genetic testing a thorough history and physical exam to identify any noncardiac manifestations of possible syndromes and a detailed, a three-generation family history with attention to heart disease and other birth defects, consanguinity, and spontaneous abortions should be performed. Central to this process is the collaboration between primary care clinicians ACHD cardiologists, and, when available, cardiovascular geneticists testing.

Sexual Dysfunction

Sexual dysfunction and anxiety around sexual activity may impact adolescents and adults of all ages with CHD. Sexual dysfunction, including diagnosis and management, is discussed in Chap. 7, Sexual Dysfunction. In this section we discuss specifically how CHD can impact sexual function as well as the treatment options available for sexual dysfunction.

The impact of CHD on sexual function can be quite debilitating, even in patients with relatively mild disease (NYHA I or II) [14]. Patients with CHD may complain about their sexual dysfunction in various ways. The most frequent complaints that patients report during sexual activity are dyspnea, perceived arrhythmia, increased fatigue, and syncope [19]. Additionally, cis-gender men may complain of erectile dysfunction [12]. The proportion of patients experiencing sexual dysfunction increases dramatically with worsening functional class. An increased degree of severity of these symptoms are also related to the severity of the underlying lesion [19]. Although the American Heart Association (AHA) recommends that "sexual activity is reasonable for most CHD patients who do not have decompensated or advanced heart failure, severe and/or significantly symptomatic valvular disease, or uncontrolled arrhythmias," little data exist to help guide clinicians on counseling ACHD regarding sexual activity and sexual dysfunction [14]. We recommend taking into account the patient's chronologic age and developmental status, the severity of his or her underlying CHD lesion from both an anatomical and a physiological perspective and any other non-CHD physical and mental conditions.

The above discussion focused on intrinsic factors that may affect sexual dysfunction related to the severity of the underlying cardiac lesion. However, external factors, foremost of these are medications, may contribute to sexual dysfunction in CHD patients. It is possible that treatment with medications for CHD may increase the incidence and severity of sexual dysfunction [22]. Several diuretics, especially chlorthalidone and hydrochlorothiazide, have been associated with impaired sexual function [21]. Beta-blockers such as propranolol have been associated with sexual dysfunction, but the literature is more conflicted on the sexual impact of beta-blockers as opposed to diuretics [16]. The evidence is also mixed for ACE inhibitors and ARBs, as there is some evidence that suggests these drugs actually improve sexual function [22].

Management of Perimenopausal Symptoms

The use of hormone replacement therapy for management of perimenopausal symptoms remains controversial but is generally accepted for patients with low cardiovascular risk, and approximately age 50–59 for a period of 5 years or less [15]. For patients with ACHD, any additional risk of venous thromboembolism (VTE) due to their CHD must be taken into account. For patients with lesions considered high-risk for VTE, estrogen-containing HRT should be avoided. Instead, clinicians may offer a variety of therapies to target specific symptoms. Vaginal estrogen creams and nonhormonal lubricants help with vaginal dryness and selective serotonin reuptake inhibitors help with mood disorders and vasomotor symptoms. For patients with lesions at lower risk for VTE, the lowest dose of estrogen for the shortest period of time is recommended [3], with transdermal estrogen preparations deliver lower, more consistent doses of estrogen than oral preparations.

Gender-Affirming Treatments for Transgender and Gender Nonbinary Patients with CHD

Part 3 of this book details several gender-affirming therapeutic options available to transgender and gender nonbinary patients. With appropriate monitoring, the vast majority of gender-affirming medications are safe for patients with even the most complex congenital heart disease. Only three situations exist wherein special considerations should be made for patients with CHD: androgen suppression in patients at risk for prolonged QTc, spironolactone in patients at risk for hyperkalemia, and estrogen in patients at increased risk for thromboembolism.

Gonadotropin-releasing hormone (GnRH) analogues such as leuprolide are often used to delay puberty, giving the adolescent more time to explore gender identity. While androgen deprivation therapy in adults with coronary artery disease has been shown to increased risk of sudden cardiac death, stroke, and prolonged QT/QTc interval [13], these data cannot be extrapolated to adolescent and pediatric patients with CHD. However, it is reasonable to monitor QTc intervals in pediatric and adolescent patients receiving androgen deprivation therapy who have a baseline prolonged QTc or are on medications that prolong the QTc.

Spironolactone is commonly used in conjunction with estrogens to suppress the development of male secondary sex characteristics. It may raise potassium levels in susceptible individuals, including patients with renal dysfunction or those already on angiotensin converter enzyme inhibitors (ACEi) or angiotensin receptor blocker (ARB) regimen. Adjustments in ACEi or ARB therapy may need to be made to avoid the cumulative impact on potassium levels. Patients may also experience polyuria, polydipsia, or orthostasis due to the diuretic properties of high dose spironolactone, which may be problematic for patients with reduced ejection fraction [4].

Patients on trans feminine regimens may experience a higher incidence of venous thromboembolism than non-transgender controls, although extension to heart disease is less clear [7]. For patients at significant risk for thrombus, such as patients with Fontan procedures, cyanotic lesions, or significant pulmonary hypertension, discussions regarding estrogen should include their adult-congenital cardiologist. No such negative connection to trans masculine regimens has been made.

Conclusion

Sexual and reproductive health are important aspects of life for all patients, including patients with congenital heart disease. Primary care clinicians are in a unique position to improve this often-neglected domain of health.

References

1. Balci A, Sollie-Szarynska KM, van der Bijl AGL, Ruys TPE, Mulder BJM, Roos-Hesselink JW, et al. Prospective validation and assessment of cardiovascular and offspring risk models for pregnant women with congenital heart disease. Heart. 2014;100(17):1373–81. https://doi.org/10.1136/heartjnl-2014-305597.
2. Beauchesne LM, Warnes CA, Connolly HM, Ammash NM, Grogan M, Jalal SM, Michels VV. Prevalence and clinical manifestations of 22q11.2 microdeletion in adults with selected conotruncal anomalies. J Am Coll Cardiol. 2005;45(4):595–8. https://doi.org/10.1016/j.jacc.2004.10.056.
3. Canobbio MM, Perloff JK, Rapkin AJ. Gynecological health of females with congenital heart disease. Int J Cardiol. 2005;98(3):379–87. https://doi.org/10.1016/j.ijcard.2003.11.021.

4. Center of Excellence for Transgender Health. Guidelines for the primary and gender-affirming care of transgender and gender nonbinary people. University of California, San Francisco, 199. 2016. Retrieved from http://transhealth.ucsf.edu/pdf/Transgender-PGACG-6-17-16.pdf.
5. Cowan JR, Ware SM. Genetics and genetic testing in congenital heart disease. Clin Perinatol. 2015;42(2):373–93. https://doi.org/10.1016/j.clp.2015.02.009.
6. Drenthen W, Hoendermis ES, Moons P, Heida KY, Roos-Hesselink JW, Mulder BJM, et al. Menstrual cycle and its disorders in women with congenital heart disease. Congenit Heart Dis. 2008;3(4):277–83. https://doi.org/10.1111/j.1747-0803.2008.00202.x.
7. Getahun D, Nash R, Flanders WD, Baird TC, Becerra-Culqui TA, Cromwell L, Hunkeler E, Lash TL, Millman A, Quinn VP, Robinson B, Roblin D, Silverberg MJ, Safer J, Slovis J, Tangpricha V, Goodman M. Cross-sex Hormones and Acute Cardiovascular Events in Transgender Persons: A Cohort Study. Ann Intern Med. 2018 Jul 10. https://doi.org/10.7326/M17-2785. [Epub ahead of print] PubMed PMID: 29987313
8. Guiahi M, Davis A. Clinical guidelines first-trimester abortion in women with medical conditions. 2012. https://doi.org/10.1016/j.contraception.2012.09.001.
9. Hargrove A, Penny DJ, Sawyer SM. Sexual and reproductive health in young people with congenital heart disease: a systematic review of the literature. Pediatr Cardiol. 2005;26(6):805–11. https://doi.org/10.1007/s00246-005-0950-3.
10. Horner T, Liberthson R, Jellinek MS. Psychosocial profile of adults with complex congenital heart disease. Mayo Clin Proc. 2000;75(1):31–6. https://doi.org/10.4065/75.1.31.
11. Khajali Z, Ziaei S, Maleki M. Menstrual disturbances in women with congenital heart diseases. Res Cardiovasc Med. 2016;5(3):e32512. https://doi.org/10.5812/cardiovascmed.32512.
12. Lee TH, Marcantonio ER, Mangione CM, Thomas EJ, Polanczyk CA, Cook EF, et al. Derivation and prospective validation of a simple index for prediction of cardiac risk of major noncardiac surgery. Circulation. 1999;100(10):1043–9. https://doi.org/10.1161/01.cir.100.10.1043.
13. Levine GN, D'Amico AV, Berger P, Clark PE, Eckel RH, Keating NL, et al. Androgen-deprivation therapy in prostate cancer and cardiovascular risk: a science advisory from the American Heart Association, American Cancer Society, and American Urological Association: endorsed by the American Society for Radiation Oncology. Circulation. 2010;121(6):833–40. https://doi.org/10.1161/CIRCULATIONAHA.109.192695.
14. Moons P, Van Deyk K, De Bleser L, Marquet K, Raes E, De Geest S, Budts W. Quality of life and health status in adults with congenital heart disease: a direct comparison with healthy counterparts. Eur J Cardiovasc Prev Rehabil. 2006;13(3):407–13. Retrieved from http://www.ncbi.nlm.nih.gov/pubmed/16926671.
15. Santen RJ, Allred DC, Ardoin SP, Archer DF, Boyd N, Braunstein GD, et al. Postmenopausal hormone therapy: an endocrine society scientific statement. J Clin Endocrinol Metabol. 2010;95(7_supplement_1):s1–s66. https://doi.org/10.1210/jc.2009-2509.
16. Schwarz ER, Rastogi S, Kapur V, Sulemanjee N, Rodriguez JJ. Erectile dysfunction in heart failure patients. J Am Coll Cardiol. 2006;48(6):1111–9. https://doi.org/10.1016/J.JACC.2006.05.052.
17. Siu SC, Sermer M, Colman JM, Alvarez AN, Mercier LA, Morton BC, et al. Prospective multicenter study of pregnancy outcomes in women with heart disease. Circulation. 2001;104(5):515–21. Retrieved from http://www.ncbi.nlm.nih.gov/pubmed/11479246.
18. Thorne S, MacGregor A, Nelson-Piercy C. Risks of contraception and pregnancy in heart disease. Heart. 2006;92(10):1520–5. https://doi.org/10.1136/hrt.2006.095240.
19. Vigl M, Kaemmerer M, Niggemeyer E, Nagdyman N, Seifert-Klauss V, Trigas V, et al. Sexuality and reproductive health in women with congenital heart disease. Am J Cardiol. 2010;105(4):538–41. https://doi.org/10.1016/j.amjcard.2009.10.025.
20. Vigl M, Kaemmerer M, Seifert-Klauss V, Niggemeyer E, Nagdyman N, Trigas V, et al. Contraception in women with congenital heart disease. Am J Cardiol. 2010;106(9):1317–21. https://doi.org/10.1016/j.amjcard.2010.06.060.

21. Wassertheil-Smoller S, Blaufox MD, Oberman A, Davis BR, Swencionis C, Knerr MO, et al. Effect of antihypertensives on sexual function and quality of life: the TAIM study. Ann Intern Med. 1991;114(8):613–20. Retrieved from http://www.ncbi.nlm.nih.gov/pubmed/2003706.
22. Westlake C, Dracup K, Walden JA, Fonarow G. Sexuality of patients with advanced heart failure and their spouses or partners. J Heart Lung Transplant. 1999;18(11):1133–8. https://doi.org/10.1016/S1053-2498(99)00084-4.
23. Wilson W, Taubert KA, Gewitz M, Lockhart PB, Baddour LM, Levison M, et al. Prevention of Infective Endocarditis: guidelines From the American Heart Association: a guideline from the American Heart Association Rheumatic Fever, Endocarditis, and Kawasaki Disease Committee, Council on Cardiovascular Disease in the Young, and the Council on Clinical Cardiology, Council on Cardiovascular Surgery and Anesthesia, and the Quality of Care and Outcomes Research Interdisciplinary Working Group. Circulation. 2007;116(15):1736–54. https://doi.org/10.1161/CIRCULATIONAHA.106.183095.

Chapter 10
Patients with Cancer and Survivors

Linda Overholser and Anne Franklin

Contents

Introduction

As of January 1, 2016, the estimated prevalence of individuals living with a history of cancer in the United States was over 15.5 million [1]. This number is anticipated to rise, due to a combination of advances in treatment, cancer screening, and an aging population [1]. Though these individuals have survived cancer, many will be left with lingering physical and psychosocial effects from their cancer experience and from cancer treatment itself. Among the unmet needs of cancer survivors, gaps in addressing sexual health and reproductive concerns are significant [2, 3]. As a result, intimate partner relationships in particular can suffer if sexual health concerns are not adequately addressed, contributing to the burden of stress and morbidity in partners who are also primary caregivers. This chapter will provide an overview of some of the late and long-term effects that can result from cancer treatment, challenges in addressing sexual health concerns, and some strategies for overcoming barriers to care for survivors of adult and childhood onset cancers.

L. Overholser (✉)
University of Colorado Denver Anschutz Medical Campus, Division of General Internal Medicine, Aurora, CO, USA
e-mail: Linda.Overholser@cuanschutz.edu

A. Franklin
University of Colorado, Children's Hospital Colorado, Center for Cancer and Blood Disorders, Aurora, CO, USA

Adult Survivors of Adult Cancers

Sexual function in individuals who have been diagnosed with and treated for cancer is often not assessed especially in the primary care setting [2], yet sexual dysfunction is known to be a significant concern for many survivors, impacting both individual quality of life and intimate relationships. The estimated prevalence of sexual dysfunction in adult cancer survivors is difficult to summarize given the heterogeneity of cancer and treatment; however, it has been reported to affect at least 40% and up to 100% in studies of the most common cancers of men and women [4–6]. Thus, a first step in addressing sexual dysfunction in cancer survivors is to systematically and routinely inquire about sexual health and sexual functioning as a part of comprehensive care. This approach necessitates skill in collecting a sexual history, regardless of sexual orientation, sexual practices, or gender identity. Individuals in sexual minority groups, defined as those who identify as lesbian, gay, bisexual, transgender or gender nonbinary, and queer (LGBTQ) who also have a history of cancer report lower satisfaction with care [7] and may be at risk for disparities in care across the cancer spectrum [8], including underrepresentation in national clinical practice guidelines [9]. Challenges and stresses exist in the transition from active treatment to long-term follow-up for any individual. This is especially true with regard to the development of sexual side effects and may be magnified in individuals from sexual minority groups [10].

Screening for Sexual Dysfunction

A variety of screening tools are available to assist clinicians interested in opening up conversations with cancer survivors about sexual function. Sexual function is included as part of a comprehensive assessment that is recommended to be performed annually on all adult cancer survivors from the National Comprehensive Cancer Network (NCCN) Survivorship Guidelines (available at www.nccn.org). Examples of specific screening instruments include the NIH Patient-Reported Outcome Measurement Information System® Sexual Function and Satisfaction Measure [11], the Sexual Symptom Checklist for Female Patients After Cancer [12], the Female Sexual Function Index [13], and the Sexual Health Inventory for Men [14]. A 2013 review of selected instruments highlights the wide range with regards to the specific features of sexual function being addressed (e.g., sex drive, arousal, orgasm, ejaculatory function, satisfaction); the method in which they may be administered (e.g., via healthcare personnel interview or self-administered); and the target gender (male/female) [15].

However helpful patient-reported outcome instruments may be in any given setting, it is very important to remember that they are intended to be an approach that complements but does not replace, a clinical interview [15]. Many barriers can exist to screening and assessing sexual dysfunction in patients both at the patient and the provider level. With a history of cancer, an additional confounding factor can be a lack of clarity as to which specialist is best suited to address sexual complaints: the oncologist, the primary care clinician, or another specialist (e.g., urology, gynecology, behavioral health). While the treating oncology team may be expected to take on the primary responsibility of educating patients about how treatment could affect sexual function, primary care clinicians can help to meet the needs of their patients by being prepared to address these concerns during clinical visits that address any aspect of cancer follow-up care, which begins at the time of diagnosis. Strategies that can help include the use of normalization of sexual concerns and of open-ended questions. Examples of this would be: "Many individuals who have been treated for breast cancer experience sexual problems; how about you?" [15] or "Many individuals going through cancer treatment experience negative impacts on their sexual relationships; what has this been like for you?".

Sexual dysfunction encompasses a wide variety of symptoms, and it is helpful to try to more specifically characterize the nature of the dysfunction. For example, it helps to get the perspective of the patient in regard to the type of sexual dysfunction described (e.g., loss of sexual desire versus difficulties achieving orgasm), when the concern started in relation to cancer treatment, whether or not pain is a factor, and how pain relates to other symptoms [15]. The etiologies of sexual dysfunction in cancer survivors is quite varied, ranging from direct physical effects of specific treatment modalities (surgery, radiation, chemotherapy, hormonal therapy), psychosocial morbidity associated with cancer (e.g., depression, anxiety, diminished libido, altered body image), or medications used to manage other nonsexual side effects of treatment (e.g., SSRI medications, tricyclic medications, opioid medications). It is also important to recognize that more than one of these etiologies could be present at any given time and may overlap. Not all sexual dysfunction may be attributable to cancer treatment and a thorough evaluation is necessary to rule out other potentially reversible or contributing causes, such as comorbidity (diabetes, cardiovascular disease, substance abuse) or other medications (antihistamines, beta-blockers).

Fertility Concerns

For individuals of childbearing age, an additional layer of distress may arise if fertility is affected. Thus, it is especially important to assess family planning status and wishes in regard to starting a family in adolescents and young adults diagnosed with cancer. This discussion may initially happen with caregivers in the case of pediatric cancer. A more detailed description of fertility in this population follows later in this chapter. Even if these individuals may not be in a position to immediately consider child-bearing, their plans may change over time, and it is important to prepare them with adequate information and resources. Counseling should occur ideally prior to treatment, but if it did not occur, it does not preclude assessment and counseling in the posttreatment phase.

It is equally important to counsel sexually active survivors, regardless of their gender, to take precautions to avoid conception if it is not desired and they are not aware of their fertility status, as there is a chance that reproductive function could recover with time. The use of contraception should be assessed for any cancer survivor of childbearing age who is sexually active with a partner where pregnancy could occur. A 2014 study demonstrated that young female survivors may be at three times the risk of unintended pregnancy than women of similar age without a history of cancer, despite having received counseling prior to treatment [16]. Additionally, loss of fertility does not equate to protection against sexually transmitted infections.

Late and Long-Term Effects of Therapy Are Dependent on Treatment Modality

Because sexual side effects can often be dependent on specific treatment modalities, we will first review common treatment modalities with selected examples of late and long-term effects that impact sexual function:

- Radiation: Radiation therapy (RT) causes toxicity to cells in the field of radiation. The potential effects of RT on any organ are dependent upon many factors, including the tissue being irradiated, the sensitivity of the tissue to radiation, cumulative dose of radiation, and the age of the individual being treated. For example, cranial RT can disrupt normal functioning of the hypothalamic-pituitary axis and associated reproductive hormones through either direct toxicity or through damage to the vascular supply. Cells in the pituitary gland are differentially sensitive to RT, such that deficiencies in gonadotropins (LH and FSH) are less common than deficiencies in somatotropin (Growth Hormone, GH) in adult cancer survivors [17, 18]. It is uncommon to see deficiencies of gonadotropins at a dose of cranial RT below 40 Gy [18].
- Women who have received radiation therapy to breast tissue can experience significant scarring, pain, and/or disfigurement that adversely affects body image. Others may be left with diminished sensation that impairs the ability to experience pleasurable sensations. Patients with cancer treated with RT to the reproductive organs (ovaries, uterus, testes, prostate) may experience either loss of normal function of these organs and/or scarring of proximate tissues that affect the ability to engage fully in sexual activity. Patients with female sex organs may experience dyspareunia, vaginal fibrosis, decreased sensitivity, atrophy, decreased arousal, and difficulties achieving orgasm either through direct end-organ effects or secondarily through ovarian failure. In particular, younger patients diagnosed with breast cancer in recent years may be treated with ovarian suppression/radioablation in addition to hormonal therapies, and the associated side effects may be more distressing and permanent [19, 20]. Patients with male sex organs may experience primary hypogonadism with resultant loss of sexual desire, the possibility of gynecomastia, and erectile dysfunction occurring through effects on the penile vasculature. In both genders, total body irradiation (TBI) used as a conditioning regimen for hematopoietic stem cell transplantation has been described as having adverse effects on sexual functioning [21].

- Chemotherapy: The chemotherapeutic agents most closely associated with sexual dysfunction in cancer survivors include alkylating agents such as cyclophosphamide, ifosfamide, busulfan, carboplatin, cisplatin, dacarbazine, melphalan, oxaliplatin, carmustine, lomustine, melphalan, and thiotepa. Sexual dysfunction is primarily related to the effects of premature ovarian failure and hypogonadism. Importantly, fertility can also be adversely affected by these therapies. The psychological effects of infertility can overlap with the physical effects of gonadal dysfunction and potentially contribute to difficulties with sexual desire, performance, and intimate relationships.
- Hormonal therapy: Much of what we know about hormonal effects of cancer therapy derive from experiences of breast and prostate cancer survivors, where the use of antiestrogen therapies and androgen deprivation therapy (ADT), respectively, are used most commonly. Though other therapies can result in similar end effects mediated through changes in hormone levels, the use of hormonal agents is reviewed here.
  - Androgen deprivation therapy (ADT) may be a component of treatment for more advanced prostate cancer. Although surgical and radiation treatments may have a more direct impact on sexual dysfunction, patients with a history of prostate cancer on ADT can experience symptoms similar to menopause [22], including hot flashes, mood swings, cognitive dysfunction, fatigue, and hair thinning. These symptoms can adversely affect sexual desire, intimacy, arousal, and body image, all of which interfere with sexual performance, while ADT and resulting hypogonadism can further contribute to erectile dysfunction and diminished libido.
  - Treatment for breast cancer often includes hormonal treatments such as tamoxifen, aromatase inhibitors (anastrozole (Arimidex), letrozole (Femara) exemestane (Aromasin)), and fulvestrant (Faslodex). These agents can lead to a variety of symptoms that are mediated through the induction of a menopausal state. Symptoms may include hot flashes, vaginal dryness, vaginal/ urogenital atrophy, vaginal discharge, dyspareunia, and vulvar irritation in addition to decreases in sexual desire and libido [23].
- Surgery: Surgical treatments in cancer can impact sexual function as a direct result of damage to tissues involved, including skin and nerves that can affect function or sensitivity. While this is particularly true for surgeries that involve pelvic organs, reproductive organ function may sometimes be affected by surgery elsewhere. For example, with testicular cancer, surgery to remove retroperitoneal lymph nodes can impact nerve bundles that affect ejaculatory function. Newer techniques are becoming available that can reduce sexual side effects without sacrificing survival [24] . Surgical treatments in individuals with a history of colorectal cancer can have a range of effects, such as the development of adhesions involving sex organs or erectile dysfunction [25]. Data on the impact of stomas on sexual function is mixed, though the potential for interference is certainly present [25]. Patients with ovarian cancer may face repeated surgeries and the loss of ovarian function in addition to extensive

adhesions, leading to multifactorial causes for sexual dysfunction. Here again it is important to recognize the potential contribution of the psychological effects of surgery on body image and sexual desire in addition to sexual dysfunction.

- Bone marrow transplantation: Hematopoietic stem cell transplantation (HSCT) can also lead to a variety of sexual disorders. Conditioning regimens can include a combination of total body irradiation (TBI) and chemotherapy, both of which have been described above to have impacts on sexual well-being. Graft versus host disease (GVHD) can affect tissues of the genital tract and can involve the use of high-dose steroids to help manage symptoms, which can affect mood [26]. Sexual dysfunction in individuals having received HSCT is highly prevalent in all genders, but women may be at higher risk [27].

To be able to predict with certainty any individual's likelihood of developing any specific sexual side effect once a cancer diagnosis has been made would be beyond the scope of this review, but it may be helpful to consider a summary of selected common cancers and consideration of how various treatments have potential to impact sexual function. Table 10.1 below describes the types of issues to consider, though should not be considered comprehensive:

Hormonally Mediated Symptoms and Menopause

A couple of treatment-related late and long-term effects that impact sexual health deserve a mention here due to their prevalence and cross cutting effects on overall health. Premature ovarian failure (POF) can induce a menopausal state in women, and hypogonadism in men can similarly result in changes that mimic menopause [22]. Clinical practice guidelines for survivorship available from the National Comprehensive Cancer Network distinguish menopause, defined as the "absence of menses for one year in the absence of prior chemotherapy or tamoxifen use or no menses after surgical removal of all ovarian tissue" [26] from menopausal symptoms, and thus all genders are included in the consideration of treatment for menopausal symptoms. All genders may experience hot flashes, urinary difficulties, disruption of sleep and mood, fatigue, cognitive decline, and musculoskeletal complaints in addition to sexual dysfunction. If individuals are not complaining of menopausal symptoms at the time of initial assessment, it is recommended to reassess patients at regular intervals in follow-up, as new symptoms could occur over time [15, 22]. If the clinician is suspicious of treatment-related hormonal changes as the cause of symptoms, and if other causes have been ruled out (comorbidities, medication, thyroid disease), then a first step would include an FSH, LH, and prolactin level as well as estradiol levels in women and morning testosterone levels in men. Of note, current data tend to focus on cisgender patients, and the language used in these two sections follow from the available data. However, we believe it is reasonable, until newer data are available, applying these data to patients of all genders based on the sex organs each patient may have.

Table 10.1 Common cancer treatment modalities and associated side effects related to sexual and reproductive health

Cancer type	Treatment modality			
	Surgery	Chemotherapy	Radiation therapy	Hormonal therapy
Breast	Breast removal, disfigurement, scarring can lead to negative body image, decreased desire Diminished tissue/nipple sensitivity Pain Oophorectomy in those at increased hereditary risk can lead to menopausal symptoms Lymphedema can cause pain, swelling	Can affect ovarian function Hair loss/body image concerns Fatigue can affect desire, confidence	Scarring, disfigurement Possible pain, scarring, swelling	Can induce menopausal symptoms Vaginal dryness, pain
Ovarian/uterine/cervical cancer	Adhesions, scarring can lead to pain Removal of ovaries leads to drop in hormone levels Potential adverse effects on fertility Diminished vaginal/cervical and/or clitoral sensitivity which may impact ability to achieve orgasm Possible bowel/bladder dysfunction from nerve involvement	Fatigue, loss of interest in sex	Can lead to loss of ovarian function (menopausal symptoms) May affect fertility status Could lead to vaginal scarring, shortening	
Testicular cancer	Removal of testes and resulting hypogonadism Potential for nerve damage effecting ejaculation		Loss of testicular function	
Prostate cancer	Surgery can lead to erectile dysfunction		Can affect vascular supply; lead to erectile dysfunction At risk for radiation cystitis, proctitis	Androgen deprivation can lead to hypogonadism, decreased sexual desire, arousal Development of gynecomastia leading to body image concerns

(continued)

Table 10.1 (continued)

Cancer type	Treatment modality			
	Surgery	Chemotherapy	Radiation therapy	Hormonal therapy
Colorectal cancer	*Adhesions, scarring can lead to pain* *Potential for damage to nerves affecting ability to achieve orgasm, ejaculation* *Stomas could lead to body image/intimacy concerns*	*Fatigue can affect sexual desire/ confidence* *Mucositis could affect oral or vaginal tissue* [25]	*Potential for scarring* *Could lead to vaginal dryness/ irritation, erectile dysfunction*	
Leukemia/ lymphoma[a]		*Fatigue* *Potential adverse effects on heart, lungs, fertility, ovarian function*	*Chest radiation could increase risk for breast cancer*	

[a]Additional consideration for leukemia/lymphoma is the use of bone marrow/stem cell transplant, which can lead to graft versus host disease (GVHD), which could affect vaginal mucosa [28]

Considerations to Manage Hormonally Mediated Symptoms in Patients with Female Sex Organs

In general patients who are premenopausal at the time of cancer diagnosis and receive treatment that induces a menopausal state will experience more intense menopausal symptoms than women who have already entered into menopause at the time of diagnosis and treatment. For women who have received chemotherapy, who are on tamoxifen or who have had radiation affecting the ovaries, FSH may not be helpful to confirm menopause [22], but estradiol levels can be used to follow hormone levels and to help assess ovarian function; anti-mullerian hormone (AMH) may be another marker useful for the latter purpose [22]. The presence of irregular menses alone after cancer treatment does not confirm loss of ovarian function and therefore does not rule out the possibility of becoming pregnant.

For the treatment of hot flashes in women, considerations include both nonhormonal medications, hormone therapy, and strategies that do not involve the use of medications:

- Serotonin-specific reuptake inhibitors (SSRIs) or serotonin norepinephrine reuptake inhibitors (SNRIs) may be considered and generally can be given in lower doses than those required for the treatment of depression or anxiety. The use of SSRIs for the treatment of hot flashes in women who are also on tamoxifen therapy has been controversial. Because SSRI medications can block the cytochrome P450 2D6 (CYP2D6) pathway, the concern is that the activity of tamoxifen could be lowered through blockage of the conversion of tamoxifen to its active metabolite through this pathway. In 2006 the Food and Drug Administration (FDA) issued a warning on the label of tamoxifen indicating that postmenopausal women with breast cancer who are concomitantly using medications that block CYP2D6 activity may be at increased risk for breast cancer recurrence. Since that time, a large cohort study of early stage breast cancer patients on tamoxifen followed for up to 14 years did not find any statistically significant association with the use of any antidepressant, and specifically paroxetine and fluoxetine, with breast cancer recurrence [29]. However caution is still advised and if available, alternatives to SSRI therapy for the use of hot flashes in those on tamoxifen therapy should be considered [22, 30].
- Other nonhormonal therapies that could be considered, though with limited data in cancer survivors, include gabapentin [31, 32] and pregabalin [33], both anticonvulsants, and clonidine, an alpha-agonist blood pressure-lowering medication [34–36].
- In general, hormone therapy, including use of estrogen and/or progesterone, should be avoided for women who have a history of hormonally mediated cancers [22, 30]. For women who do not have a history of hormonally mediated cancers, use can be considered but the same contraindications (history of blood clot, history of abnormal vaginal bleeding, chronic liver disease, pregnancy) and precautions (smoking, cardiovascular disease, genetic predisposition to cancer).
- Acupuncture, yoga, regular exercise, loss of weight for individuals that are overweight/obese, and cognitive behavioral therapy could be considered.

- The use of dietary supplements such as vitamin E and black cohosh, and phytoestrogens have not been extensively studied in cancer survivors [22].

The vaginal atrophy that results from antiestrogen-directed therapies can not only cause discomfort interfering with sexual activity but increase risk for lichen sclerosus, which can cause not only irritative symptoms and tearing but can ultimately increase the risk for vulvar cancer [27]. This condition can be managed with topical corticosteroids or calcineurin inhibitors, and referral to a specialist could be considered. Periodic pelvic examinations are therefore an important part of the clinical assessment for women experiencing vaginal or vulvar symptoms related to hormonal changes:

- Therapies for vaginal dryness include vaginal moisturizers and lubricants. Whereas vaginal lubricants are intended to be used to increase comfort during sexual activity, vaginal moisturizers work best when used regularly to maintain the integrity of the vaginal mucosa [27].
- The use of localized vaginal hormonal therapy (estrogen, progesterone, and testosterone) may be appropriate to treat localized vaginal symptoms, with input of the primary oncology team.
- Vaginal dilators may be helpful if scarring, stenosis, or pain has occurred as a result of therapy (i.e., radiation therapy or adhesions related to surgery) [23].

Pelvic physical therapy can be helpful across multiple domains of sexual function, including arousal and physical functioning. Some treatments are available for the general population but have not been adequately studied in cancer, such as ospemifene, an estrogen receptor modulator approved for the treatment of postmenopausal dyspareunia, and flibanserin, a mixed $5\text{-}HT_{1A}$ agonist/$5\text{-}HT_{2A}$ antagonist that has been approved to treat hypoactive sexual desire disorder in premenopausal women.

Considerations to Manage Hormonally Mediated Symptoms in Patients with Male Sex Organs

Men receiving androgen deprivation therapy (ADT) are the most likely to experience symptoms directly related to a drop in circulating hormone levels, chiefly testosterone, resulting in hypogonadism. Hypogonadism can also develop in men who have received pelvic/testicular radiation or orchiectomy (primary hypogonadism) as well as cranial radiation which can affect the hypothalamic-pituitary axis (secondary hypogonadism):

- If hot flashes are problematic, androgen (testosterone replacement) as well as estrogen therapy can be used, but these are contraindicated in men with hormonally mediated cancers (prostate, breast cancer). Androgen replacement therapy can be considered in patients who are considered disease free from prostate cancer, as well as in those who were treated for other types of cancers and experience hypogonadism as a late effect. Men on active surveillance for prostate cancer or who are on ADT should **not** be considered for testosterone replacement therapy [22].

- In men eligible for testosterone replacement therapy (in general testosterone levels less than 300 ng/dL and not otherwise contraindicated as described above), this can help with physical sexual function:

  - Blood counts need to be monitored regularly as testosterone therapy can increase serum hematocrit levels to a dangerous level in approximately 2–20% of cases, depending on the formulation used [23].
  - Those who have expressed a desire to have children in the future testosterone therapy may have a suppressive effect on the hypothalamic pituitary axis [23]. Consultation with a reproductive medicine specialist may be appropriate.

- Erectile dysfunction (erectile dysfunction) is just one of the possible symptoms of hypogonadism. It is important first to rule out and treat other potential causes of ED, such as diabetes or vascular disease, and to provide counseling to reduce risk factors (e.g., hypertension, smoking):

  - Phosphodiesterase type 5 inhibitors (PDE5i) (examples include sildenafil (Viagra), tadalafil (Cialis), or vardenafil (Levitra)) are considered first-line therapies and can be used either on an as-needed basis or in low daily doses.
  - The efficacy of PDE5i therapy may be reduced in individuals who have diabetes or have undergone extensive pelvic surgery, as both can affect nerve function [23].
  - Testosterone replacement therapy may be used along with PDE5i therapy [23].
  - Other therapies to consider include vacuum devices, penile injection therapy, or intraurethral prostaglandin suppositories [23, 27].

- Similar to women who experience symptoms of hot flashes, nonhormonal and non-pharmacologic therapies may also be considered for relief of vasomotor symptoms in men, with the same caveats as to the limited evidence base for effectiveness for many treatments such as supplements. Venlafaxine and gabapentin are the only therapies that have been studied for this purpose in males [26].
- For gynecomastia, surgery or RT can be considered (though RT should be discussed as a preventive measure).

Relationship and Body Image Concerns [30]

Cancer treatment can lead to many changes in a survivor's appearance, including weight changes decreased muscle mass, scarring, hair loss, and limb amputation. Survivors with pre-existing depression and or body image issues may be at higher risk of developing body image issues that affect their quality of life.

Healthcare providers should ask about body image concerns early in the treatment and then reassess concerns often throughout the cancer care continuum. Such discussions should account for social, cultural, and religious variations. The most effective intervention when concerns arise is psychosocial counseling for the survivor. If partnered, couples-based interventions are also very effective. However, permission from the survivor should be sought prior to any discussions with the partner by the healthcare provider.

Survivors Diagnosed with Cancer as a Child, Adolescent, or Young Adult (CAYA)

Though CAYA survivors make up a minority of overall cancer survivors in the United States [1], we now know a great deal about the long-term impact of cancer in this population. As a result, guidelines specific to this population are available and speak to the potential risks to overall health and need for ongoing surveillance long after cancer treatment is finished [37, 38]. Sexual health concerns are an important consideration for CAYA survivors and merit a discussion distinct from that of older cancer survivors due to unique phase of life activities for each of these groups. Here we will consider issues around the development of sexual identity, fertility, and surveillance for premature morbidity.

Development of Sexual Identity

An individual's sense of self and of sexual identity occurs through a series of important developmental stages beginning in childhood. For CAYA survivors, progression through these developmental stages can be significantly impacted by their cancer diagnosis and treatment [39]. Many factors contribute to this developmental process, including the building of personal relationships, learning about sexual issues and sexual health, physical development of sexual characteristics, educational attainment, and family relationships. A cancer diagnosis and associated treatment could generate disruptions in relation to any or all of these factors; CAYA survivors may have limited or even no experience with sexuality before their cancer diagnosis While receiving treatment, young people in school may miss out on opportunities to learn about sexual health with their peers or engage in romantic or intimate relationships, but at the same time may be presented with information about fertility, fertility preservation, or side effects that impact sexual development [39]. They may suffer from perceived social isolation if treatment requires missing peer social events or leaves them with scars, physical limitations, or neurocognitive changes. Comorbidities related to their cancer diagnosis, such a depression or body image concerns, may also affect the development of their sexual identity. Likewise, peers who have not had any personal experience with cancer may struggle with how to interact with CAYA survivors due to fear or misinformation about the disease [39]. Well-intentioned parents who became accustomed to having to speak and make decisions for their younger children may have difficulty letting go of this function as that child grows up or may persist in a protective role. This may interfere with an emerging adult's sense of independence and ability to fully explore his or her self-identity [39].

As primary care clinicians play an important role in the care of CAYA survivors once cancer treatment is completed and take on comprehensive aspects of care, it is vital for these providers to be prepared to recognize, assess, and provide assistance for sexual health concerns when appropriate. Strategies to help address sexual health and identify development concerns in CAYA survivors may include [39, 40]:

- Asking about the past cancer diagnosis and treatments received, including obtaining records to confirm treatment modalities and any complications or known late effects.
- Gaining an understanding of current sociodemographic status, including sexual activity and relationship status.
- Ensuring a safe, confidential atmosphere to discuss sexual concerns and invite questions.
- Validating and normalizing concerns if a CAYA survivor indicates distress about sexual inexperience.
- Providing opportunities for the CAYA survivor to practice decision making if not already doing so. This includes decisions about who they want to share information with, if of legal age.
- Providing education about sexual and reproductive health, including fertility preservation options, in a consistent and culturally appropriate manner regardless of sexual orientation. Fertility preservation options and information about contraception should be provided to eligible CAYA patients prior to the start of treatment [22].
- Referring for neuropsychological testing to identify potential deficits and consider appropriate strategies to address them.
- Offering opportunities to share stories or for peer mentoring. Mentoring relationships can help model adaptive coping behaviors and provide a sense of self-worth [39].

Fertility

The treatment of cancer may impact a survivor's fertility. Knowledge of fertility status after cancer treatment empowers patients to be able to have informed discussions with partners about family planning and the need for contraception to prevent unwanted pregnancies. Uncertainty about fertility status can impair social and sexual identity development in CAYA survivors.

The current data on the risk of infertility after cancer treatment is suboptimal. Most data in women is based on the surrogate marker of resumption of normal menses, for example, which we now know is not predictive of fertility. There is very limited data on the effects of novel agents and newer chemotherapy regimens.

Male cancer survivors tend to have recovery of spermatogenesis by 1 year off therapy, if they are going to recover. However, a small proportion of males may continue to have recovery over several years. Semen analysis is the gold standard to assess the effects of cancer therapy on spermatogenesis. The recommended time for semen analysis is 2 years since completion of therapy as well as sexually mature (at least Tanner Stage IV).

Female fertility continually declines over time as women age. Younger women may retain fertility after completion of therapy but then develop premature ovarian insufficiency before desired family building has been completed. With more frequent monitoring of women at high risk of infertility, oocytes could be harvested and cryopreserved as fertility is declining to allow for desired family building when the survivor is ready.

Recently, the International Late Effects of Childhood Cancer Guideline Harmonization Group (IGHG) developed consensus guidelines for gonadotoxicity surveillance for both male and female CAYA survivors [41, 42] which are summarized below.

Impaired Spermatogenesis

Patients exposed to alkylating agents or radiation to the testicles are at increased risk of impaired spermatogenesis. Semen analysis is the primary and direct surveillance modality and, as such, is the gold standard. Secondary surveillance modalities are indirect measures of spermatogenesis and include measurement of testicular volume, FSH, and inhibin B. For survivors unable to ejaculate, testicular sperm extraction or aspiration (TESE or TESA) are methods to evaluate for spermatogenesis within the testis.

Semen analysis after completion of therapy should allow for adequate time for recovery of spermatogenesis. The kinetics of spermatogenesis vary based on both the schedule and cumulative doses of chemotherapy and radiation [43]. As such, survivors are advised to delay semen analyses until at least 12 months from completion of therapy. Sperm count and quality often continue to improve as more time passes since completion of therapy. Childhood cancer survivors should be at least Tanner stage IV and report the ability to ejaculate before being referred for a semen analysis after completion of therapy. For males who have sperm-banked, assessing residual fertility may prevent the need to pay annual storage fees for the banked specimens.

Premature Ovarian Insufficiency (POI)

A study from the Childhood Cancer Survivor Study showed the cumulative incidence of nonsurgical premature menopause is 8% by age 40 years and is markedly increased compared to sibling controls. Independent risk factors for POI include procarbazine dose $\geq$4000 mg/m^2, any ovarian RT, and stem cell transplantation. Survivors with POI were less likely to ever be pregnant or have a live birth between the ages of 31 and 40 years of age [44].

The IGHG recommendations define POI as a clinical condition in any adult female at age <40 years characterized by absence of menstrual cycles for $\geq$4 months and 2 elevated FSH levels in the menopausal range. However, definitions of POI vary from study to study and between groups.

Surveillance for POI is recommended for female survivors who received any RT to the ovaries or any alkylating agents but particularly cyclophosphamide and procarbazine. Pre- or peripubertal survivors should be assessed for linear growth and pubertal development and progression. The menstrual history is important in postpubertal survivors, specifically asking about the presence and regularity of cycles. Unfortunately, regular menstrual cycles do not ensure fertility, just as an abnormal menstrual cycle does not translate into infertility.

Assessment of various hormone levels are used to monitor for POI. For postpubertal survivors, FSH and estradiol are recommended by the IGHG. However, these tests are an indirect measure of ovarian function. In addition, survivors must be off any hormone therapy (including hormone-based birth control) and are best interpreted on day 3 of a menstrual cycle, which can be challenging logistically.

Anti-mullerian hormone (AMH) is not recommended as the primary surveillance modality, although it may be reasonable to include in conjunction with FSH and estradiol. The benefits of AMH include its stability throughout the menstrual cycle, less cycle-to-cycle variability than FSH, and that it is a direct measure of oocytes remaining in the ovary. While AMH is widely used in infertility clinics to test ovarian reserve and guide IV management, the role of AMH in the general population is less clear [45, 46].

Testosterone Deficiency

Patients who have undergone RT exposing the testicles to more than 12 Gy (including TBI) are at risk of testosterone deficiency. CAYAs should be monitored for linear growth and pubertal development. A referral to a pediatric endocrinologist should be made if there are no signs of puberty by age 14. An early morning testosterone level may be monitored for those at risk. Luteinizing hormone (LH) levels may provide additional information in conjunction with a testosterone for survivors with clinical hypogonadism or previous low normal testosterone. There is a paucity of systematic data on when and how to replete testosterone so a referral to a male reproductive specialist (andrologist, endocrinologist, or urologist) should be made.

For the general population, infertility is defined as the inability to conceive after 12 months of regular unprotected intercourse. However, cancer survivors exposed to gonadotoxic therapy should be referred to reproductive endocrinologists after only 6 months of attempting to achieve pregnancy.

Conclusion

Among the unmet needs of individuals diagnosed with cancer, sexual health and fertility concerns are the most prevalent. The multiple modalities used to treat cancer can impact sexual health development and functioning in different ways and not only impact survivors but their intimate and romantic relationships as well. It is crucial that clinicians be proactive and screen their patients for symptoms related to sexual dysfunction, for distress around sexual functioning, and for late effects on reproductive health as support and resources are available to help.

Resource List

1. NCCN Guidelines: AYA & Supportive Care guidelines, www.nccn.org
2. American Society of Clinical Oncology, Patient & Survivor Care guidelines, https://www.asco.org
3. The Oncofertility Consortium: oncofertility.northwestern.edu
4. The Sexual Medicine Society of North America: www.sexhealthmatters.org
5. International Society for the Study of Women's Health: www.isswsh.org
6. American Association of Sexuality Educators, Counselors and Therapists: www.aasect.org
7. American Society for Clinical Oncology resources for patients: www.cancer.net
8. National LGBT Cancer Project: https://Lgbtcancer.org

References

1. Miller KD, Siegel RL, Lin CC, et al. Cancer treatment and survivorship statistics, 2016. CA Cancer J Clin. 2016;66(4):271–89.
2. Park E, Bober S, Campbell E, Recklitis C, Kutner J, Diller L. General internist communication about sexual function with cancer survivors. J Gen Intern Med. 2009;24(2):407–11.
3. Bober SL, Varela VS. Sexuality in adult cancer survivors: challenges and intervention. J Clin Oncol. 2012;30(30):3712–9.
4. Derogatis LR, Kourlesis SM. An approach to evaluation of sexual problems in the cancer patient. CA Cancer J Clin. 1981;31(1):46–50.
5. Stanford JL, Feng Z, Hamilton AS, et al. Urinary and sexual function after radical prostatectomy for clinically localized prostate cancer: the prostate cancer outcomes study. JAMA. 2000;283(3):354–60.
6. Ganz PA, Rowland JH, Desmond K, Meyerowitz BE, Wyatt GE. Life after breast cancer: understanding women's health-related quality of life and sexual functioning. J Clin Oncol. 1998;16(2):501–14.
7. Jabson J, Kamen CS. Sexual minority cancer survivors' satisfaction with care. J Psychosoc Oncol. 2016;34(1–2):28–38.
8. Obedin-Maliver J. Time to change: supporting sexual and gender minority people—an underserved, understudied cancer risk population. J Natl Compr Canc Netw. 2017;15(11): 1305–8.

9. Hudson J, Schabath MB, Sanchez J, et al. Sexual and gender minority issues across NCCN guidelines: results from a national survey. J Natl Compr Canc Netw JNCCN. 2017;15(11):1379–82.
10. Kamen C. Lesbian, Gay, Bisexual, and Transgender (LGBT) Survivorship. Semin Oncol Nurs. 2018;34(1):52–59. https://doi.org/10.1016/j.soncn.2017.12.002. Epub 2017 Dec 21. PMID: 29275016; PMCID: PMC5811352
11. Flynn KE, Lin L, Cyranowski JM, Reeve BB, Reese JB, Jeffery DD, Smith AW, Porter LS, Dombeck CB, Bruner DW, Keefe FJ, Weinfurt KP. Development of the NIH PROMIS ® Sexual Function and Satisfaction measures in patients with cancer. J Sex Med. 2013;10 Suppl 1(0 1):43–52. https://doi.org/10.1111/j.1743-6109.2012.02995.x. PMID: 23387911; PMCID: PMC3729213.
12. Bober SL, Reese JB, Barbera L, Bradford A, Carpenter KM, Goldfarb S, Carter J. How to ask and what to do: a guide for clinical inquiry and intervention regarding female sexual health after cancer. Curr Opin Support Palliat Care. 2016;10(1):44–54. https://doi.org/10.1097/SPC.0000000000000186. PMID: 26716390; PMCID: PMC4984532.
13. Rosen R, Brown C, Heiman J, Leiblum S, Meston C, Shabsigh R, Ferguson D, D'Agostino R Jr. The Female Sexual Function Index (FSFI): a multidimensional self-report instrument for the assessment of female sexual function. J Sex Marital Ther. 2000;26(2):191–208. https://doi.org/10.1080/009262300278597. PMID: 10782451.
14. Cappelleri JC, Rosen RC. The Sexual Health Inventory for Men (SHIM): a 5-year review of research and clinical experience. Int J Impot Res. 2005;17(4):307–19. https://doi.org/10.1038/sj.ijir.3901327. PMID: 15875061.
15. Althof SE, Parish SJ. Clinical interviewing techniques and sexuality questionnaires for male and female cancer patients. J Sex Med. 2013;10 Suppl 1:35–42.
16. Quinn MM, Letourneau JM, Rosen MP. Contraception after cancer treatment: describing methods, counseling, and unintended pregnancy risk. Contraception. 2014;89(5):466–71.
17. Appelman-Dijkstra NM, Kokshoorn NE, Dekkers OM, et al. Pituitary dysfunction in adult patients after cranial radiotherapy: systematic review and meta-analysis. J Clin Endocrinol Metab. 2011;96(8):2330–40.
18. Darzy KH. Radiation-induced hypopituitarism. Curr Opin Endocrinol Diabetes Obes. 2013;20(4):342–53.
19. Ribi K, Luo W, Bernhard J, et al. Adjuvant tamoxifen plus ovarian function suppression versus tamoxifen alone in premenopausal women with early breast cancer: patient-reported outcomes in the suppression of ovarian function trial. J Clin Oncol. 2016;34(14):1601–10.
20. Frechette D, Paquet L, Verma S, et al. The impact of endocrine therapy on sexual dysfunction in postmenopausal women with early stage breast cancer: encouraging results from a prospective study. Breast Cancer Res Treat. 2013;141(1):111–7.
21. Armenian SH, Hudson MM, Mulder RL, et al. Recommendations for cardiomyopathy surveillance for survivors of childhood cancer: a report from the international late effects of childhood cancer guideline harmonization group. Lancet Oncol. 2015;16(3):e123–36.
22. Denlinger CS, Sanft T, Baker KS, et al. Survivorship, version 2.2017, NCCN clinical practice guidelines in oncology. J Natl Compr Canc Netw. 2017;15(9):1140–63.
23. Goldfarb S, Mulhall J, Nelson C, Kelvin J, Dickler M, Carter J. Sexual and reproductive health in cancer survivors. Semin Oncol. 2013;40(6):726–44.
24. Pettus JA, Carver B, Masterson T, Stasi J, Sheinfeld J. Preservation of ejaculation in patients undergoing nerve-sparing post-chemotherapy retroperitoneal lymph node dissection for metastatic testicular cancer. Urology. 2009;73(2):328–32.
25. Averyt JC, Nishimoto PW. Addressing sexual dysfunction in colorectal cancer survivorship care. J Gastrointest Oncol. 2014;5(5):388–94.
26. Denlinger CS, Barsevick AM. The challenges of colorectal cancer survivorship. J Natl Compr Canc Netw. 2009;7(8):883–94.
27. Zhou ES, Frederick NN, Bober SL. Hormonal changes and sexual dysfunction. Med Clin North Am. 2017;101(6):1135–50.

28. Guida M, Castaldi MA, Rosamilio R, Giudice V, Orio F, Selleri C. Reproductive issues in patients undergoing hematopoietic stem cell transplantation: an update. J Ovarian Res. 2016;9:72.
29. Haque R, Shi J, Schottinger JE, et al. Tamoxifen and antidepressant drug interaction among a cohort of 16 887 breast cancer survivors. JNCI J Natl Cancer Instit. 2016;108(3):djv337.
30. Carter J, Lacchetti C, Andersen BL, et al. Interventions to address sexual problems in people with cancer: American Society of Clinical Oncology clinical practice guideline adaptation of Cancer Care Ontario guideline. J Clin Oncol:JCO.2017.2075.8995.
31. Butt DA, Lock M, Lewis JE, Ross S, Moineddin R. Gabapentin for the treatment of menopausal hot flashes: a randomized controlled trial. Menopause. 2008;15(2):310–8.
32. Pandya KJ, Morrow GR, Roscoe JA, et al. Gabapentin for hot flashes in 420 women with breast cancer: a randomised double-blind placebo-controlled trial. Lancet. 2005;366(9488):818–24.
33. Loprinzi CL, Qin R, Baclueva EP, et al. Phase III, randomized, double-blind, placebo-controlled evaluation of pregabalin for alleviating hot flashes, N07C1. J Clin Oncol. 2010;28(4):641–7.
34. Using the medicine clonidine to treat hot flashes in breast cancer patients taking tamoxifen. Ann Intern Med. 2000;132(10):788.
35. L'Espérance S, Frenette S, Dionne A, Dionne J-Y. Pharmacological and non-hormonal treatment of hot flashes in breast cancer survivors: CEPO review and recommendations. Support Care Cancer. 2013;21(5):1461–74.
36. Goldberg RM, Loprinzi CL, O'Fallon JR, et al. Transdermal clonidine for ameliorating tamoxifen-induced hot flashes. J Clin Oncol. 1994;12(1):155–8.
37. Landier W, Bhatia S, Eshelman DA, et al. Development of risk-based guidelines for pediatric cancer survivors: the Children's Oncology Group long-term follow-up guidelines from the Children's Oncology Group Late Effects Committee and Nursing Discipline. J Clin Oncol. 2004;22(24):4979–90.
38. Kremer LCM, Mulder RL, Oeffinger KC, et al. A worldwide collaboration to harmonize guidelines for the long-term follow-up of childhood and young adult cancer survivors: a report from the International Late Effects Of Childhood Cancer Guideline Harmonization Group. Pediatr Blood Cancer. 2013;60(4):10.1002/pbc.24445.
39. Evan EE, Kaufman M, Cook AB, Zeltzer LK. Sexual health and self-esteem in adolescents and young adults with cancer. Cancer. 2006;107(7):1672–9.
40. Aubin S, Perez S. The clinician's toolbox: assessing the sexual impacts of cancer on adolescents and young adults with cancer (AYAC). Sex Med. 2015;3(3):198–212.
41. Skinner R, Mulder RL, Kremer LC, et al. Recommendations for gonadotoxicity surveillance in male childhood, adolescent, and young adult cancer survivors: a report from the International Late Effects of Childhood Cancer Guideline Harmonization Group in collaboration with the PanCareSurFup Consortium. Lancet Oncol. 2017;18(2):e75–90.
42. van Dorp W, Mulder RL, Kremer LCM, et al. Recommendations for premature ovarian insufficiency surveillance for female survivors of childhood, adolescent, and young adult cancer: a report from the International Late Effects of Childhood Cancer Guideline Harmonization Group in Collaboration with the PanCareSurFup Consortium. J Clin Oncol. 2016;34(28):3440–50.
43. Meistrich ML. The effects of chemotherapy and radiotherapy on spermatogenesis in humans. Fertil Steril. 2013;100(5). https://doi.org/10.1016/j.fertnstert.2013.1008.1010.
44. Levine JM, Whitton JA, Ginsberg JP, et al. Nonsurgical premature menopause and reproductive implications in survivors of childhood cancer: a report from the Childhood Cancer Survivor Study. Cancer. 2018;124:1044–52.
45. Tobler KJ, Shoham G, Christianson MS, Zhao Y, Leong M, Shoham Z. Use of anti-mullerian hormone for testing ovarian reserve: a survey of 796 infertility clinics worldwide. J Assist Reprod Genet. 2015;32(10):1441–8.
46. Steiner AZ, Pritchard D, Stanczyk FZ, et al. Association between biomarkers of ovarian reserve and infertility among older women of reproductive age. JAMA. 2017;318(14):1367–76.

Chapter 11
Patients with Physical, Intellectual and Developmental Disabilities

Jennifer M. LeComte and Alexis Tchaconas

Contents

Introduction

Sexual and reproductive health needs should be incorporated into routine care for patients across their lifespan. Unfortunately, sexual and reproductive health needs are often neglected for individuals with physical, intellectual, and developmental disabilities. Primary care clinicians have an opportunity to provide comprehensive care to this vulnerable population in order to optimize their overall health and wellness. This chapter will address the needs of this complex population by offering insight into the problems of limited sexuality education, understanding the risk of

J. M. LeComte (✉)
RISN/GIM, Rowan University School of Osteopathic Medicine, Sewell, NJ, USA
e-mail: lecomte@rowan.edu

A. Tchaconas
Internal Medicine/Pediatrics, The Mount Sinai Hospital, New York, NY, USA
e-mail: alexis.tchaconas@mountsinai.org

© Springer Nature Switzerland AG 2022
J. Truglio et al. (eds.), *Sexual and Reproductive Health*,
https://doi.org/10.1007/978-3-030-94632-6_11

abuse, addressing alternative approaches to ensuring access to preventative sexual health and routine screenings, and maximizing the opportunities for healthy relationships.

Physical, Intellectual, and Developmental Disabilities

This chapter focuses on patients living with physical, intellectual, and developmental disabilities that manifest initially in childhood and are often part of a genetic syndrome. Chapter 12 of this book focuses on acquired physical disabilities.

Disabilities are a spectrum of conditions that impact the functioning of the body or mind in ways that limit an individual's ability to perform certain activities or engage with their surroundings [1]. Generally, disabilities are categorized into the domains of function that they impact – physical, intellectual, and developmental. The CDC reports that one in four adults in the United States has a disability, with intellectual disability being the most common among younger adults and physical disability being the most common for middle age to older adults [1]. It is important to note that there are wide ranges of ability and impairment in each domain of function among different disabilities. Accordingly, clinicians should avoid making assumptions about patients with disabilities and thoroughly evaluate each patient to assess their level of functioning.

A physical disability is any impairment of the body that affects mobility, coordination, or sensation. These disabilities are multifactorial in etiology, including genetic and acquired. In the United States, about 16% of the population has a physical disability [2].

Intellectual disability is characterized by significant impairment in intellectual functioning, which includes reasoning, learning, and problem solving, as well as adaptive behavior, which involves social and practical skills, presenting before 18 years of age [3]. About 1–3% of the general population has significant intellectual disability, with a predominance of cases affecting males [4]. Intellectual disability can be associated with various disorders including Down syndrome, cerebral palsy, autism, and spina bifida. Approximately 85% of youth with intellectual disability are classified as mild intellectual disability, defined as an intelligence quotient (IQ) between 50 and 69 [5]. These individuals tend to only require intermittent support during times of uncertainty [3]. About 10% of youth with intellectual disability are in the moderate range with IQ scores between 36 and 49 [3]. They can perform basic self-care and simple chores, socialize appropriately, and typically remain with the family but in some cases can live independently with moderate support in group home settings [5]. About 5% of individuals with intellectual disability require substantial support for daily activities, which constitute severe (IQ 20–35) and profound (IQ < 20) intellectual disability [5].

Developmental disabilities are a broad category of chronic impairments in physical and/or intellectual function, including intellectual disability, which present before age 22 during the "developmental period" [6].

Education and Anticipatory Guidance for Sexual and Reproductive Health

Sexuality is an expansive topic that incorporates both physical and emotional health with underlying tones of personal and societal values and expectations. Sexual development unfolds throughout childhood, adolescence, and adulthood in a variety of ways, drawing on portrayals of relationships and sexuality in their environment [7]. The Position Statement published in 2008 and reaffirmed in 2013 by The Arc, a national community-based organization serving people with intellectual and developmental disabilities and their families, and the American Academy for Intellectual and Developmental Disabilities (AAIDD) powerfully articulated the issues around sexuality for people with intellectual and/or developmental disabilities. It states:

> For decades, people with intellectual and/or developmental disabilities have been thought to be asexual, having no need for loving and fulfilling relationships with others. Individual rights to sexuality, which is essential to human health and well-being, have been denied. This loss has negatively affected people with intellectual disability in gender identity, friendships, self-esteem, body image and awareness, emotional growth, and social behavior. People with intellectual or developmental disabilities frequently lack access to appropriate sex education in schools and other settings. At the same time, some individuals may engage in sexual activity as a result of poor options, manipulation, loneliness or physical force rather than as an expression of their sexuality. [8]

As children age and mature, clinicians routinely provide them and their families with anticipatory guidance about the next stages of development. Just before the adolescent stage, clinicians begin to use various tools to address the impending changes with the onset of puberty and the social challenges that accompany those changes. Unfortunately, for patients with special healthcare needs, including those with chronic conditions and physical and cognitive disabilities, the standard of care is often delayed or avoided completely. However, education about sexuality should be comprehensive for all.

The role of the primary care clinician is to help patients with intellectual and developmental disabilities understand and respond appropriately to the changes, challenges, and feelings that they encounter. Clinicians should encourage families and community members to provide education and opportunities to develop confidence and self-esteem to help build healthy relationships [9]. This can be achieved using developmentally appropriate communication techniques, supporting patient privacy to provide appropriate autonomy, and promoting safe expression of sexuality.

Developmentally Appropriate Communication

While clinicians must recognize the physical development of each patient with regard to their chronologic age, communication methods should be geared towards the developmental age of the patient. For example, clinicians can direct families to initiate changes in hygiene routine using social stories. There are several resources available including a puberty and adolescence toolkit for parents of children with autism from Autism Speaks that can help start discussions about sexual maturity related to body parts, changes in hygiene needs and routines, as well as the social consequences of neglecting such tasks which are often misunderstood by patients with intellectual and developmental disabilities [9]. Picture exchange communication systems and guidance from allied health professionals like occupational therapists can help patients embrace privacy and promote additional opportunities for developing healthy relationships.

Supporting Patient Privacy and Appropriate Autonomy

For people with a disability or chronic condition, limited privacy and a high degree of physical intrusion seem to be routine. If a patient uses attendant services, lives in a group home, or is not able to maintain personal care independently, privacy is viewed very differently, and intrusion is often inappropriately tolerated. Individuals with disabilities may also experience invasions of privacy and personal space by family members and acquaintances, often due perceptions of being affectionate or requiring more affection than their typical peers [10]. Such experiences can be traumatic and can also interfere with the development of an appropriate understanding of privacy.

Clinicians can model respect for patient privacy during each encounter, much the same way this is modeled for typically developing younger children and adolescents. Simple examples include asking for permission before performing physical exam maneuvers and the appropriate use of drapes. Teaching about private parts is introduced early but needs to be reiterated throughout adolescence and beyond using developmentally appropriate language. Given the limited opportunities for patients to practice self-advocacy in their daily lives, clinicians need to reinforce modesty skills in the office, which can be taught via modeling behaviors that exhibit a respect for privacy and sharing information. Families, caregivers, and allied health professionals can continue to support respect for privacy by teaching patients to take care of their own private parts (i.e., bathing, wiping after bathroom use) so they do not have to rely on adults or older children for help; this requires reinforcement throughout the lifespan for many individuals with intellectual and developmental disabilities.

Promoting Safe Expression of Sexuality

Patients with intellectual and/or developmental disabilities are at times assumed to be asexual and at other times assumed to by hypersexual. Both assumptions are inaccurate and ignore the need for appropriate development and expression of sexuality for all patients.

The Position Statement on sexuality from The Arc and the AAIDD [8] highlights the rights of patients with respect to sexuality, stating individuals have a right to:

- Sexual expression and education, reflective of their own cultural, religious, and moral values and of social responsibility.
- Individualized education and information to encourage informed decision-making, including education about such issues as reproduction, marriage and family life, abstinence, safe sexual practices, sexual orientation, sexual abuse, and sexually transmitted diseases.
- Protection from sexual harassment and from physical, sexual, and emotional abuse.

People with intellectual, developmental, and physical disabilities have the desire and the right to develop and express their sexuality. Some studies have shown the level of sexual activity is not significantly related to the severity of disability [11]. All are capable of having relationships and "enjoying the sensation that comes from being respected and loved" [12]. They have the right to be emotionally and physically involved with an appropriate partner. Issues involving informed consent and guardianship need to be addressed when supporting patients with intellectual and developmental disabilities. When partners mutually agree to pursue a more intimate relationship, they should expect those around them to facilitate that by offering as much privacy as needed when asked. In addition, people with disabilities often need to plan for romantic physical experiences as they may need to alter their bowel or bladder regimens or modify medication to reduce spasticity prior to the activity. While this decreases the ability to be spontaneous, it does not reduce the need for privacy and intimacy. When limits or restrictions are placed on private sexual expression, sexual activity can move into inappropriate settings. Research conducted by the Center for Research on Women with Disabilities (CROWD) through the National Study of Women with Physical Disabilities found that 41% of the women with disabilities believed that they did not have adequate information about how their disability affects their sexual functioning [11]. Sexual functioning and behavior should be addressed not just to prevent pregnancy and sexually transmitted infections (STIs), but to reassure individuals that they can be sexually active by providing them with the knowledge, resources and dignity afforded to their typically developing peers [13].

Inherent in this approach is assessing for and reducing the risk of sexual abuse and exploitation. An approach to sexual abuse and intimate partner violence in patients in various age groups is presented in Part I of this book. This approach may need to be modified for patients with intellectual or physical disabilities. People with a physical or intellectual disability are up to four times more likely of being sexually abused than peers without disability, regardless of their gender or age [10, 14–16]. Adolescents with developmental disabilities seem to be at the highest risk of sexual assault and acquaintance rape [14]. The risk of abuse is due to many factors including limited education and decision making, dependence on others for basic care including care that often results in public exposure, increased exposure to a large number of caregivers and settings, inappropriate social skills, inability to seek help or report abuse, and lack of strategies to defend themselves against abuse [15]. The realization of such vulnerability may lead parents to increase protection of their children, both young and old, from unsupervised social contacts and even from knowledge about sex. In order to protect and prevent abuse, clinicians and caregivers need to be aware of the problem of abuse and report any concerns or signs of abuse. The Abuse Assessment Screen-Disability (AAS-D) form, which was developed by McFarlane in 2001 and is available on the American College of Obstetrics and Gynecology (ACOG) website [17], uses the following questions:

1. Within the last year, have you been hit, slapped, kicked, pushed, shoved, or otherwise physically hurt by someone?
2. Within the last year, has anyone forced you to have sexual activities?
3. Within the last year, has anyone prevented you from using a wheelchair, cane, respirator, or other assistive devices?
4. Within the last year, has anyone you depend on refused to help you with an important personal need, such as taking your medicine, getting to the bathroom, getting out of bed, bathing, getting dressed, or getting food or drink?

    If yes to any of the questions above, who? Intimate partner, care provider, health professional, family member, other (e.g., stranger, clergy)?

In addition to screening, clinicians can provide education and opportunities to promote and enhance self-determination and self-preservation [16]. These practices will ultimately support healthy and safe sexual development for patients with intellectual disabilities and developmental delays.

Reproductive Health Exams

An approach to age-appropriate cancer screening and screenings for sexually transmitted infections are presented in Part I and Chap. 6 of this book, respectively. Such reproductive health assessments and preventative care should be offered to patients with intellectual disabilities and developmental delays. Unfortunately, there are many barriers to appropriate screening for patients with disabilities, including accessibility, a lack of prioritizing routine screening in patients with seemingly complex conditions as well as patient and families' concerns regarding symptoms during the exam such as anxiety, spasticity, imbalance, and autonomic dysreflexia.

Clinicians who assume patients with disabilities are not sexually active may not screen for sexually transmitted infections (STIs) or educate them about safe sex practices. Patients with disabilities may not detect signs and symptoms of STIs, or they may mistake the symptoms for other common complications of their chronic conditions like urinary tract infections. For these reasons and more, primary care clinicians must be intentional in enhancing access to reproductive health exams for patients with disabilities. ACOG has an interactive site for clinicians serving women with disabilities. The site includes a recorded slide show, *Reproductive Health Care for Women with Disabilities*, to guide physicians to provide the preventative care that all women need while addressing the unique approaches one might need to accommodate women with physical, developmental, and cognitive disabilities [18].

Cervical Cancer Screening

Cervical cancer screening, when performed at recommended intervals, can prevent at least 70% of cervical cancers [19]. Current guidelines for screening patients at average risk for cervical cancer are discussed in Parts I and III of this book. These guidelines apply to all patients with a uterus and cervix, regardless of gender identity, sexual practices, or presence of an intellectual or physical disability. Patients with disabilities are just as likely to get cervical cancer as the general population and yet are less likely than those without a disability to receive appropriate screening [20]. Clinicians need to be aware of accommodations and possible complications when performing pelvic exams, but these factors should not preclude doing the exam.

Patients with mobility issues may need accommodations in order to perform a pelvic exam. They may require adjustable exam tables or need assistance in getting into a comfortable position. The typical pelvic exam position may increase spasticity for some patients with mobility disabilities. Variations for the pelvic exam includes the knee-chest position, which is good for patients who need to lie on their side, and the diamond-shaped position and V-shaped position, in which women lie on their backs and the speculum is inserted with the handle up. Physicians can also use the lithotomy position to provide increased support [21].

If accommodations for positioning and the performance of the pelvic exam are not discussed ahead of time, patients with a spinal cord injury or other neurologic impairments may be at increased the risk for experiencing autonomic dysreflexia. Autonomic dysreflexia is a response to painful stimuli below the spinal cord lesion. The patient is not able to feel pain, but the body recognizes it as painful. Signs and symptoms of autonomic dysreflexia include headache, sweating, and piloerection above the level of the lesion, nasal stuffiness, facial flushing, papillary dilatation, rapid heart rate, arrhythmias, and labile hypertension that could be life-threatening.

CROWD has information [22] to prepare clinicians for examining patients at risk for autonomic dysreflexia. For some patients with mobility impairments, there is an increased need to monitor for organ prolapse because it can occur at a younger age. Some patients may require a referral for genetic counseling depending on their chronic condition. In general, it may take additional accommodations and more time to obtain a history and examine a patient with physical, intellectual or developmental disabilities, but anticipating the patient's needs will improve the experience for all involved.

For patients who are unable to speak, nonverbal communication techniques and gestures can be established so that the patient can inform the clinician when to "wait" or "stop."

For those rare circumstances for when an exam cannot be performed, for example, when congenital strictures in the vaginal opening prevent the ability to safely perform a speculum exam, HPV testing and/or pelvic ultrasound may be considered as alternatives. Data suggest that when a speculum cannot be used, the blind technique with liquid cytology and/or HPV testing could be an alternative approach [23].

Screening for Breast Cancer

Breast cancer is the most common cancer in women, projected to account for 30% of new cancer diagnoses in American women this year [24]. This is also true for women with disabilities, yet they are less likely to receive appropriate screening for breast cancer [25]. According to data from the Office on Disability of the US Department of Health and Human Services, 68% of women older than 40 years without disabilities have had a mammogram, as compared to only 54% of women in that age group with a disability [26]. Studies also show higher mortality rates related to breast cancer among women with a disability, even when diagnosed at the same stage as women without a disability. Women with disabilities were less likely to undergo standard therapy after breast-conserving surgery than other women. Differences in treatment did not explain the differences in breast cancer mortality rates [27].

Barriers to breast cancer screening for women who have physical disabilities included lack of perceived susceptibility to cancer, preoccupation with other health issues, lack of accessible screening facilities and adaptable equipment, difficulty with positioning due to physical disability or sensory sensitivities, and provider knowledge and attitudes [28]. Primary care clinicians are in a unique position to overcome these barriers for their patients with intellectual and developmental disabilities. The American Association on Health and Disability developed a handout for women to be prepared for a mammogram including how to advocate for accommodations for specific disabilities [29]. The CDC also lead a campaign called "Breast Cancer Screening: *The Right to Know,*" which offers stories and resources to promote higher rates of screening among patients with disabilities [28].

Menstruation

A discussion about menstruation should happen prior to onset of menses. For patients with intellectual and developmental disabilities and their families, there can be significant anxiety about the impact menstruation will have on daily functioning. Autism Speaks addresses some of the sensitivity issues young women on the autism spectrum and/or with intellectual disabilities may encounter:

> Menstrual management for patients typically centers around family planning or treatment of symptoms such as dysmenorrhea and abnormal uterine bleeding. In patients with cognitive impairment and developmental delay additional considerations include hygiene, potential impact of menses on mood, and worsening of seizure disorders around the time of menses. [9]

Therapeutic amenorrhea is a common reason for patients with intellectual disability to seek sexual and reproductive health care, with some studies finding that over 60% of women with intellectual disability seek therapeutic amenorrhea at some point in their lives. When pursuing a treatment for menstrual management in patients with intellectual disability and developmental delay, there are several scenarios to consider. These include issues related to intellectual disability, issues related to physical comorbidities, and issues related to medication interactions. Chapter 5 of this book discusses contraception options in patients of all genders.

Patients with intellectual disability may find daily medications burdensome or difficult to remember. For these patients, longer-acting formulations may be preferred. These include depo-medroxyprogesterone acetate (DPMA) injectable and various patch, ring, and implantable forms of progesterone-only and estrogen-containing contraceptives. DPMA is easy to use and can achieve high rates of amenorrhea but can result in bone density loss in healthy adolescents, which may not reverse completely after discontinuation of the medication. Because of the risk to bone health, patients with mobility impairments, or exposures to certain medications, clinicians should consider evaluating baseline bone density with a dual energy X-ray absorptiometry (DEXA) scan and supplementation with calcium and vitamin D. Given the high prevalence of obesity across the population with disabilities, the risk of weight gain on DPMA should also play a role in the decision as to whether to use this agent [30].

Intrauterine devices (IUDs) represent another long-term option for many patients. Some patients with spinal cord injuries or neuromuscular conditions which effect sensation may consider avoiding the use of IUDs because of decreased ability to detect movement of the device away from its appropriate location in the uterus and autonomic dysreflexia. Spasticity of the lower extremities may also increase the difficulty of insertion of an IUD. Patients or their partners or caregivers must be able to assess the presence of the IUD string weekly [30].

Oral contraceptives pills (OCPs) are another common option for therapeutic amenorrhea. However, given that seizure disorders and epilepsy are common comorbidities in this population, it is important to remember that antiepileptic drugs

(AEDs) are the most common class of medications that interact with OCPs. In fact, the failure rate for standard oral contraceptive pills is estimated at 0.7 per 100 years in the general population and 3.1 per 100 years in women taking AEDs [31]. OCPs may also impact AED levels, with several studies finding that lamotrigine levels were reduced by up to 50% in women who take OCPs concurrently [32–35]. The mechanism appears to be that OCPs increase glucuronidation in the liver, which is the main metabolic pathway for elimination of lamotrigine and several other anti-epileptic drugs [36].

Contraception and Family Planning

The medical, social, and psychological issues related to pregnancy and a disability or chronic condition should be assessed prior to conception. All patients of reproductive age, including those with disabilities, should receive counseling about the potential effects of their chronic medical conditions, any medications, and their emotional/mental health may have on pregnancy-related outcomes. Discussion about options to alter dosages or switch to safer medications prior to conception and optimizing health conditions are essential before embarking on a pregnancy.

The choice and safety of effective contraception varies from person to person. As discussed above, patients with disabilities are sexually active and need to be offered contraception keeping in mind their unique needs. The World Health Organization (WHO) created the medical eligibility criteria to offer guidance on the safety of various contraceptive methods for use in specific health conditions to improve the quality of care in family planning [37]. The CROWD website also offers education about choice of contraceptive methods [38].

Considerations for hormone-containing contraception is discussed above. The condom is the only contraceptive method proven to be highly effective protection against both pregnancy and STIs. Barrier contraception requires intact balance, physical dexterity, and hand coordination or the willingness of both partners to assume responsibility for its use. Patients at risk for latex allergies, such as women with spina bifida, need to be cautioned to select products accordingly. The diaphragm increases the frequency of urinary tract infections [39], so patients who have disabilities that impact bladder function may require an alternative contraceptive method.

Conclusion

As the population of patients with physical, intellectual, and developmental disabilities ages, attention to their longitudinal health care needs will need to be addressed including their reproductive healthcare needs. The WHO, who has long been working in the area of sexual health, developed a working definition of sexual health as "a state of physical, mental, and social well-being in relation to sexuality. It requires a positive and respectful approach to sexuality and sexual relationships, as well as the possibility of having a pleasurable and safe sexual experience, free of coercion, discrimination and violence" [40]. Access to care with sensitivity to the unique needs of this vulnerable population will optimize the mental health, safety, and general health outcomes across the spectrum. As primary care clinicians become more educated about the needs of this complex population, they will also be able to partner with patients, families, communities, and appropriate specialists to provide comprehensive care.

References

1. Centers for Disease Control and Prevention (CDC). Disability and health overview. 2020. [online] Available at: https://www.cdc.gov/ncbddd/disabilityandhealth/disability.html. Accessed 29 Oct 2020.
2. FastStats - Disabilities or Limitations. Centers for Disease Control and Prevention. https://www.cdc.gov/nchs/fastats/disability.htm. Published June 24, 2020. Accessed 10 Feb 2021.
3. American Association on Intellectual and Developmental Disabilities (AAIDD). 2020. Faqs on intellectual disability. [online] Available at: https://www.aaidd.org/intellectual-disability/definition/faqs-on-intellectual-disability#:~:text=Intellectual%20disability%20is%20a%20disability,before%20the%20age%20of%2018. Accessed 29 Oct 2020.
4. Zablotsky B, Black LI, Blumberg SJ. Estimated prevalence of children with diagnosed developmental disabilities in the United States, 2014–2016, NCHS Data Brief, no 291. Hyattsville: National Center for Health Statistics; 2017.
5. Committee to Evaluate the Supplemental Security Income Disability Program for Children with Mental Disorders; Board on the Health of Select Populations; Board on Children, Youth, and Families; Institute of Medicine; Division of Behavioral and Social Sciences and Education; The National Academies of Sciences, Engineering, and Medicine; Boat TF, Wu JT, editors. Mental disorders and disabilities among low-income children. Washington, DC: National Academies Press (US); 2015. 9, Clinical Characteristics of Intellectual Disabilities. Available from: https://www.ncbi.nlm.nih.gov/books/NBK332877/.
6. Centers for Disease Control and Prevention. 2020. Facts about developmental disabilities. [online] Available at: https://www.cdc.gov/ncbddd/developmentaldisabilities/facts.html. Accessed 29 Oct 2020.
7. Holland-Hall C, Quint EH. Sexuality and disability in adolescents. Pediatr Clin N Am. 2017;64(2):435–49. https://doi.org/10.1016/j.pcl.2016.11.011. Epub 2017 Feb 13. PMID: 28292457.
8. The Arc Position Statement: Sexuality [Internet]. Washington, DC. Adopted c2008. Available from: http://www.thearc.org/who-we-are/position-statements/life-in-the-community/sexuality.
9. Autism Speaks [Internet] Puberty and adolescence resource. Available from: https://www.autismspeaks.org/sites/default/files/documents/atn/puberty_tool_kit.pdf.
10. Couwenhoven T. Sexuality education: building a foundation for healthy attitudes. [Internet] Lake Oswego: Disability Solutions; 2001;4(5). Available from: https://dsagsl.org/wp-content/uploads/2019/02/Sexuality-Education-Building-on-a-Foundation-of-Healthy-Attitudes-Part1.pdf.
11. Nosek MA, Howland CA, Rintala DH, Young ME, Chanpong GF. National study of women with physical disabilities: final report. Sex Disabil [Internet]. 2001;19(1):5–39. Available from: https://www.bcm.edu/research/centers/research-on-women-with-disabilities/topics/sexuality-and-reproductive-health/national-study-executive-summary.

12. Murphy NA, Elias ER. Sexuality of children and adolescents with developmental disabilities. Pediatrics. 2006;118:398–403. https://doi.org/10.1542/peds.2006-1115. Available from: http://www.pediatrics.org/cgi/content/full/118/1/398.

13. Tulloch T, Kaufman M. Adolescent sexuality. Pediatr Rev. 2013;34(1):29–38. https://doi.org/10.1542/pir.34-1-29. Available from: http://pedsinreview.aappublications.org/content/34/1/29.

14. Harrell E. Crime against persons with disabilities, 2009–2015 - statistical tables. Washington, DC: US Department of Justice, Office of Justice Programs, Bureau of Justice Statistics; 2012. Available at: https://www.bjs.gov/index.cfm?ty=pbdetail&iid=5986. Accessed 24 June 2018.

15. Sullivan PM, Knutson JF. Maltreatment and disabilities: a population-based epidemiological study. Child Abuse Negl. 2000;24(10):1257–73.

16. Davis LA. People with intellectual disabilities and sexual violence. [Internet] rev2011. Washington, DC. Available from: http://www.thearc.org/what-we-do/resources/fact-sheets/sexual-violence.

17. McFarlane J. Abuse assessment screen-disability (AAS-D): measuring frequency, type, and perpetrator of abuse toward women with physical disabilities. [Internet] J Womens Health Gend Based Med. 2001;10(9):861–6.

18. Cox RL, Caroline Signore C, Quint E. Reproductive health care for women with disabilities. Available from: http://www.acog.org/About-ACOG/ACOG-Departments/Women-with-Disabilities/Interactive-site-for-clinicians-serving-women-with-disabilities.

19. Landy R, Pesola F, Castañón A, et al. Impact of cervical screening on cervical cancer mortality: estimation using stage-specific results from a nested case–control study. Br J Cancer. 2016;115:1140–6. https://doi.org/10.1038/bjc.2016.290.

20. Armour BS, Thierry JM, Wolf LA. State-level differences in breast and cervical cancer, 2008. Womens Health Issues. 2009;19(6):406–14. https://doi.org/10.1016/j.whi.2009.08.006.

21. Simpson KM, editor. Table manners and beyond: the gynecological exam for women with developmental disabilities and other functional limitations. [Internet] Oakland 2001. Available from: http://lurie.brandeis.edu/pdfs/TableMannersandBeyond.pdf.

22. Spinal Cord Injury Model System. Autonomic dysreflexia [Internet]. 2015. Available from: https://media.bcm.edu/documents/2016/58/sci-autonomic-dysreflexia.pdf.

23. Kayoussi SK, Smith YR, et al. Cervical cancer screening with liquid cytology in women with developmental disabilities. J Women's Health. 2009;18(1). https://doi.org/10.1089/jwh.2008.0795.

24. Breastcancer.org. 2021. U.S. breast cancer statistics. [online] Available at: https://www.breastcancer.org/symptoms/understand_bc/statistics. Accessed 10 Feb 2021.

25. CDC. Behavioral risk factor surveillance system survey data. Atlanta: U.S. Department of Health and Human Services, CDC; 2008.

26. US Dept of Health and Human Services, Office on Disability Access to quality health services and disability—a companion to chapter 1 of Healthy People 2010. Available at: http://hhs.gov/od/about/fact_sheets/healthypeople2010.html. Accessed 5/8/2016.

27. McCarthy EP, Ngo LH, Roetzheim RG, et al. Disparities in breast cancer treatment and survival for women with disabilities. Ann Intern Med. 2006;145(9):637–45.

28. CDC [Internet] The right to know health campaign 2008. Available from: http://www.cdc.gov/ncbddd/disabilityandhealth/righttoknow/documents/new/234117_rtkdisseminationguide_v5_508_v1.pdf.

29. Delaware Breast Cancer Coalition. [Internet] Tips for women with disabilities (WWD): getting your mammogram c2014. Available from: http://debreastcancer.org/index.php/information/mammography_sites_wwd/.

30. Quint EH. Adolescents with special needs: clinical challenges in reproductive health care. J Pediatr Adolesc Gynecol. 2016;29(1):2–6. https://doi.org/10.1016/j.jpag.2015.05.003. Epub 2015 May 16. PMID: 26542013.

31. Minagar A, Kevill JW, Gonzalez-Toledo E. Neurological disorders and pregnancy. London: Elsevier; 2011. p. 96.
32. FSRH CEU guidance: drug interactions with hormonal contraception (January 2017, last reviewed 2019). FSRH CEU guidance: drug interactions with hormonal contraception (January 2017, last reviewed 2019) – Faculty of Sexual and Reproductive Healthcare. https://www.fsrh.org/standards-and-guidance/documents/ceu-clinical-guidance-drug-interactions-with-hormonal/. Accessed 18 Feb 2021.
33. Gebbie A, Sadler C, Raine S, et al. FSRH CEU guidance: drug interactions with hormonal contraception (January 2017, last reviewed 2019). FSRH CEU guidance: drug interactions with hormonal contraception (January 2017, last reviewed 2019) - Faculty of Sexual and Reproductive Healthcare. https://www.fsrh.org/standards-and-guidance/documents/ceu-clinical-guidance-drug-interactions-with-hormonal/. Accessed 18 Feb 2021.
34. Sabers A, Ohman I, Christensen J, Tomson T. Oral contraceptives reduce lamotrigine plasma levels. Neurology. 2003;61(4):570–1. https://doi.org/10.1212/01.wnl.0000076485.09353.7a. PMID: 12939444.
35. Wegner I, Edelbroek PM, Bulk S, Lindhout D. Lamotrigine kinetics within the menstrual cycle, after menopause, and with oral contraceptives. Neurology. 2009;73(17):1388–93. https://doi.org/10.1212/WNL.0b013e3181bd8295. PMID: 19858461.
36. Milosheska D, Lorber B, Vovk T, Kastelic M, Dolžan V, Grabnar I. Pharmacokinetics of lamotrigine and its metabolite N-2-glucuronide: influence of polymorphism of UDP-glucuronosyltransferases and drug transporters. Br J Clin Pharmacol. 2016;82(2):399–411. https://doi.org/10.1111/bcp.12984.
37. World Health Organization [Internet] 2015 Medical eligibility criteria for contraceptive use. e5. Available from: http://apps.who.int/iris/bitstream/10665/181468/1/9789241549158_eng.pdf?ua=1.
38. Center for Research on Women with Disabilities (CROWD). [Internet] Contraception. Available from: https://www.bcm.edu/research/labs-and-centers/research-centers/center-for-research-on-women-with-disabilities/a-to-z-directory/reproductive-health/contraception.
39. Fihn SD, Latham RH, Roberts P, Running K, Stamm WE. Association between diaphragm use and urinary tract infection. JAMA. 1985;254(2):240–5. https://doi.org/10.1001/jama.1985.03360020072027.
40. Sexual health. World Health Organization. http://www.who.int/topics/sexual_health/en/. Accessed 18 Feb 2021.

Resources

A Provider's Guide for the Care of Women with Physical Disabilities and Chronic Health Conditions. http://fpg.unc.edu/sites/fpg.unc.edu/files/resources/other-resources/NCODH_ProvidersGuide.pdf.
Autism Speaks. https://www.autismspeaks.org/sites/default/files/documents/atn/puberty_tool_kit.pdf.
Baylor College of Medicine - Center for Research on Women with Disabilities (CROWD). https://www.bcm.edu/research/centers/research-on-women-with-disabilities.
CDC. http://www.cdc.gov/ncbddd/disabilityandhealth/women.html.
Massachusetts Department of Public Health - Healthy Relationships, Sexuality and Disability Resource Guide. http://www.mass.gov/eohhs/docs/dph/com-health/prevention/hrhs-sexuality-and-disability-resource-guide.pdf.

Sexuality and Disability: A Guide for Parents. http://www.srcp.org/pdf_versions/Alberta.pdf.

Sexuality Resource Center for Parents (SRCP). http://www.srcp.org/for_some_parents/physical_disabilities/generalPD.html, http://www.srcp.org/for_some_parents/developmental_disabilities/additional_resources/index.html.

University of Michigan - YourChild is a Website especially for parents about kids' development and behavior. Sexuality Education for Youth with Disability or Chronic Illness - A Resource List. http://www.med.umich.edu/yourchild/topics/disabsex.htm.

Villanova – Nurse Practitioner's Guide to Disability. https://www1.villanova.edu/villanova/nursing/community/npsknowdisabilitycare.html.

Chapter 12
Orthopedic and Physical Ability Issues

Robyn Gisbert and Dana Judd

Contents

Introduction

The World Association for Sexual Health posits sexuality as a basic human right and an essential part of healthy life [1]. Sexual activity can be an indicator of quality of life and functional status [2]. Further, the World Health Organization's Classification of Functioning, Disability, and Health considers participation in sexual relationships as a major factor to describe and measure health and disability [3]. Acute and chronic health conditions to varying degrees may diminish quality of life and abilities to engage in meaningful activity.

R. Gisbert (✉) · D. Judd
Physical Therapy Program, Department of Physical Medicine and Rehabilitation, University of Colorado Anschutz Medical Campus, Aurora, CO, USA
e-mail: Robyn.Gisbert@cuanschutz.edu; Dana.Judd@cuanschutz.edu

© Springer Nature Switzerland AG 2022
J. Truglio et al. (eds.), *Sexual and Reproductive Health*,
https://doi.org/10.1007/978-3-030-94632-6_12

The approach to patients with physical or cognitive disabilities from congenital and genetic conditions is discussed in Chap. 11. This chapter will focus on acquired physical conditions and non-congenital chronic illness. Additionally, discussions of sexual positions that limit pain and discomfort for patients with musculoskeletal positions will be described in this chapter.

Events such as joint replacement surgeries, spinal cord injury, stroke, or myocardial infarction can result in impairments of body structure and function including muscle weakness, decreased range of motion, pain, balance deficits, and limited activity tolerance. These impairments can lead to difficulty performing daily tasks and alter participation in life, including sexual activity. Similarly, chronic health conditions such as osteoarthritis and coronary artery disease may result in adaptive changes that limit physical abilities. Whether affected temporarily or chronically with disability, people remain sexual beings. Sexual problems are common and associated with a myriad of health conditions [4]. Patients and partners have concerns about sexual activity in the context of health care. However, the topic of sexual activity is often overlooked and clinicians are underprepared for conversations that would best serve their patients [5–10].

There is a lack of materials available for counseling on physical ability and sexual activity. Those which exist are predominately considered from a heteronormative point of view with very little literature available in relation to same-sex couples [10]. There is a clear and important need for the development of clinician knowledge, skills, and materials for education regarding sexual functioning and disability. Clinicians should take an active role in investigating the impact of health conditions on sexual health and make recommendations to address concerns. In addition to clinician recommendations, peer support and guidance have been effective in some health populations with persons benefitting from learning about sexual functioning from individuals with similar injuries [11].

In order to meet the best needs of patients, providers should consider strategies around history taking, physical examination, and interventions related to sexual health. Several models exist (e.g., PLISSIT, PLEASURE, ALARM, BETTER) to prepare clinicians for therapeutic conversations about sexual health [12]. The models elucidate the importance for primary care clinicians to have the capacity to build rapport, giving permission for patients to share sexual health concerns in a nonjudgmental and confidential environment. This requires providers consider their own knowledge, comfort, and biases as related to sex and disability. Two models most commonly referred to in the literature to initiate conversations around sexual health and physical activity are the PLISSIT and BETTER models. The PLISSIT (*P*ermission, *L*imited *I*nformation, *S*pecific *S*uggestions, *I*ntensive *T*herapy) model developed by JS Annon, in 1976 [13], expects that all primary care clinicians be able to validate that sexual health is a legitimate concern and topic to discuss and, as such, be able to provide preliminary information on the topic limited information that, when shared, can empower patients to understand their conditions and potentially remedy problems. The BETTER (*B*ring up the topic, *E*xplain your concerns, *T*ell patients you can help, consider *T*iming of conversation, provide *E*ducation, document in medical *R*ecord) model, developed and utilized largely for use in oncology, echoes the communication strategy and education components of the PLISSIT model. In addition, the BETTER model reminds primary care clinicians to consider the timing of sexual counseling and the importance of recording assessments and interventions about sexual health in patients' medical records [12]. Both models can be reasonably applied to other populations and patients.

Patients with physical limitations affecting daily life and mobility may also present to providers with challenges for physical examination procedures for sexual health, such as a pelvic examination. Evidence suggests that patients with disabilities are less likely to have a full and complete physical examination due accessibility of the examination room and physician training [14]. To improve access and care, clinicians may benefit from learning from persons with disabilities and rehabilitation therapists about safe transfers to a standard examination table. Patients with mobility issues may need more time, physical assistance, or adaptive equipment such as a step stool to safely transfer to a traditional examination table. To ensure patient safety during an exam, other considerations may include use of a lower table, a wider table to facilitate rolling, or use alternate positions to the traditional dorsal lithotomy position, such as side lying, or altering the position of the legs while supine. Modified footrest positions, such as placing footrest under the knees or lower legs, rather than the feet, will lessen the amount of hip and knee flexion and may be more comfortable for patients with back pain from lumbar disc herniation who may have symptom exacerbation in spinal flexion. Additionally, modifying the footrest position to allow the patient to have one leg up and one leg down may achieve a more extended spine position, while also providing access to pelvic area for examination. Alternatively, providing modifications to allow for a neutral or flexed lumbar spine may be helpful for patients with lumbar spine stenosis, who have more comfort in spinal flexion. If footrest position modification is not possible, wedges and towels under the sacrum to facilitate spinal flexion, or rolled and placed under the lumbar spine to facilitate spinal flexion may offer support and comfort. These may also be used for other patient populations who need accommodations to the traditional position. For patients with neurological injuries, clinicians will want to use an integrated knowledge of the patient's sensory and motor status during the physical examination. Patients with impaired sensory and motor status may be at increased risk for tissue damage of insensate areas from positioning and from examination procedures. It is recommended that clinicians visualize vulnerable bony prominences and inspect skin and internal tissues before and after procedures. Providers may also need to modify the sexual health physical examination for patients with medical conditions. Specifically, patients with gastroesophageal reflux disease and related gastrointestinal disorders should be examined in a modified supine position with the trunk and head supported in flexion. Likewise, individuals recovering from cardiac procedures may have similar restrictions to avoid a full supine position. Access to adjustable tables will aid in achieving this semi-reclined position, as can the use of wedges, towels, and pillows.

In addition to considerations for communicating and examining patients, providers should be prepared to offer specific advice that is individualized to a patient's needs and concerns regarding sexual health. This may include advice for positioning to protect joints, care for neurogenic bladder and bowel functioning, or use of adaptive equipment. Finally, there are specialty clinicians that can provide intensive therapy. These include sex therapists, psychiatrists, urologists, surrogates, and other licensed practitioners with unique training in sexual health for additional and targeted interventions. Primary care clinicians, as part of the team with the patient at the center, can apply these models and the specific suggestions that follow to address sexual functioning when physical ability is impaired.

Orthopedic Conditions: Considerations and Suggestions

Pain from muscle, joints, and bones, including arthritis, is a common complaint among adults. In a recent survey, more than half of adults in the United States reported musculoskeletal pain [15] and estimates suggest that between 60% and 77% of all injuries involve the musculoskeletal system. Most commonly, adults report low back pain, knee pain, and neck pain, in that order [16]. Further, almost 24 million adults report a diagnosis of arthritis [17]. Living with musculoskeletal pain and injury is often accompanied by changes in joint mobility, muscle strength, balance, and flexibility and, therefore, results in limitations in activity. These limitations include difficulty carrying out basic self-care, and home- and work-related activities of daily living. It has been widely reported that chronic low back pain is associated with considerable disability and that an estimated 44% of individuals living with arthritis report activity limitations related to their diagnosis [17]. Included in these reported activity limitations are reports of decreased sexual activity due to pain with sex, decreases in libido, and decreases in satisfaction in sex [18–20]. Although it is likely that most musculoskeletal injuries and musculoskeletal pain effects participation in sexual activity, patients with lower extremity pain and spinal pain are reporting more difficulties participating in sexual activity. For example, patients with low back pain report more difficulty with sex that those with neck pain [21] and a higher percentage of patients with hip arthritis and hip arthroplasty report disruptions in their sexual activity compared to patients who have arthritis in other areas of the body [19, 20]. Therefore, the following information will provide common presentations and specific suggestions related to lower extremity and spine pain and injuries; however, the principles behind the suggestions can be extrapolated to any individual living with musculoskeletal pain or injury.

Lower Back Pain

Low back pain is among the most common medical conditions for adults over the age of 18 such that almost one third of adults in the United States are currently experiencing back pain [15]. It is also the most common condition for which patient seek medical care and negatively affects individuals' ability to participate in work and activities of daily living [15]. Individuals with low back pain report interruption of regular domestic chores, recreation and exercise, sleep, and social and leisure activities. Additionally, individuals suffering from low back pain report changes in work productivity, from modifying regular tasks at work, to not being able to participate in work altogether [22]. Not only does low back pain result in challenges with physical function, but it also results in challenges with social relationships. Individuals often report difficulty with relationships due to changes in their social roles due to pain, difficulty with social interactions, and in maintaining sexual function [22].

Studies suggest that half to three-quarters of patients with low back pain report a negative impact on their sexual activity, resulting in decreased satisfaction, sexual drive, and frequency [5, 21]. Yet, less than one-third of individuals report discussing sex with their healthcare provider. This is despite the fact that individuals with low back pain expect their clinician to provide ways improve their sexual activity and feel that it should be a routine part of managing low back pain [5]. A large proportion of patients report pain during intercourse—position was a major concern, and women more often report pain during sex than men [5, 21]. However, there is variability in the literature as to the specific influence of position on pain.

A potential source of this variability lies in the complexity of low back pain, its etiology, and the way it manifests in individuals. Each person likely experiences low back pain differently; therefore, it would be impossible to provide one single recommendation to patients regarding their sexual activity. One approach to managing the variable presentations of low back pain is determining the motions and positions which provoke a patient's pain, which is a critical part of the successful subgrouping for treatment method, which is considered best practice currently [23]. This can be done as a part of a physical examination or could also be elucidated with a thorough patient interview in which patients could be able to report activities or positions that worsen pain. Clinicians should ascertain whether their patients' pain is exacerbated in positions of spinal flexion or spinal extension, the two most common joint motions identified during sex. In some case, patients may report exacerbation in both positions, making recommendations more difficult. This information is imperative for the clinician to provide meaningful advice on coital positions for comfort.

The following discussion will provide specific suggestions on coital position for individuals with low back pain, depending on their position of exacerbated symptoms. For this discussion, positions for those in position for penetration and those in position to receive will be provided.

Recommended Positions for Patients in Position for Penetration

For individuals whose pain is exacerbated in flexion, two rear entry methods are recommended, with the patient tall-kneeling behind the partner, who would be in quadruped, as it requires little flexion range of motion. The least amount of flexion is required with the quadruped partner leaning forward on their arms. It has been noted that even small changes in a partner's position is likely to change the mechanics for the patient in this position, so advising on their partners position is also important [24]. In addition, face-to-face position with the individual in a push-up position, is also recommended due to the fact that the spine will remain mostly in extension [24]. Face-to-face position in which the person's position is lower and weight is on the forearms, and side-lying positions would be contraindicated for patients whose symptoms are aggravated in flexion due the range of motion into flexion in these positions. However, for individuals whose symptoms are aggravated in extension, these positions are likely to be positions of comfort, while the tall-keeling and extended face-to-face positions would be contraindicated. For individuals whose symptoms are exacerbated in both flexion and extension, it will be important to think about advising patients on their mechanics of penetration, since all positions may be potentially aggravating. Specifically, counseling individuals to maintain a neutral spine (neither flexion nor extension) during penetration by moving through hip flexion, rather than spinal flexion, will decrease pain since the spine remains relatively still [24].

Recommendations for Those in Position to Receive

For patients whose pain is exacerbated in spinal flexion, three rear-entry methods are recommended as they place the individual in a position of more spinal extension, thus avoiding the painful spinal range of motion. Those positions are quadruped, side-lying, and quadruped with weight on the forearms [25]. Alternatively, face-to-face positions are contraindicated, as they promote spinal flexion. In fact, the more a person's hips are flexed, the more the spine will flex. Therefore, any face-to-face position in which the patient's feet leave the surface would be further contraindicated due to the extreme amounts of spinal flexion range of motion that position would induce. However, for patients whose pain is exacerbated in extension, a face-to-face position would be recommended, particularly with more spinal flexion, and the rear-entry methods, especially quadruped, would be contraindicated. Patients with pain in both flexion and extension should be counseled to move more from their hips than their spine to maintain comfort [25].

It is not reasonable to think that all patients seeking advice for sexual position would be limited to the positions suggested above. Therefore, it will be important for clinicians to have honest conversations with patients about their sexual activity and advise accordingly. A key principle guiding the advice for patients will be to avoid coital positions which would put patients' spines in positions of pain provocation, regardless of their desired position. This discussion may also include alterations to their practiced positions or use of pillows, wedges, or other props to achieve a comfortable spinal posture for sex.

Arthritis and Total Joint Replacement

Arthritis should be considered a major heath concern as the population continues to age, as it will negatively affect the quality of life for more than 34 million individuals [26]. The consequences of living with arthritis are multifactorial. Negative effects on both physical and mental health have been documented [27]. In particular, deficits in muscle strength and muscle mass [28, 29] and range of motion [30], and difficulty with activities of daily living are common [31]. Further, due to high pain levels and significant stiffness [30], many individuals are physically inactive [32]. In addition, difficulties in sexual activity have been reported due to hip and knee arthritis in the literature, negatively effecting participation and satisfaction in sex [7, 20]. Difficulties with sexual activity is correlated with poor reported quality of life for individuals with arthritis, as patients with sexual activity limitations report poorer general function compared with peers who do not report sexual activity limitations due to their arthritis [33].

A large percentage of individuals with hip arthritis report difficulty participating in sexual activity and report difficulty with sex more often than patients with knee arthritis [19, 20, 34]. Importantly, decline in sexual activity due to symptoms of their arthritis has been reported to occur as early as the fourth decade [33]. Two major consequences of arthritis are joint stiffness and pain, which are both likely contributing to declines in sexual activity and satisfaction in patients with arthritis. However, it is possible that stiffness affects patients with hip arthritis to a greater degree. In a study of patients with diagnosed hip arthritis, patients who reported limitations in their sexual activity also reported higher levels of pain and stiffness and had more limited range of motion compared to those with hip arthritis who didn't report sexual activity limitations [34]. Of patients who report declines in sexual activity, stiffness due to their hip arthritis was the primary impairment associated with difficulty during sex [19]. While stiffness was also reported as a factor interfering with sexual activity with those with knee arthritis, pain also played a large role in declining sexual activity. In particular, patients reported the necessity to change positions during sex, primarily due the inability to kneel during sex due to pain [20]. The impact of hip and knee arthritis on sexual activity is a major factor, as between 66% and 82% of patients with hip arthritis, more women than men, and 45% of patients with knee arthritis report difficulty with sex [19, 20, 34], and of those who report difficulties engaging in sex, tension in their relationships is also reported [33]. However, a large percentage of physicians report that they do not discuss sex with their patients [7].

Commonly, patients will undergo total hip or total knee arthroplasty to ameliorate the pain and disability of their arthritis. Total hip and total knee arthroplasty are considered successful surgeries and typically result in improved quality of life for individuals with end-stage arthritis. Generally, undergoing total hip or knee arthroplasty also improves sexual activity; however, some limitations in sexual activity remain [19, 20]. The largest reduction in sexual activity occurs in the first year after surgery, especially in the first few months following surgery. Most patients report ability to return to sexual activity 1–4 months after surgery, with patients after total knee arthroplasty able to return sooner than those with total hip arthroplasty [7, 19, 20]. Kneeling remains an issue for patients after total knee arthroplasty, which potentially affects sexual activity as it did before surgery. However, patients after total hip arthroplasty have larger concerns regarding pain, stiffness, and risks of dislocation, complicating their return to normal sexual activity. To date, the postero-lateral approach remains the most common approach to performing total hip arthro-plasty [35]. This approach incises and divides the posterior hip musculature, leaving the hip particularly vulnerable to dislocation when in position of extreme flexion, internal rotation, and adduction. To decrease the risk of dislocation following sur-gery, range of motion precautions are often prescribed which likely interfere with sexual activity. Despite this, most surgeons believe patients can safely resume sex-ual activity 1 month following surgery.

To account for pain, stiffness, and postsurgical precautions, specific suggestions for positioning during sex can be provided. Finding positions to ease pain, accom-modate stiffness, and promote safety will provide patients with the necessary tools to avoid declines in sexual activity due to these factors. While these suggestions come primarily from the postoperative literature, they can easily be translated to patients with arthritis of the hip or knee.

Knee Pain

The most common pain complaint during sex in individuals with knee pain is in a kneeling position. Pain during kneeling could be due to pressure in the anterior part of the knee that is painful or could be due to stiffness in the knee, where complete knee flexion is not possible. While it could be simple to advise patients to avoid kneeling positions during sex, it's worthwhile to note that of patients with knee pain and stiffness who reported declines in sexual activity, a primary reason noted was that a change in position led to less satisfying sex, and changed their participation in sexual activity [20]. Therefore, it is important to be able to provide specific sugges-tions that would allow patients to more comfortably assume a kneeling position during sex, thus allowing them to participate as they desire.

For patients reporting pain with kneeling, either in a tall-kneeling or quadruped position, additional padding under the knees will provide a softer surface to kneel on, thus decreasing pain and pressure in a kneeling position. Additionally, consider-ing positions that unweights the knees could be helpful. For example, individuals who are in a position of receiving their partner in a quadruped position, using a rounded bolster under the torso will shift weight away from the knees, decreasing pressure and pain on the anterior surface of the knee. Alternatively, for patients with difficulty kneeling due to stiffness and inability to assume full knee flexion, assuming a position in which the receiving partner is on top may be difficult. Patients may need to adjust their body position to be more upright in their torso to decrease the demand in knee flexion or consider using small pads or bolsters behind the knees to rest on, thus decreasing the angle of knee flexion while in this position. Finally, for patients willing to alter their position during sex, positions in which the individual and partner are standing, or seated, or in supine or prone positions will also be protective for a painful or stiff knee.

Hip Pain

The presence of hip arthritis often leads to pain and stiffness, which arguably has a larger impact than knee pain and stiffness on sexual activity due to the mechanics of engaging in sex. Often, individuals voluntarily self-limit sexual activity due to pain and stiffness but also due to fear of injury or insufficient knowledge about safe positions and options for participation [33]. Individuals engaging in vaginal receptive sex with hip pain report more difficulties with sexual activity and report difficulties with sex sooner after the onset of pain [33, 34]. Individuals with hip arthritis who report difficulty with sex also demonstrate limitations in hip flexion, abduction, and external rotation range of motion, limiting options for positions during sex [34]. This makes supine positions in which they would receive their partner painful or impossible and may also eliminate the option to assume a position on top of a supine partner, due to the same range of motion concerns. Therefore, information regarding positions which do not require large amounts of hip flexion, abduction, and external rotation range of motion will be helpful to patients wishing to maintain their sexual activity. Positions which have been identified as safe for individuals with hip pathology and that also minimize hip flexion, abduction, and external rotation are likely a rear entry method such as both partners standing, both partners supine or in partial side-lying positions, which require little range of motion in these difficult positions [36]. The requirement of large amounts of hip flexion, abduction, and external rotation to participate in sex appears to be unique to cisgender women and transgender women engaged in vaginal intercourse, which could be why cisgender men with hip arthritis do not typically report difficulties with sex or often need to alter positions to participate in sex [33].

As mentioned previously, patients often choose to undergo total hip arthroplasty to treat the pain and stiffness due to hip arthritis. Undergoing hip arthroplasty improves participation in sexual activity for a good percentage of patients, but not for all patients [7, 19, 33]. Resumption of sexual activity following hip arthroplasty is safe as early as 1 month after surgery [19], although the timeframe to resume sexual activity can vary anywhere from 1 to 4 months after [7, 19]. However, careful consideration for safety in resuming sexual activity is imperative to avoid injury, particularly hip dislocation, which has occurred during sex [7]. In particular, individuals often have range of motion limitations of hip flexion greater than 90°, hip

adduction, and internal rotation, mandated by the surgeon to protect from dislocation. These precautions need to be acknowledged when providing advice regarding
return to sexual activity—all individuals should avoid coital positions with large
amounts of hip flexion, whether they are in position to receive or in position of penetration. As is the case in those with hip arthritis, cisgender women more often
report needing to change their position during sex than cisgender men, as cisgender
men can more often use similar positions to before surgery [33, 36]. However, in
opposition to comfortable positions suggested above for patients with hip arthritis,
positions which promote hip abduction and external rotation are actually preferred
to place the hip joint in a more stable position and thus, lessen the risk for dislocation. Taking these principles into consideration, several positions are considered
safe for individuals after hip arthroplasty [36]. The most recognized safe coital position after surgery is a position where both partners are standing, either upright, or
with the receiving partner flexed slightly forward from the trunk, supported by their
upper extremities [33, 36]. Other safe positions include rear entry positions such as
both partners prone and, both partners sitting, with the receiving partner facing
away. Some supine positions may also be safe and comfortable after surgery, such a
missionary, or with the vaginal receptive individual on top facing the partner.
However, some modifications for these positions need to be considered. For example, for a vaginal receptive individual in a traditional, face-to-face position, a pillow
or wedge under the pelvis will work to raise the pelvis, placing the hips in more relative hip extension, thus avoiding a hip flexion position. In addition, for the insertive
partner in this position, it will helpful to counsel individuals to extend their legs
while on top of their partner to avoid hip flexion positions that are more likely to
occur while on the knees. Some individuals may find that changing positions or the
use of supports, such as pillows or wedges, may initially change the sexual experience for one or both partners, so it is also important to counsel patients to communicate with their partners during and after sex. In addition, the first sexual encounter
after surgery or any sexual encounters early after surgery may be anxiety provoking
for the partner who just had surgery. Again, encouraging individuals to communicate with their partners to communicate concerns will be paramount, and acknowl-
edging that many patients have difficulty returning to sexual activity may provide
needed comfort.

Millions of adults are living with low back pain, arthritis, and other injuries or
diseased affecting the musculoskeletal system. Of these adults, nearly three quarters
report that their injury or disease affects their sexual health and activity. Therefore,
sex is a topic that cannot be overlooked during clinical encounters and should be
part of routine care. We have described specific suggestions to guide such discussions. The principle of advising patients to find positions that avoid pain provocation through changing preferred positions, or using props to change positioning can
be extrapolated to any individual living with pain or injury. However, it is also
important to note that for some patients with musculoskeletal pain, intercourse may
not always be possible. It may also be prudent to discuss with patients and have
patients discuss with their partners, the idea of other means of sexual intimacy
including oral sex, manual stimulation, and masturbation.

Neurologic Conditions: Considerations and Suggestions

Neurological disorders can alter sensory, integrative and motor abilities affecting capacities for self-care, functional mobility, work, and recreation. Ultimately, neurological disorders may alter relationships and quality of life. Neurological disease frequently alters sexual response and activity, often to devastating degrees for patients and their partners. There are many neurological conditions known to alter sexual functioning, including but not limited to epilepsy, stroke, multiple sclerosis, Parkinson's disease, neuropathies, traumatic brain, and spinal cord injury [4, 6]. Here we will focus on spinal cord injury, stroke, and the degenerative condition of Parkinson's disease. These conditions will collectively serve to illustrate problems of physical ability and sexual activity. Clinicians may relate the suggestions to other pathologies and associated impairments.

Spinal Cord Injury

Spinal cord injury (SCI) prevalence is relatively low. However, its impact is profound. Currently, an estimated 282,000 persons are living with the consequences of SCI in the United States. The average age at time of injury has increased from 29 to 42 years, with males representing 80% of persons with SCI. Motor vehicle accidents account for the vast majority of SCI, followed by injury from falls, violence, and sports/recreational activity [37]. Much has been learned about sex and disability from this population due of the nature of the injury and the demographics predominately affected. SCI, primarily a traumatic event, leaves those affected with varying degrees of sensory loss, paralysis, and autonomic dysfunction from damage to the white and grey matter of the spinal cord. This consequentially affects multiple systems and participation in life [38]. During rehabilitation for SCI, common pressing questions arise about return to activity, namely, walking, self-care, sexual function, and reproductive abilities.

The Consortium for Spinal Cord Medicine has developed Clinical Practice Guidelines to comprehensively address rehabilitation and life after SCI, including sexuality [38]. The consortium recommends the use of the PLISSIT framework to encourage open and respectful communication. The guidelines emphasize maintaining dignity while matching the patient's readiness to learn about sexual function across the continuum of care. Evidence has shown that for people with SCI, there is an ideal time period that exists for sexual counseling between inpatient rehabilitation and 6 months after discharge. It is important to include sexual partners in these intervention sessions [39].

The level of a person's SCI correlates to a degree with the physiologic effects on sexual function. In the general population, cisgender men experience psychogenic, reflexogenic, and spontaneous erections. For cisgender men with complete upper motor neuron SCI above the level of T11, psychogenic erection typically does not occur, but they may experience reflexogenic and spontaneous erections. For those with lower motor neuron injuries below T11, psychogenic arousal may be possible, but reflexive arousal typically is not. Clinicians can counsel about expectations, remind patients that actual abilities with physiologic sexual functioning will be unique, and advise about alternate forms of sexual expression—touching on sensate areas, masturbation, and the use of adaptive equipment for pleasure. Clinicians, including rehabilitation therapists, can help identify safety and appropriateness given hand function, general motor, sensory, and mobility abilities. Intensive therapy may be indicated for counseling, and to address fertility and reproduction.

SCI has an impact on the persons psychological, physiological, and physical abilities which may all have an impact upon sexual functioning. Individuals with SCI may have problems assuming positions for sex, physiologic disturbances with arousal, and changes in body image that interfere with sexuality [40]. Here we include specific suggestions, emphasizing those relating to physical activity. Early in rehabilitation, spinal precautions associated with fracture and surgical decompression and stabilization need be maintained to allow for healing and prevent injury. Clinicians can help identify and translate these precautions as related to sexual activity. As persons with SCI may require assistance with functional mobility and transfers, it is important to educate caregivers and patients about optimal positioning. This may include use of alternate positions for coitus in bed with accommodations for weakness and to protect skin and joints from injury. Additionally, this may include expanding activities for pleasure (i.e., mutual masturbation, oral sex, and the use of adaptive sexual aids). Positions that offer the most support and stability for the individual with SCI are recommended. Supine in bed and seated in the person's wheelchair can both allow for maximum stability and therefore safety. Optimally, persons with SCI and their partners can collaborate with health care providers to find solutions facilitating sexual participation. Rehabilitation therapists are encouraged to examine and understand a person's neurological and mobility status, readiness for sexual counseling, and individual goals related to sexual function. When appropriate, written educational materials may provide a tool for important collaborative conversations to address sexual wellbeing, positioning, equipment needs, and special considerations [41, 42].

Special considerations of skin integrity, care of bladder and bowel, and risk of autonomic dysreflexia are important in this population. Providers can help individuals with SCI identify and understand safety and risks related to skin integrity. It is important to protect and inspect areas of insensate skin that are potentially exposed to friction and shear during sexual activities. Things to consider include surfaces that allow for stability and mobility while also protecting skin and joints. Firm mattresses, while facilitating transfers and bed mobility, may be uncomfortable for a person with sensory loss and joint pain. Adaptive equipment such as wedges and thigh slings can help compensate for paralysis and make the physical activity of sex more accessible. Rehabilitation specialists can help to ascertain weight limits and safety precautions for couples engaging sexually in the wheelchair, provide examples of wedges for position, and link an individual's neurological status and mobility skills to the physical abilities involved in sexual activity.

Primary care clinicians should discuss the risk of autonomic dysreflexia and functioning of bowel and bladder as related to sexual activity with individuals with

SCI. During sexual activity, able-bodied persons are known to experience moderate increases in blood pressure, but those with SCI particularly at higher levels (above T6) with intense stimulation have increased likelihood for the hyperreflexive response known as autonomic dysreflexia (AD) wherein blood pressure quickly escalates to life threatening levels [43]. AD can by managed by couples recognizing symptoms (goosebumps, headache, lightheadedness) and contributing factors (UTI, full bowel or bladder, presence of aggressive, or noxious sensory stimuli). Most importantly, couples need to know how to manage AD should it occur. To manage the symptoms of AD, sit the individual with SCI upright, and remove or decrease any contributing factors.

Incontinence is a concern for individuals with SCI, but does not necessarily restrict sexual activity [44]. Bladder management options after SCI include self-catheterization, the use of an indwelling catheter, and suprapubic catheters. Sexual activity is possible with all types, and as such, providers should work to assist the individual with SCI in choosing the option that maximizes health, function, and personal desires. Suprapubic catheters can make sexual activity easier, as they provide an alternate route to the bladder, leaving the genitals free for sexual stimulation. For those who self-catheterize, voiding prior to sex may be helpful. However, some cis-gender men with SCI find a full bladder assists with achieving erection, while others report it impairs erectile function [44]. In this case clinicians should caution patients that a full bladder may increase likelihood of AD. Clinicians should encourage persons with SCI to explore to determine their best individual practice and to have contingency plans in place to address incontinence and AD should either or both occur.

Stroke

Stroke is a leading cause of death and disability. With an aging population and advanced medical treatments, large numbers of adults survive stroke [45]. Following stroke an individual may be left with weakness, sensory loss, spasticity, and fatigue making mobility and activities of daily living difficult. Studies have shown that sexual functioning is also impaired. Many persons with even mild stroke report problems with sexual functioning and consequences increase with severity [46]. While the majority of couples experience decreases in their sexual life after stroke, some identified a positive impact from learning slow down and to be mindful and more accepting of their partner [8]. Barriers to sexual function following stroke may be physical, psychosocial, or psychological in nature. Further, problems with sexual functioning may be the result of medication side effects or comorbid conditions. Frequently, multiple domains need to be addressed [47–49]. Examples of psychosocial barriers after stroke include loss of identity and shifts in relational or caretaking roles. Depression, a known frequent consequence of stroke, and the medications used to treat depression can diminish sex drive. Likewise, antihypertensive and lipid-lowering medications are known to have similar side effects. Regardless of causation, survivors of stroke and their partners desire counseling about sexual dysfunction and activity [9].

Approaches by healthcare professionals to addressing these needs are varied but mostly lacking [48]. Studies have identified personal level of comfort, lack of knowledge, perceptions and fears of patient responses to talking about sex, and unsupportive rehabilitative environments as barriers to effectively engaging with patients to address sexual health following stroke [49]. Primary care clinicians caring for patients after stroke should consider timing regarding inquiry about and counseling for sexual function. There are mixed reports with some persons wanting this information readily in acute care and others with preferences for later in outpatient settings. However, 71% of patients wish to receive counseling within 1-year post stroke [9]. Primary care clinicians can use the PLISSIT model discussed above to initial conversations about sexual activity after stroke. As with other populations, giving permission to discuss sexual health and providing preliminary information that helps patients understand the relationship of their current health condition to sexual functioning is helpful. Encourage patients to assess their own attitudes and feelings about sex after stroke and to talk with their partner(s) and to clinicians. One general recommendation is to plan ahead for sex and allow more time. This may be an adjustment for patients and their partners who have previously enjoyed spontaneity with sex but can address many of the known and potential problems such as fatigue, pain, and incontinence that can occur following stroke.

Commonly following stroke, individuals experience hemiplegia, balance problems, and decreased endurance for activity. Ninety-four percent of people with stroke identify these types of physical limitations as limiting sexual activity [9]. Positions of supine and side lying are recommended as compensatory to provide stability and safety. Bolsters and pillows may be helpful to protect limbs and joints while positioning for comfort and pleasure. Both the individual with stroke and their partner(s) should be aware of insensate areas and counseled to inspect skin that is subject to shear and friction from sexual activity.

In general, a willingness of providers to address sexual activity and provide any written materials has been demonstrated as effective as specific and structured sexual rehabilitation programming [50]. This is promising as providers may be most comfortable with giving permission and limited information but health systems don't always allow time for specific recommendations. Some examples of printable educational materials available online are included (Table 12.1) [48].

Table 12.1 Printable online materials for stroke survivors and caregivers

Website	Document title	Year	Weblink
National Stroke Association	Recovery After Stroke: Redefining Sexuality	2006	http://www.stroke.org/stroke-resources/library/redefining-sexuality
United States Department of Veterans Affairs	RESCUE Resources and Education for Stroke Caregivers Understanding and Empowerment	2016	http://www.stroke.org/stroke-resources/library/redefining-sexuality
The Stroke Association	Sex After Stroke	2017	https://www.stroke.org.uk/sites/default/files/sex_after_stroke.pdf

Adapted from Hamam et al. [48]

Degenerative Neurological Conditions

Degenerative neurological conditions such as Parkinson's disease (PD), multiple sclerosis (MS), and Alzheimer's disease (AD) systematically progress in morbidity, typically with advancing degrees of disability. Persons with such neurodegenerative disorders may experience progressive loss of abilities with locomotion, transfers, mobility, communication, independence with self-care, and ability to carry out activities of daily living changes. Similarly, sexual responses and abilities are altered [11].

Parkinson's disease (PD) affects approximately 1% of Americans older than 60 years, and an estimated 4% of the oldest Americans are now diagnosed with PD. This prevalence is anticipated to double by 2030 [51]. Sexual function may be affected directly by PD, made difficult by the condition's motor impairments (bradykinesia, tremor, rigidity, loss of dexterity) or secondarily by non-motor symptoms of the disease. Non-motor symptoms such as drooling (hypersalivation), pain, fatigue, sleep disturbances, and autonomic dysfunction are known to be troublesome to people with PD. Further, consequences of comorbid conditions and/or side effects of medications can impair sexual functioning. Cisgender men with PD report erectile dysfunction with studies identifying 50–70% having difficulty maintaining an erection. Cisgender women with PD, when compared to aged matched controls, experience more vaginal tightness, decreased lubrication, involuntary urination, and overall a dissatisfaction with sex [4]. Clinicians can help individuals with PD by normalizing conversations about sexual health, considering medication therapies, recommending the use of lubricants and reminders to void prior to sex. Clinicians should investigate complicating factors and be prepared to refer for intensive therapies if indicated. The motor symptoms of PD (rigidity, bradykinesia, decreased fine motor control) tend to be worse in the evening and subject to medication on-off times and may interfere with sexual activity. Encouraging couples to plan for intimacy in relationship to these fluctuations may be helpful. Additionally, suggestions about outercourse (experiencing sexual pleasure without concern for erection, orgasm or intercourse) are also advised for those seeking intimacy but with impaired genital functioning. Satisfaction with sexual activity is negatively affected by the presence of motor symptoms, anxiety, and depression [4]. It is important, then, that primary care clinicians address motor symptoms and mood in PD. Physical therapy and exercise are known to benefit people with PD [52]. Recommending therapy and activity can enable individuals with PD to manage their health condition and improve physical mobility for activity and participation, including sexual activity.

Medical Conditions: Considerations and Suggestions

Individuals with cardiovascular disease (CVD) face challenges with endurance and exercise tolerance, which includes sexual activity. A concern that arises in patients with medical conditions and their partners is the fear that sexual activity can cause another event such as stroke, heart attack, or death. However, the link between coitus and stroke is not well established [47]. A known patent foramen ovale, post-coital headache, and severe headache with orgasm are associated with an increased risk for stroke with sexual activity. In an analysis of love-death (death associated with sexual activity), several risk factors were identified—preexisting coronary heart disease and myocardial infarction, high body mass index, and elevated heart rate [53].

The American Heart Association recommends that patients with cardiovascular disease (CVD) wishing to resume sexual activity undergo a physical examination, including exercise stress testing, if indicated [54]. Sexual activity is considered safe for patients who are able to exercise at a level of 3–5 METS, which is equivalent to walking up a flight of stairs, without angina or dyspnea. Encouraging cardiac rehabilitation and regular cardiovascular exercise is recommended to reduce risk of cardiovascular complications during sex. Clinicians should engage in conversations with patients about sexual activity and can counsel about engaging in sexual activities that are less energy demanding. One suggestion is to begin with lower level energy expending activities and progressively increase tolerance to all activity including sex. Activities of hugging, kissing, and sexual touching have the lowest energy expenditures, whereas vaginal and anal intercourse have the highest energy expenditures [55]. Lastly, patients may need to be counseled to defer resumption of sexual activity until their medical condition is stable [54].

Conclusion

Sexual health, an important component of whole health, is affected by physical abilities. Many adults are dealing with health conditions that impair physical activity. It is estimated that one-half of adults are affected by chronic conditions, such as arthritis, stroke, or heart disease [56]. These conditions, degenerative neurological conditions and traumatic injuries, are all known to have deleterious effects on sexual health and activity.

Primary care clinicians should include conversations about sexual health in caring for the whole individual.

References

1. Council WAfSHA. Declaration of sexual rights. 2014. http://www.worldsexology.org/wp-content/uploads/2013/08/declaration_of_sexual_rights_sep03_2014.pdf. Accessed 21 Dec 2017.
2. Stock SR, Cole DC, Tugwell P, Streiner D. Review of applicability of existing functional status measures to the study of workers with musculoskeletal disorders of the neck and upper limb. Am J Ind Med. 1996;29(6):679–88.

3. Organization WH. ICF browser. 2017. http://apps.who.int/classifications/icfbrowser/. Accessed 10 Jan 2018.
4. Bronner G, Aharon-Peretz J, Hassin-Baer S. Sexuality in patients with Parkinson's disease, Alzheimer's disease, and other dementias. Handb Clin Neurol. 2015;130:297–323.
5. Bahouq H, Allali F, Rkain H, Hajjaj-Hassouni N. Discussing sexual concerns with chronic low back pain patients: barriers and patients' expectations. Clin Rheumatol. 2013;32(10):1487–92.
6. Courtois F, Gerard M, Charvier K, Vodusek DB, Amarenco G. Assessment of sexual function in women with neurological disorders: a review. Ann Phys Rehabil Med. 2018;61(4):235–44.
7. Dahm DL, Jacofsky D, Lewallen DG. Surgeons rarely discuss sexual activity with patients after THA: a survey of members of the American Association of Hip and Knee Surgeons. Clin Orthop Relat Res. 2004;(428):237–40.
8. Nilsson MI, Fugl-Meyer K, von Koch L, Ytterberg C. Experiences of sexuality six years after stroke: a qualitative study. J Sex Med. 2017;14(6):797–803.
9. Stein J, Hillinger M, Clancy C, Bishop L. Sexuality after stroke: patient counseling preferences. Disabil Rehabil. 2013;35(21):1842–7.
10. Steinke EE, Jaarsma T, Barnason SA, et al. Sexual counselling for individuals with cardiovascular disease and their partners: a consensus document from the American Heart Association and the ESC Council on Cardiovascular Nursing and Allied Professions (CCNAP). Eur Heart J. 2013;34(41):3217–35.
11. Rees PM, Fowler CJ, Maas CP. Sexual function in men and women with neurological disorders. Lancet. 2007;369(9560):512–25.
12. Mick J, Hughes M, Cohen MZ. Using the BETTER model to assess sexuality. Clin J Oncol Nurs. 2004;8(1):84–6.
13. Annon JS. The PLISSIT model: a proposed conceptual scheme for the behavioral treatment of sexual problems. J Sex Educ Ther. 1976;2(1):1–15.
14. Pharr JR. Accommodations for patients with disabilities in primary care: a mixed methods study of practice administrators. Glob J Health Sci. 2013;6(1):23–32.
15. Andersson G. Spine: low back and neck pain. 2014. http://www.boneandjointburden.org/2014-report/ii0/spine-low-back-and-neck-pain. Accessed 11 Jan 2018.
16. Pollack AN. Injuries. 2014. http://www.boneandjointburden.org/2014-report/vi0/injuries. Accessed 11 Jan 2018.
17. Barbour KE, Helmick CG, Boring M, Brady TJ. Vital signs: prevalence of doctor-diagnosed arthritis and arthritis-attributable activity limitation - United States, 2013-2015. MMWR Morb Mortal Wkly Rep. 2017;66(9):246–53.
18. Campbell P, Jordan KP, Dunn KM. The role of relationship quality and perceived partner responses with pain and disability in those with back pain. Pain Med. 2012;13(2):204–14.
19. Issa K, Pierce TP, Brothers A, Festa A, Scillia AJ, Mont MA. Sexual activity after total hip arthroplasty: a systematic review of the outcomes. J Arthroplast. 2017;32(1):336–40.
20. Kazarian GS, Lonner JH, Hozack WJ, Woodward L, Chen AF. Improvements in sexual activity after total knee arthroplasty. J Arthroplast. 2017;32(4):1159–63.
21. Maigne JY, Chatellier G. Assessment of sexual activity in patients with back pain compared with patients with neck pain. Clin Orthop Relat Res. 2001;385:82–7.
22. Froud R, Patterson S, Eldridge S, et al. A systematic review and meta-synthesis of the impact of low back pain on people's lives. BMC Musculoskelet Disord. 2014;15:50.
23. Brennan GP, Fritz JM, Hunter SJ, Thackeray A, Delitto A, Erhard RE. Identifying subgroups of patients with acute/subacute "nonspecific" low back pain: results of a randomized clinical trial. Spine (Phila Pa 1976). 2006;31(6):623–31.
24. Sidorkewicz N, McGill SM. Male spine motion during coitus: implications for the low back pain patient. Spine (Phila Pa 1976). 2014;39(20):1633–9.
25. Sidorkewicz N, McGill SM. Documenting female spine motion during coitus with a commentary on the implications for the low back pain patient. Eur Spine J. 2015;24(3):513–20.

26. Hootman JM, Helmick CG, Barbour KE, Theis KA, Boring MA. Updated projected prevalence of self-reported doctor-diagnosed arthritis and arthritis-attributable activity limitation among US adults, 2015–2040. Arthritis Rheumatol. 2016;68(7):1582–7.
27. Salaffi F, Carotti M, Grassi W. Health-related quality of life in patients with hip or knee osteoarthritis: comparison of generic and disease-specific instruments. Clin Rheumatol. 2005;24(1):29–37.
28. Rydevik K, Fernandes L, Nordsletten L, Risberg MA. Functioning and disability in patients with hip osteoarthritis with mild to moderate pain. J Orthop Sports Phys Ther. 2010;40(10):616–24.
29. Rasch A, Dalen N, Berg HE. Muscle strength, gait, and balance in 20 patients with hip osteoarthritis followed for 2 years after THA. Acta Orthop. 2010;81(2):183–8.
30. van Dijk GM, Veenhof C, Spreeuwenberg P, et al. Prognosis of limitations in activities in osteoarthritis of the hip or knee: a 3-year cohort study. Arch Phys Med Rehabil. 2010;91(1):58–66.
31. Vissers MM, Bussmann JB, de Groot IB, Verhaar JA, Reijman M. Walking and chair rising performed in the daily life situation before and after total hip arthroplasty. Osteoarthr Cartil. 2011;19(9):1102–7.
32. Veenhof C, Huisman PA, Barten JA, Takken T, Pisters MF. Factors associated with physical activity in patients with osteoarthritis of the hip or knee: a systematic review. Osteoarthr Cartil. 2012;20(1):6–12.
33. Laffosse JM, Tricoire JL, Chiron P, Puget J. Sexual function before and after primary total hip arthroplasty. Joint Bone Spine. 2008;75(2):189–94.
34. Lavernia CJ, Villa JM. High rates of interest in sex in patients with hip arthritis. Clin Orthop Relat Res. 2016;474(2):293–9.
35. Kelmanovich D, Parks ML, Sinha R, Macaulay W. Surgical approaches to total hip arthroplasty. J South Orthop Assoc. 2003;12(2):90–4.
36. Charbonnier C, Chague S, Ponzoni M, Bernardoni M, Hoffmeyer P, Christofilopoulos P. Sexual activity after total hip arthroplasty: a motion capture study. J Arthroplast. 2014;29(3):640–7.
37. Center NSCIS. Spinal cord injury facts and figures at a glance. 2016. www.nscisc.uab.edu/Public/Facts%202016.pdf. Accessed 13 Dec 2017.
38. Medicine CfSC. Clinical practice guidelines. 2010. www.pva.org/publications/clinical-practice-guidelines. Accessed 13 Dec 2017.
39. Fisher TL, Laud PW, Byfield MG, Brown TT, Hayat MJ, Fiedler IG. Sexual health after spinal cord injury: a longitudinal study. Arch Phys Med Rehabil. 2002;83(8):1043–51.
40. Connell KM, Coates R, Wood FM. Sexuality following trauma injury: a literature review. Burns Trauma. 2014;2(2):61–70.
41. Naphtali K. pleasureABLE. In: Network DHR, ed2009.
42. Baer RW. Is Fred dead? A manual on sexuality for men with spinal cord injuries. First ed. Pittsburgh: Dorrance Publishing Co; 2003.
43. Davidson R, Elliott S, Krassioukov A. Cardiovascular responses to sexual activity in able-bodied individuals and those living with spinal cord injury. J Neurotrauma. 2016;33(24):2161–74.
44. Anderson KD, Borisoff JF, Johnson RD, Stiens SA, Elliott SL. Long-term effects of spinal cord injury on sexual function in men: implications for neuroplasticity. Spinal Cord. 2007;45(5):338–48.
45. Prevention CfDCa. Stroke facts. 2017. www.cdc.gov/stroke/facts.htm. Accessed 14 Dec 2017.
46. Seymour LM, Wolf TJ. Participation changes in sexual functioning after mild stroke. OTJR (Thorofare N J). 2014;34(2):72–80.
47. Boller F, Agrawal K, Romano A. Sexual function after strokes. Handb Clin Neurol. 2015;130:289–95.
48. Hamam N, McCluskey A, Cooper Robbins S. Sex after stroke: a content analysis of printable educational materials available online. Int J Stroke. 2013;8(7):518–28.
49. Richards A, Dean R, Burgess GH, Caird H. Sexuality after stroke: an exploration of current professional approaches, barriers to providing support and future directions. Disabil Rehabil. 2016;38(15):1471–82.

50. Ng L, Sansom J, Zhang N, Amatya B, Khan F. Effectiveness of a structured sexual rehabilitation programme following stroke: a randomized controlled trial. J Rehabil Med. 2017;49(4):333–40.
51. Gisbert R, Schenkman M. Physical therapist interventions for Parkinson disease. Phys Ther. 2015;95(3):299–305.
52. Tomlinson CL, Herd CP, Clarke CE, et al. Physiotherapy for Parkinson's disease: a comparison of techniques. Cochrane Database Syst Rev. 2014;(6):Cd002815.
53. Lange L, Zedler B, Verhoff MA, Parzeller M. Love death-a retrospective and prospective follow-up mortality study over 45 years. J Sex Med. 2017;14(10):1226–31.
54. Levine GN, Steinke EE, Bakaeen FG, et al. Sexual activity and cardiovascular disease: a scientific statement from the American Heart Association. Circulation. 2012;125(8):1058–72.
55. Steinke EE, Johansen PP, Dusenbury W. When the topic turns to sex: case scenarios in sexual counseling and cardiovascular disease. J Cardiopulm Rehabil Prev. 2015;36(3):145–56.
56. Prevention CfDCa. Chronic disease overview. 2017. https://www.cdc.gov/chronicdisease/overview/index.htm. Accessed 15 Jan 2018.

Chapter 13
Religiosity and Spirituality

Jo Hirschmann

Contents

Introduction

This chapter explores how primary care clinicians can most effectively explore, assess, and respond to patients' religious and spiritual (R/S) needs, as they intersect with sexual and reproductive health (SRH) in the primary care setting. Section "Religion, Spirituality, and Health: Setting the Scene" provides definitions of key terms, describes the sometimes uneasy relationship between religion and sexual/

J. Hirschmann (✉)
Center for Spirituality and Health, Icahn School of Medicine at Mount Sinai,
New York, NY, USA
e-mail: jo.hirschmann@mountsinai.org

© Springer Nature Switzerland AG 2022
J. Truglio et al. (eds.), *Sexual and Reproductive Health*,
https://doi.org/10.1007/978-3-030-94632-6_13

reproductive health priorities, and looks at the history of the emergence of the field of spirituality and health over the past 25 years. Section "Clinical Practice" offers practical guidance for integrating spiritual care into medical practice. It defines the terms *spiritual care generalist* and *spiritual care specialist*, offers an example of a screening tool clinicians can use, and lists barriers to, and facilitators of, spiritual care within primary care settings. Section "Considerations Specific to Demographic Groups, Stages of the Life Cycle, and/or Targeted Health Promotion Efforts" looks at R/S themes in five clinical areas: screening for prostate cancer, screening for cervical and breast cancer, neonatology and infertility, adolescent sexual health, and LGBTQ healthcare. This section aims to help clinicians identify the kinds of concerns, support, and struggles that may be present for their patients. In this section and throughout the chapter, a recurrent theme is the ways in which R/S beliefs and practices can play both supportive and harmful roles in patients' lives, leading to both positive and negative effects on health. Section "Case Studies" pulls together content from the earlier sections into two cases that illustrate salient themes and offer a guide to practice.

Religion, Spirituality, and Health: Setting the Scene

In 2014, an international panel of physicians, psychologists, and chaplains developed the following consensus definition of spirituality: "Spirituality is a dynamic and intrinsic aspect of humanity through which persons seek ultimate meaning, purpose, and transcendence, and experience relationship to self, family, others, community, society, nature, and the significant or sacred. Spirituality is expressed through beliefs, values, traditions, and practices" [41]. In this definition, religion is a subset of spirituality; it is one means by which people find meaning and transcendence in their lives. Koenig provides us with a helpful working definition of religion as "beliefs, practices and rituals related to the transcendent" that are "designed (a) to facilitate closeness to the transcendent and (b) to foster understanding of one's relationship and responsibility to others in living together in a community" [29].

In 2015, the Pew Research Center published a study entitled "America's Changing Religious Landscape," which reported on findings from surveys conducted with more than 25,000 Americans in 2014. Compared to the Pew Research Center's prior survey, which was conducted in 2007, the key findings of the second survey were that the proportion of Christians in the US population has declined, while the proportion of those who do not identify with any organized religion is growing. The decline of the Christian share of the population is driven primarily by drops in the number of Catholics and mainline Protestants. Meanwhile the number of "nones" – i.e., those who do not claim any religious affiliation – in the population now exceeds both the number of Catholics and the number of mainline Protestants. The Pew study also found that Americans frequently switch religions and that Evangelical Christians and the "nones" have experienced the greatest gains as the result of people switching into their groups. Overall, 25% of Americans identify as

Evangelical Protestants, 15% as mainline Protestants, 21% as Catholic, 1.9% as Jewish, and less than 1% each as Buddhist, Muslim, and Hindu. Twenty-three percent identified as unaffiliated, a category that included atheist, agnostic, and "nothing in particular" [39]. Based on the 2014 consensus definition of spirituality offered above, this unaffiliated category may include those who identify as "spiritual" or as "spiritual but not religious."

Sociologist Ellen Idler describes people who share religious beliefs and practices as "populations, whose health may be influenced in various ways by their religious beliefs and practices." In this way, religion is a social determinant of health like other demographic factors. According to the Centers for Disease Control (CDC) definition, social determinants of health (SDOH) refers to "conditions in the places where people live, learn, work, and play [that] affect a wide range of health risks and outcomes." Noting that religion has not been studied nearly as extensively as other SDOHs, Idler identifies *social support*, *social control*, and *social capital* as key themes. With regard to *social support*, which Idler defines as the "critical support and nurturance" that religious institutions may provide to their members, the research "shows a net benefit of social ties, religious or otherwise, for health." Additionally, Idler describes how "communities are... composed of political, economic, educational, religious, and social institutions, resources collectively referred to as *social capital*" (italics in original). She points out that religious communities have the ability to "creat[e] social capital in their communities, by establishing schools, hospitals, and clinics and providing health and social services, often to the neediest members of their communities" and that this plays a supportive and protective role for community members [27].

At the same time, religion can function as a form of *social control*, defined by Idler as religious groups' ability to "regulate behavior" of its members. While these effects on behavior can be beneficial, social control mechanisms can also have harmful effects on vulnerable populations. This is especially true with regard to sexual and reproductive health. This category includes LGBTQ healthcare, HIV/AIDS public health efforts, contraception, and abortion, all of which are religiously contentious topics. For example, Lynn and Carol Hogue trace the history of the Comstock Law, "the first comprehensive, federal, anti-obscenity law," which was enacted in 1873 and not fully struck down until 1983. Ostensibly an effort to combat "vice," the Comstock Law affected the dissemination of information about sexual and reproductive health. In their telling of the story, Hogue and Hogue describe how "sin codified as crime" shaped the history of sexual and reproductive health in the United States for more than a century [23].

While a full exploration is beyond the scope of this chapter, Table 13.1 summarizes the stances of major religious groups on contraception and abortion. This table provides a useful overview but should be used with the caveat that there is enormous diversity of belief and practice among people who claim the same religious affiliation. Taking a spiritual history, as described later in this chapter, helps clinicians draw out the nuances and complexities of patients' beliefs and practices. While earlier approaches to culturally competent care emphasized the need to learn and memorize how different cultural groups may approach healthcare, culturally

Table 13.1 Religious groups' stances on contraception and abortion

Religious denomination/ group	Stance on contraception (Much of the information in this column is adapted from [17].)	Stance on abortion (Some of the information in this column is adapted from www. pewforum.org/2013/01/16/religious-groups-official-positions-on-abortion. Accessed March 3, 2018.)
Afro-Caribbean religious traditions, including Santeria [a]	Not a centralized religion so no official stance and a great variety of practices and beliefs	Not a centralized religion so no official stance and a great variety of practices and beliefs
American Baptist Church	Supports full range of contraceptive options	Opposes abortion in many circumstances but does not condemn it outright; encourages those considering the procedure to seek spiritual counsel
Bahá'í	Preference given to methods that prevent conception	Prohibited to Bahá'ís for the purpose of terminating an unplanned pregnancy, but the decision of medical necessity is left to the conscience of those concerned. No official position on the abortion issue for the general public because Bahá'ís do not seek to impose their beliefs on others[b]
Buddhism	Preference is given to contraception options that prevent conception or implantation	No official position, although many Buddhists have a moral aversion to abortion
Chinese religions including Taoism and Confucianism[c]	Preference is given to contraception options that prevent conception or implantation	No official position, although many Taoists and Confucianists have a moral aversion to abortion
Church of Jesus Christ of Latter-day Saints	No official stance on the use of contraception options; deems contraception a matter of personal conscience	Generally opposes abortion with the caveat that certain circumstances, such as a pregnancy that is life-threatening or results from rape or incest, can justify an abortion
Conservative Judaism	Supports full range of contraceptive options	Advocates for the right to safe and accessible abortions
Episcopal Church	Supports full range of contraceptive options	Recognizes the right to terminate a pregnancy but condones abortion only following rape or incest, when a pregnancy poses a threat to physical or mental health, or if there are fetal abnormalities
Evangelical Lutheran Church in America	Supports full range of contraceptive options	Official position states that "abortion prior to viability [of a fetus] should not be prohibited by law or by lack of public funding" but that abortion after the point of fetal viability should be prohibited except when the pregnancy is life-threatening or there are potentially fatal fetal abnormalities

Table 13.1 (continued)

Religious denomination/ group	Stance on contraception (Much of the information in this column is adapted from [17].)	Stance on abortion (Some of the information in this column is adapted from www. pewforum.org/2013/01/16/religious-groups-official-positions-on-abortion. Accessed March 3, 2018.)
Greek Orthodox Archdiocese of America	Defines abstinence as only acceptable method of contraception	Opposes abortion in all circumstances[d]
Hinduism	Support for contraceptive options remains varied. No evidence of public opposition to contraception in general	Unless the pregnancy is life-threatening, traditional Hindu teachings oppose abortion on the grounds that it violates the religion's teachings of nonviolence
Islam	Support for contraceptive options varies, with nonhormonal/barrier methods most widely accepted. Sterilization is generally considered unacceptable	Most Islamic scholars agree that the termination of a pregnancy after 4 months – the point at which a fetus is thought to become a living soul – is not permissible. Many Islamic scholars argue that, prior to 4 months of gestation, abortion is permissible only in instances in which the pregnancy is life-threatening or following rape or incest
National Association of Evangelicals	Generally open to all methods of contraception[e]	Opposes abortion, although may make exceptions following rape/incest or if the pregnancy is life-threatening
Native American religions	Supports full range of contraceptive options. Preference is given to natural methods/remedies	No unified position. Abortions cannot be performed on reservations so access to abortions is sometimes more limited for Native Americans[f]
Orthodox/Hasidic Judaism	Hormonal methods are preferred because they are temporary and, unlike barrier methods, do not result in "wasting of seed." Sterilization is generally prohibited. Religious authority is not centralized, and Orthodox Jews typically consult with their own rabbi on questions related to contraception[g]	Abortion is generally prohibited, although there is a significant variety of opinions among individual rabbis. Religious authority is not centralized, and Orthodox Jews typically consult with their own rabbi on questions related to abortion[h]
Presbyterian Church (USA)	Supports full range of contraceptive options	Views abortion as a personal decision
Reform/ Reconstructionist Judaism	Supports full range of contraceptive options	Advocates for the right to safe and accessible abortions
Roman Catholic	Forbids all artificial means of contraception	Opposes abortion in all circumstances

(continued)

Table 13.1 (continued)

Religious denomination/ group	Stance on contraception (Much of the information in this column is adapted from [17].)	Stance on abortion (Some of the information in this column is adapted from www. pewforum.org/2013/01/16/religious-groups-official-positions-on-abortion. Accessed March 3, 2018.)
Seventh-day Adventist	Supports full range of contraceptive options	Generally opposes abortion but regards it as a personal matter that is allowable under certain circumstances, such as a life-threatening pregnancy or following rape or incest[i]
Southern Baptist Church	Supports the use of some forms of contraceptive options by married couples as long as contraception prevents conception, rather than destroying a fertilized egg or preventing implantation	Opposes abortion unless the pregnancy is life-threatening
Unitarian Universalist Association of Congregations	Supports full range of contraceptive options	Advocates for the right to safe and accessible abortions
United Church of Christ	Supports full range of contraceptive options	Advocates for the right to safe and accessible abortions
United Methodist Church	Supports full range of contraceptive options	Opposes abortion but sanctions "the legal option of abortion under proper medical procedures." Encourages women and couples considering the procedure to seek spiritual and medical counsel
Wicca/ Paganism	Highly decentralized religions that allow for diversity of belief and practices. Contraception not generally a controversial question	Highly decentralized religions that allow for diversity of belief and practices. Wicca and Pagan communities include adherents who are pro-life and pro-choice[j]

[a]The Rev. Carlos Alejandro offered guidance on Afro-Caribbean religious traditions. Personal email correspondence, March 29, 2018
[b]Email correspondence with Jan Mauras on behalf of the Spiritual Assembly of the Bahá'ís of the City of New York, April 19, 2018
[c]Lucia Sau Chan, Senior Director of the Asian Services Center at Mount Sinai Beth Israel, offered guidance on the sections on Buddhism and Chinese religions
[d]www.oca.org/parish-ministry/familylife/common-pro-abortion-cliches-and-the-pro-life-response. Accessed March 6, 2018
[e]www.nae.net/evangelical-leaders-are-ok-with-contraception. Accessed March 3, 2018
[f]https://carafem.org/native-americans-and-access-to-abortion/. Accessed March 6, 2018
[g]www.yoatzot.org/womens-health-and-halacha. Accessed April 30, 2018
[h]www.halachipedia.com/index/php?title=Abortion. Accessed April 30, 2018
[i]www.adventist.org/en/information/official-statements/guidelines/article/go/-/abortion/. Accessed March 6, 2018
[j]https://www.thoughtco.com/abortion-in-paganism-and-wicca-2561713. Accessed March 6, 2018

effective care invites providers to ask open-ended questions to learn about what is important to individual patients. This approach is guided by the understanding that R/S, like other social structures, can affect the health of individuals and communities; therefore, providers should seek to understand how it shapes their patients' approaches to healthcare and decision-making.

To build on Idler's work, religion can function as a form of social control for LGBTQ patients. Researchers at the Fenway Institute in Boston have documented how the current wave of so-called "religious exemption" bills, legislation introduced in state legislatures since 2012, could exacerbate LGBTQ health disparities. These bills have explicitly targeted LGBTQ people's access to healthcare and, according to the Fenway Institute, threaten to exacerbate health disparities and undermine the provision of "affirming and competent care for LGBTQ patients" [50]. At the same time and despite the sometimes uneasy relationship between religion and LGBTQ rights, LGBTQ people continue to claim and create places for themselves within religious life. As Copeland and Rose [10] describe, these approaches include the reinterpretation of scripture, the creation of new rituals, special ministries oriented toward LGBTQ inclusion, and the actions of lay and ordained leadership.

Kenneth Pargament, a psychologist who studies the relationship between religion and health, distinguishes between positive and negative coping. These concepts help explain the ways in which religion can be both a supportive and a harmful force in people's lives, especially with regard to sexual and reproductive health. According to Pargament, positive religious coping – for example, benefiting from the support of a religious community or using the concept of God's will as a framework for understanding unwanted change – is generally associated with better health outcomes. In contrast, negative religious coping – for example, believing that God is punitive or that one is unlovable by God – is generally predictive of declines in health [38]. Pargament's work points to the need to understand how R/S are nuanced and complex dynamics in patients' lives that cannot be understood by means of simple formulae. In addition, the impact of religion and spirituality upon patients' health may be mediated by race, ethnicity, sexual orientation, and gender identity. Against this backdrop, clinicians have the opportunity to inquire about patients' R/S lives as part of the overall medical care they offer. Indeed, the imperative to provide culturally and structurally effective care requires this – because it is increasingly recognized that spirituality is an aspect of culture that may affect patients' healthcare decisions [28].

The past 25 years have seen the development of clinical practices, research articles, and medical education curricula about spirituality and health. Christina Puchalski, MD, is a palliative care physician with the George Washington University School of Medicine and Health Sciences and leader in the development of the field of spiritual care within medicine. She and her colleagues write that "the close connection between spirituality and health has been acknowledged for centuries," but the technological advances of the early twentieth century "overshadowed the more human element of medicine." Beginning in the early 1990s with an initiative at George Washington University spearheaded by Puchalski and her colleagues, some medical schools began incorporating spirituality into their curricula, and by 2011 more than 75% of medical school curricula included topics related to spirituality [42].

In 2004, the National Consensus Conference for Palliative Care included patients' spiritual, religious, and existential concerns among its domains of care. Currently in its fourth edition, which was published in 2018, the Clinical Practice Guidelines for Quality Palliative Care incorporate the expectation that the IDT will assess the spiritual, religious, existential, and emotional dimensions of a patient's illness and facilitate appropriate spiritual, religious, or cultural rituals, especially at the time of death [48]. The Joint Commission's requirements for inpatient settings include the provisions that providers address patients' right to access religious and spiritual services and, to the extent possible, accommodate patients' spiritual needs during end-of-life care (The Joint Commission, Standards RI.01.01.01 EP9 and PC.02.02.13 EP1). At this time, there are no Joint Commission standards related to patient care in outpatient settings [48].

Much of the conversation about spirituality and health has focused on palliative and critical care contexts [28]. Healthcare chaplains frequently work in these kinds of inpatient settings, which means that when palliative and critical care clinicians encounter patients with complex R/S needs, chaplains may be part of the interdisciplinary team working with the patient. While hiring practices vary, healthcare chaplains are typically well-trained professionals with specialized chaplaincy training and an advanced degree in theology (Handzo and Koenig 2014). Most bodies that certify chaplains require a Master of Divinity degree or its equivalent, four 400-hour units of Clinical Pastoral Education (CPE) training provided by an Association for Clinical Pastoral Education (ACPE)-accredited training center, and 2000 hours of work experience. For more information, refer to the websites of the Association of Professional Chaplains, the oldest and largest chaplaincy certifying body in the United States (www.professionalchaplains.org) and the Association for Clinical Pastoral Education (www.acpe.edu).

Hiring chaplains in primary care settings may be a desirable goal, but, at the time of writing, it is not the norm. Given this reality, this chapter seeks to apply, where appropriate, themes, practices, and research findings from inpatient settings to the primary care setting. It also draws on the available outpatient and primary care literature. Section "Clinical Practice" takes a practical look at how primary care physicians might integrate spiritual care into their clinical practice.

Clinical Practice

George Handzo and Harold Koenig, a chaplain and a physician respectively, differentiate between spiritual care *generalists* and *specialists*. They propose a model in which primary care physicians conduct a basic spiritual assessment, just as they also assess patients' physical and psychological domains. Patients with R/S needs can then be referred to board-certified chaplains, who function as spiritual care specialists, diagnosing patients' spiritual states and implementing an appropriate treatment plan [22]. As already noted, primary care teams do not generally include a chaplain. Given this constraint, this section will focus on how primary care clinicians can most effectively provide their patients with spiritual care.

The first step is for clinicians to assess how patients' R/S lives may affect their health behaviors. The field of spiritual care differentiates between spiritual *screens*, *histories*, and *assessments*. A *screen* is typically used by admissions staff, nurses, or social workers who, with a few brief questions, aim to identify spiritual distress in patients. A spiritual *history*, which can be one part of an overall history taken by a physician or other primary care clinician, seeks to uncover R/S beliefs and sources of support as these relate to patients' healthcare needs. A spiritual *assessment* is conducted by a chaplain with the goal of assessing spiritual needs and resources and developing appropriate spiritual care interventions [32]. Table 13.2 summarizes these distinctions.

Over the past 25 years, physicians have developed a number of spiritual history tools; one of the most widely used is Christina Puchalski's FICA Spiritual History Tool © (see Table 13.3). Puchalski recommends using FICA not as a checklist but as a guide for conversation. She encourages clinicians to consider spirituality as a "potentially important component of every patient's quality of life" and recommends that clinicians address spirituality at each new visit, at annual office visits, and, if appropriate, at follow-up visits [40]. The FICA is appropriate for use with adult patients of all ages, including geriatric patients.

At the time of writing, there is not yet a spiritual history tool for use with pediatric patients and their parents. However, a modified version of the FICA that asks family members to describe important people and activities could be effective. When working with pediatric patients, and especially with LGBTQ children and adolescents, it is important to understand that children and their parents may not subscribe to the same belief systems [19].

Despite the existence of screens like the FICA, clinicians describe a number of barriers to the provision of spiritual care, particularly in primary care settings. In a review of earlier studies, Tanyi and colleagues identify a list that includes the following: the fear that patients don't want to discuss spirituality with primary care physicians, physicians' belief that they lack adequate training; the fear that patients

Table 13.2 Screens, histories, and assessments

Assessment	Purpose	Typically conducted by
Screen	Screen for spiritual distress	Any spiritual care generalist, including admissions staff, nurses, and social workers
History	Learn about patients' R/S beliefs and sources of support as related to healthcare needs	Physicians, nurse practitioners, physician assistants
Assessment	Assess spiritual needs and resources in order to develop appropriate spiritual care interventions	Chaplains

Table 13.3 The FICA Spiritual History Tool ©

F - Faith and Belief
"Do you consider yourself spiritual or religious?" or "Is spirituality something important to you" or "Do you have spiritual beliefs that help you cope with stress/ difficult times?" (Contextualize to reason for visit if it is not the routine history).
If the patient responds "No," the healthcare provider might ask, "What gives your life meaning?" Sometimes patients respond with answers such as family, career, or nature.
(The question of meaning should also be asked even if people answer yes to spirituality)
I – Importance
"What importance does your spirituality have in our life? Has your spirituality influenced how you take care of yourself, your health? Does your spirituality influence you in your healthcare decision-making? (e.g., advance directives, treatment, etc.)"
C – Community
"Are you part of a spiritual community? Communities such as churches, temples, and mosques, or a group of like-minded friends, family, or yoga, can serve as strong support systems for some patients. Can explore further: Is this of support to you and how? Is there a group of people you really love or who are important to you?"
A – Address in Care
"How would you like me, your healthcare provider, to address these issues in your healthcare?" (With the newer models including diagnosis of spiritual distress, A also refers to the Assessment and Plan of patient spiritual distress or issues within a treatment or care plan)

© Copyright, Christina M. Puchalski, MD, 1996

will perceive conversations about R/S as proselytizing, the perception that spirituality is a "private" topic, and clinicians' fear that they don't have enough time to adequately pursue the topic [47]. It is helpful to look in depth at each of these five barriers, along with a sixth: the need for clinicians to explore their own biases.

Perception that patients do not want to discuss spirituality with their physicians This perception is not borne out by the research literature. In a white paper published by the HealthCare Chaplaincy Network, Marin et al. cite a 2016 American Medical Association resolution that notes that 41% of patients would like to discuss religious or spiritual concerns in a healthcare setting, but less than half report being offered the opportunity to do so. Elsewhere in the white paper, the authors note that, while not all patients want to discuss religious and spiritual matters, "the majority do" [32]. In a survey of almost 1000 patients at family practice residency training sites and a private group practice in Ohio, 83% of respondents wanted their physicians to ask about spiritual beliefs in at least some circumstances. By talking to their physicians about their spirituality, patients thought physicians would be able to encourage realistic hope (67%), give medical advice (66%), and change medical treatment (62%) [34].

Lack of adequate training As noted above, the topic of spirituality is now integrated into the curricula of more than 75% of medical schools [41, 42]. However, it is likely that many physicians currently in practice have a need for ongoing training on this topic. Best et al. [4] conducted a review of the literature that includes a summary of factors that facilitate physicians asking about spirituality. They list training in communication skills and qualities such as "sensitivity, patience, tolerance for ambiguity and sensitivity to one's own spirituality." They also note that, in some studies, discussion of R/S is more common among physicians who regard medicine as a vocation, rather than as a job, and that talking to patients about spirituality is associated with increased job satisfaction. Tanyi et al. [47] conducted a qualitative study involving three physicians, five NPs, and two PAs in family practice to understand how they integrate spirituality into conversations with patients. These respondents described how "exhibiting a positive caring demeanor that was genuine and nonjudgmental" was an essential element of such conversations. They also reported that it is important to educate primary care providers about spirituality, although they "believed that educating each other about techniques that are effective in managing barriers [to asking patients about their R/S lives] can be more effective than attending conferences and relying on management to arrange seminars."

Fear that patients will perceive conversations about R/S as proselytizing; perception that spirituality is a "private" topic Both of these concerns are connected to the possible violation of ethical boundaries when physicians introduce the topic of spirituality. When talking about patients' R/S concerns, Winslow and Wehtje-Winslow [52] remind us it is essential that physicians provide respectful care to patients and attend to their own boundaries. They offer five guidelines for the ethical provision of spiritual care within the context of a medical visit. First, clinicians should conduct some kind of assessment (they propose the FICA tool) to gain a basic understanding of patients' spiritual needs, resources, and preferences. Second, clinicians must respect patient autonomy by following patients' expressed wishes regarding spiritual care. Third, clinicians should not be prescriptive by urging patients to adopt or relinquish practices, even if they suspect a practice is detrimental to a patient's health. Fourth, they should understand their own spiritual beliefs and practices, which will help them, fifth, provide spiritual care that is consonant with their professional integrity. In the two cases presented below, we will use these five guidelines as a framework for practice.

Perception of inadequate time While lack of time is a perennial challenge for all clinicians, Tanyi et al.'s [47] respondents describe how they build R/S conversations into the time they already spend with patients. These respondents also reported that they make time for such conversations because of the importance they ascribe to them.

The need for clinicians to explore their own biases Clinicians can more effectively meet their patients' R/S needs if they become familiar with their own implicit and explicit biases toward R/S in general and toward specific manifestations of R/S in their patients' lives. The cases at the end of this chapter provide examples of how clinicians might recognize and manage their own biases.

With these overarching tools and guidelines, primary care clinicians might begin integrating spiritual care into their work with patients or might deepen work they are already doing. The next section highlights key themes and considerations related to specific areas of clinical practice.

Considerations Specific to Demographic Groups, Stages of the Life Cycle, and/or Targeted Health Promotion Efforts

This section draws out key themes from research literature related to how patients' R/S concerns affect five areas of clinical practice: screening for prostate cancer, screening for cervical and breast cancer, neonatology and infertility, adolescent sexual health, and LGBTQ healthcare. A number of themes recur in one, some, or all of these areas of clinical practice:

1. R/S beliefs and practices sometimes serve a protective function with regard to sexual and reproductive health.
2. Paradoxically, R/S beliefs and practices sometimes serve a damaging function with regard to sexual and reproductive health.
3. Religious communities may serve as a venue for, and partner in, health promotion efforts. Primary care clinicians may be able to partner with houses of worship, clergy, and congregants in these efforts.
4. Religion may function as a social determinant of health, and health inequities related to religion sometimes intersect with health inequities related to race, language, and socioeconomic status.
5. The impact of religiosity on health is complex, with different aspects of religious beliefs and behaviors supporting or undermining health promotion efforts in different ways. In addition, the effect of religiosity on health is mediated by race, SES, immigration status, language, and level of acculturation, among other factors.

Screening for Prostate Cancer

In the words of Husaini et al. [26], "Racial disparities in prostate cancer incidence and mortality are a national concern." According to the National Cancer Institute of the National Institutes of Health, African American and Black men in the United States have the highest incidence of prostate cancer compared to other racial groups and are more than twice as likely as white men to die of the disease. This disproportionate burden is often explained in the literature by purported genetic factors and biologic differences between races. However, given that race is clearly a social, not a biologic construct [53], and other research shows that lack of access to healthcare services and fewer ties to primary care physicians are barriers to screening and early diagnosis,[1] there is clearly a need for structurally effective health education efforts aimed at reducing these health inequities. Some clinicians, educators, and researchers have identified Black churches as a promising venue for this. Although these studies were conducted in the context of now outdated screening guidelines, they are included here because they offer templates for utilizing existing religious networks in the service of health promotion. In addition, they are examples of strengths-based approaches to the social determinants of health.

In South Carolina, a qualitative study of 43 African-American men and 38 female spouses or family members explored barriers to talking about and being screened for prostate cancer. Respondents most often recommended churches as a location for reaching African-American men of all ages. In addition, male and female respondents recommended that churches be involved in the planning and implementation of cancer education programs [16]. Similarly, when Ross et al. [45] conducted focus groups in Alabama and Mississippi, two other southeastern states with similarly high rates of diagnosis of, and mortality from, prostate cancer, respondents identified religious leaders as people who can influence health-related behaviors.

While these two studies looked at the church and its leaders as influential forces in African-American men's lives, a study by Holt et al. [24], which also focused on men in southeastern states, investigated the relationship between religious beliefs and behaviors and prostate cancer screening. This study found that religious involvement was predictive of having had a digital rectal exam (DRE) in the past year, having an upcoming appointment for a DRE, or planning to make an appointment for a DRE within the next 6 months. While fatalism can be understood as a mediating factor that decreases the likelihood of pursuing testing and treatment, Lisa Christman et al. [9] found some evidence that intrinsic religious beliefs partially mediate the relationship between fear of prostate cancer testing and fatalism. They speculate that "[g]iving control to another may not involve a sense of helplessness and may allow the individual, through their religious beliefs, to adopt a more active stance in decision-making." As in Holt's study, Christman found that religious beliefs and behaviors can be protective factors.

Taken together, these studies suggest that religious beliefs, practices, institutions, and leaders might all play a role in reducing racially based health inequities. The following two studies illustrate how this might work in practice. Holt et al. [25] describe a health education initiative they tested at two Baptist churches in the Birmingham, AL, metropolitan area. This intervention built on this team's earlier work to encourage mammography screening among African-American women and included elements that Holt et al. describe as both "religious" (e.g., scripture) and "spiritual" (e.g., "balance of healthy body, mind, and spirit"). The researchers collaborated with pastors to identify men who were then trained as community health advisors (CHAs). Some CHAs were trained to lead a "spiritually based"

---

[1] www.cancer.gov/about-nci/organization/crchd/cancer-health-disparities-fact-sheet#q9. Accessed March 3, 2018.

educational intervention; others were trained to lead a "non-spiritually based" intervention. While both educational programs were positively received, the men who attended the spiritually based session reported they read more of the educational materials and demonstrated increased self-efficacy with regard to making informed choices about prostate cancer screening.

In another study, African-American men were recruited from seven Boston-area churches to take part in an educational program that took place in churches but didn't include any R/S content. Pre- and post-tests indicated the educational intervention was effective in disseminating knowledge that may promote informed decision-making regarding testing. The authors acknowledge that the study did not include follow-up to determine the extent to which gains were maintained over time [15]. Since these interventions both involved men who were already church-going, an ongoing question is how to reach Black men who do not attend church.

In clinical practice In the United States, there are significant racial inequities in screening, treatment, and mortality related to prostate cancer. This inequity highlights the need for structurally effective care to reduce observed health inequities. The research literature provides an example of the intersection of religious and racial social determinants and highlights the use of these determinants as a strength from which to reduce inequities.

Screening for Cervical and Breast Cancer

While the literature on prostate cancer screening points to a generally positive relationship between church involvement and the efficacy of health promotion efforts, findings about the relationship between R/S and cervical cancer screening are more ambiguous. Matthews et al. [33], in their evaluation of a CDC faith-based breast and cervical cancer early detection and prevention intervention for African-American women, reached similar conclusions to those described in the section above on prostate cancer screening. Participants described how scripture reinforced the message of caring for the body (the body is a gift from God and/or a "temple of Christ"), ministers are effective health educators because they are responsible for the physical and spiritual health of the congregation, and testimonials by church members reinforced the importance of screening. Allen et al. [2] piloted an intervention in a Latino Baptist church in Boston that focused on screening for multiple cancers. Their respondents were highly receptive to the program, but the authors note that further research is needed to assess the impact on long-term health behaviors.

Nguyen et al. [36] recruited 111 Vietnamese women from a Catholic Vietnamese church and a Buddhist temple in the Richmond, VA, metropolitan area. Seeking to understand which aspects of religiosity may increase the likelihood of screening for cervical cancer, they used the Religious Orientation Scale, which differentiates between intrinsic and extrinsic religiosity. They also measured acculturation because they hypothesized it would be positively associated with cancer screening, which was borne out by their research. For acculturated women, religiosity was associated with higher probability of a Pap screen. However, in less acculturated women, some manifestations of religiosity were associated with lower probability of a Pap screen. This is similar to the findings of a study of 254 Muslim women in the Chicago area, who were recruited through mosques and Muslim community events. Women who perceived illness as a punishment from God were less likely to have had a Pap smear. Positive predictors were having lived in the United States for 20 or more years and having a primary care physician [37]. Meanwhile, a study of Muslim immigrant women in Canada found that HPV self-sampling may be a preferable option for this community because it protects patients' modesty [30].

In clinical practice These studies demonstrate that R/S beliefs, practices, and communities affect and shape attitudes toward screening in a wide variety of ways. Given this, clinicians can provide the most culturally effective care when they are open to a wide range of responses from patients as they take spiritual histories. By inviting their patients to talk about their R/S beliefs in the context of screening, clinicians may be more likely to identify culturally effective approaches to screening, such as the option of HPV self-sampling for patients concerned about modesty.

Neonatology and Infertility

Noting that, compared to spiritual concerns at the end of life, the spiritual dynamics of childbirth have received scant attention, a number of recent articles have drawn attention to this topic [13, 20]. While primary care physicians do not typically attend births, they work with families pre- and postnatally. Belanger-Levesque et al. [3] looked at mothers' and fathers' experiences of childbirth and found that both parents experienced childbirth as an "intensification of the human experience." While this heteronormative model of parenting does not apply to all families, the authors' findings are helpful for primary care clinicians working with expectant and new parents.

Breen et al. [6] conducted a review of the literature that looks at the emotional dynamics of high-risk pregnancies and concurrent spiritual coping mechanisms. Their synthesis includes the following emotional dynamics: fear, guilt, anxiety over loss of control, uncertainty, boredom, depression, loneliness, loss of identity, grief, and fear. Spiritual coping mechanisms included prayer, visualizations, affirmations, and biblical readings. A synthesis of studies looking at the spiritual dynamics of infertility listed subthemes in the category of expression of spiritual needs, including the need for: purpose in life, meaning in life, harmonious relationships, love, forgiveness, source of hope, source of strength, trust, expression of personal beliefs and values, spiritual practices, and expression of the concept of God or Deity or Divinity [43]. Both of these studies underscore how R/S can be supportive factors in patients' lives. However, there is no neat formula in which increased religiosity translates to lower stress. In a study of 248 pregnant and postpartum Latina women at a publicly funded hospital in California, R/S was associated with increased perceived stress among respondents who completed the survey instrument in English, but not among those who completed it in Spanish. The authors note that there are contradictory findings about the impact of acculturation (in this case, choosing the English-language survey instrument) on the well-being of Latina/os and conclude that further research is needed [31].

At the time of writing, there do not appear to be studies looking at the R/S lives of LGBTQ parents as related to childbirth, but one study looks at how Catholic Hispanic lesbian mothers negotiate their relationships with the church. This includes utilizing strategies of identifying as spiritual and of redefining religious meanings [49]. This study points to the need for more research into how R/S intersect with the childbirth and parenting experiences of LGBTQ people.

In clinical practice These data show that R/S dynamics can manifest in patients' lives in the context of childbirth and/or infertility in complex ways. Primary care clinicians can invite exploration of these topics by asking their patients if they have R/S beliefs and practices that are important to them as they attempt to get pregnant and/or experience pregnancy (as the person who is pregnant and/or as a partner of someone who is pregnant). Clinicians can also ask patients if their R/S traditions include particular beliefs about pregnancy, procreation, and/or infertility.

Adolescent Sexual Health

In a summary of findings about adolescents' overall rates of religiosity and spirituality, Cotton et al. [11] state the following: approximately 95% report that they believe in God and 85–95% report that religion is important in their lives. Ninety-three percent believe that God loves them, and more than half attend religious services at least once a month. Elsewhere, Cotton and Berry [12] report that adolescent religiosity is generally associated with initiating sexual intercourse later, having fewer sexual partners, and being less likely to have unprotected sex. While there is some truth in this, the reality – as Cotton and Berry themselves report – is more complex. They explain that, although R/S is generally protective for adolescents and may be related to resilience and a capacity for meaning making, greater religiosity is also connected to less frequent use of contraceptives.

Williams et al. [51] ran focus groups with young adults and their parents in two predominantly African-American churches in Flint, MI. They found that both youth and adults wanted parents to be the primary source of sexual health information but that some adolescents found their parents' messages confusing, especially regarding the effectiveness of contraceptives. Speculating about the reasons for this, Williams et al. suggest parents may be conflating values (sex should be reserved for marriage) with facts (contraception is generally safe and effective). The authors suggest that "making intentional distinctions" between values and facts "might enhance the sexual health communication within religious families."

A few studies have looked at whether adolescents' religious beliefs and practices influence their decision making around abortion. Adamczyk [1] found that conservative Protestants appear less likely to obtain abortions than Catholics, mainline Protestants, and those from non-Christian faiths. While religious belonging does seem to influence decision making, "[a]t the individual level, personal religious importance and involvement do not appear to influence reported abortion behavior."

In clinical practice These data suggest that young people's religiosity may affect their beliefs and decision-making about sexual health in complex and contradictory ways. Clinicians who ask adolescents about their R/S beliefs and practices in the context of a conversation about sexual health may run the risk of causing their patients to feel shame or stigma. A better course of action may be for clinicians to ask open-ended questions about the people and activities that are important to their adolescent patients.

LGBTQ Healthcare

There is a small body of literature exploring the R/S lives of LGBTQ people generally and transgender and gender diverse (TGD) people specifically. These studies suggest that R/S can protect against the stressors of discrimination [5, 7, 8, 44] and can serve a protective function against risky behaviors [14, 18, 21]. Dowshen et al.'s study of HIV risk among young transgender women distinguishes between "God Consciousness" (i.e., a belief in God), which is protective, and "Formal Religious Practices" (i.e., participation in religious practices such as attending worship services or studying scripture), which are not. This distinction echoes findings in other clinical areas, cited above, in which religious beliefs and behaviors have multiple effects on people's lives.

Several qualitative studies describe what LGBTQ people's beliefs and practices look like. In a qualitative study looking at the lives of 11 transgender people, Singh and McKleroy [46] find that nontraditional spiritual practices can be a source of resilience. Buser et al.'s study [8] of seven LGBTQ people's experiences in counseling found that, despite therapists' initial assumption that their clients would experience religious discord, these subjects chose to claim R/S beliefs and practices that were concordant with their LGBTQ identities. Despite the small sample size, this study's findings are worthy of further exploration. Rosenkrantz et al.'s [44] qualitative study of 213 subjects found that positive aspects of R/S include the spiritual strength derived from coming out and from coping with stigma and prejudice.

The 2015 US Transgender Survey [35], which had more than 27,000 respondents, shows a cycle of belonging, leaving, and finding that illustrates the harmful and supportive effects of religious community in transgender people's lives. Sixty-six percent of respondents reported that they had been part of a faith community at some point in their lives and, of those, 60% belonged or do belong to a faith community in which leaders and/or members thought or knew the respondent is transgender. However, 39% of respondents had left a faith community due to the fear they would be rejected because they are transgender, and 19% reported that they had been rejected by a faith community. Of these, 42% then found a new faith community that welcomed them as a transgender person.

As the Pew Center's "America's Changing Religious Landscape" report notes, this pattern of movement between denominations is common among Americans as a whole; it may be particularly pronounced among LGBTQ people because of the homophobic and transphobic voices within some religious communities. This may point to a desire to create meaningful R/S lives, beliefs, and communities, which is reflected in the US Transgender Survey's finding that 9% of respondents identified as Pagan, 4% as Wiccan, and 6% as Buddhist, which is many times higher than in the population as a whole. (In the Pew Center's study, Buddhists account for 0.7% of respondents and Pagans/Wiccans for 0.3%.)

In clinical practice While patients in general may describe (1) movement between denominations and (2) R/S's hurtful and supportive effects, these dynamics may be particularly pronounced among LGBTQ patients. The following questions may help elicit these histories:

• Do you have any R/S beliefs or practices that are currently important to you?
• Have these beliefs and practices changed over the course of your life?

Case Studies

The following two case studies draw together themes from the earlier sections of the chapter, including our exploration of screening tools, barriers to practice, and data from studies of clinical practice. We use Winslow and Wehtje-Winslow's five practice guidelines (introduced above in the section "Clinical Practice") to frame what culturally effective care might look like in each of these cases.

Case 1[2]

"Rosario" is a 26-year-old Latina heterosexual cisgender woman who is 10 weeks pregnant. She is partnered with a 32-year-old heterosexual cisgender Filipino man and became pregnant after the condom they were using broke. Rosario practices Afro-Caribbean spiritual practices, which include consulting a *lucumi* (priest) for guidance on important matters. She has a regularly scheduled annual checkup with her primary care clinician, Dr. Iacobi, a physician who is a 37-year-old

---

[2] I am grateful to my colleague, the Rev. Carlos Alejandro, who offered guidance on the development of this case.

Italian-American cisgender heterosexual woman who describes herself as a "lapsed Catholic."

Rosario begins the appointment by telling Dr. Iacobi that she is pregnant. She says she initially considered getting an abortion because her pregnancy is unplanned and she expects to have greater financial stability a few years from now. However, following a divination reading, her *lucumi* recommended against this.

Dr. Iacobi notices that her initial reaction is confusion (she doesn't know what a *lucumi* is or what divination involves) and judgment (as a pro-choice lapsed Catholic, she wants her patient to "make up her own mind" about whether to terminate a pregnancy). Dr. Iacobi takes a breath and recognizes that she has an opportunity to listen with care and curiosity to her patient and to deepen her capacity for culturally effective care. Here is what she might do if she follows Winslow and Wehtje-Winslow's five guidelines.

1. *Conduct an assessment to gain a basic understanding of patients' spiritual needs, resources, and preferences* – Dr. Iacobi begins with the invitation, "Tell me more about your spiritual practices and the role they played in you arriving at this decision." Rosario describes spiritual practices rooted in a connection to her ancestors, the belief that the day of people's births and deaths are predetermined, and a practice of using divination to assist with decision-making. She explains that a *lucumi* is a priest, also called a *santero* or *santera*, in the Santeria religion. Dr. Iacobi has heard of Santeria and feels like she is beginning to understand what is important to her patient. Rosario's *lucumi* told her that her child will have important work to do in the world and counseled her that abortion would not be the best choice. Rosario states she is at peace with her decision and is seeking a referral to a good ob/gyn.

2. *Respect patient autonomy by following patients' expressed wishes regarding spiritual care* – Rosario isn't seeking spiritual care from a chaplain, but Dr. Iacobi senses that her patient finds meaning and affirmation in being able to describe what is important to her. This careful and respectful listening is a form of spiritual care.

3. *Avoid being prescriptive by urging patients to adopt or relinquish practices, even if they suspect a practice is detrimental to a patient's health* – While Dr. Iacobi still wonders about the wisdom of "placing so much trust" in divination, she appropriately refrains from saying this.

4. *Understand one's own spiritual beliefs and practices* – Dr. Iacobi makes a mental note that her dislike of the Catholic church's teachings on abortion may be influencing her here. She may be reacting to what she hears as a religious proscription on abortion. She makes a mental note to seek consultation on this, which she recognizes as countertransference, from a colleague.

5. *Provide spiritual care that is consonant with one's own professional integrity* – Through all of this, Dr. Iacobi has maintained her own professional integrity. She hasn't endorsed religious practices with which she is uneasy – but nor has she dismissed them. She has maintained a strong relationship with her patient, establishing herself as a clinician who can provide support throughout and after her patient's pregnancy.

Case 2

"Cameron" is a 31-year-old African-American transgender man, whose sex assigned at birth was female. He has always presented on the transmasculine spectrum, began identifying as a lesbian in his teens, and has been undergoing transgender hormone treatment since age 24. He now identifies as queer and transgender and is currently partnered with a transgender man. His hormones are prescribed by his primary care provider, Dr. Chu, a Chinese-American heterosexual atheist who was raised in a Presbyterian family.

Cameron is one of three transgender patients on Dr. Chu's panel and he prescribes hormones to all of them. Dr. Chu collaborated with an endocrinology colleague at a nearby academic medical center to educate himself on gender-affirming hormones and overcome his initial discomfort and lack of familiarity with care needs of gender diverse patients.

Cameron makes an appointment with Dr. Chu because he is interested in getting pregnant. He wants to begin a conversation about coming off testosterone in order to resume menstruation. Dr. Chu feels taken aback when he hears this because it seems to contradict all he has learned about supporting transgender patients. He has the presence of mind to tell Cameron that he will consult with his endocrinology colleague to learn more and, if appropriate, make a referral. Recognizing that he is struggling to make sense of Cameron's request, Dr. Chu asks Cameron to tell him more about his interest in getting pregnant. With this open-ended question, Dr. Chu learns about Cameron's interest in parenthood and also about his R/S values.

1. *Conduct an assessment to gain a basic understanding of patients' spiritual needs, resources, and preferences* – Cameron tells Dr. Chu that, in his family of origin, parenthood is a highly valued role. Cameron says he grew up in a Baptist family and church community, both of which advocated narrow gender roles. Cameron still feels hurt by this but is also drawn to values from his childhood around the importance of nurturing children. He is in a stable partnership with another transgender man, and they are interested in raising a child together. Their first preference for how a child would come into their family is that Cameron get pregnant and a cisgender male friend serve as their sperm donor. Cameron describes himself as someone who "believes in God but not necessarily the same God my childhood pastors preached about." He tells Dr. Chu that, as he imagines himself as a parent, he feels very connected to "what God wants for me." Without taking a formal history, Dr. Chu has learned a great deal about what motivates Cameron's desire to be a parent.

2. *Respect patient autonomy by following patients' expressed wishes regarding spiritual care* – While Cameron isn't seeking spiritual care per se, he wishes to be seen and understood by his primary care provider. Dr. Chu successfully offers this.

3. *Avoid being prescriptive by urging patients to adopt or relinquish practices, even if they suspect a practice is detrimental to a patient's health* – Dr. Chu's initial

reaction is to wonder why someone who identifies as a man would want to be pregnant. He wonders if this choice will "undermine" Cameron's male identity in some way. By asking "tell me more," rather than offering his own opinion, Dr. Chu is able to work effectively with his patient.

4. *Understand one's own spiritual beliefs and practices* – Dr. Chu thinks about his own journey from the Presbyterian church of his childhood to his current atheism. He considers how, even though he no longer practices religion, he finds comfort in his childhood memories of attending church. This helps him to imagine and connect to Cameron's religious journey.

5. *Provide spiritual care that is consonant with one's own professional integrity* – Dr. Chu successfully offers care that honors his own integrity and that of his patient.

Conclusion

Implications for Clinical Practice, Health Promotion Efforts, Research, and Medical Education

There is enormous variation in how R/S beliefs and practices manifest in patients' lives and the effects this may have on their health and their receptiveness to health promotion efforts. Clinicians will benefit from openness and curiosity when inquiring about their patients' R/S practices and how this may or may not support their health and help them cope. For physicians who are involved with health promotion efforts, there may be value in collaborating with local houses of worship, clergy, and lay leaders. While medical schools have demonstrated a move toward the integration of spirituality into their curricula, there may be a need for ongoing training, education, and support for physicians who are already in practices. Overall, there is a need for more research, especially research that elucidates R/S dynamics in underserved and hard-to-reach communities.

Resource List

- The George Washington Institute for Spirituality and Health – www.smhs.gwu. edu/gwish/
- The Center for Spirituality and Health at the Icahn School of Medicine at Mount Sinai – www.mountsinai.org/patient-care/spiritual-care-and-education
- United States Transgender Survey – www.ustranssurvey.org. Pages 77–79 discuss findings related to religion.
- Idler EL. *Religion as a social determinant of public health*. 2014: Oxford

- Copeland M, Rose D. *Struggling in good faith: LGBTQI inclusion from 13 American religious perspectives*. 2016. Woodstock, VT: Skylight Paths Publishing
- Witten TM, Eyler AE (editors). *Gay, lesbian, bisexual & transgender aging: challenges in research, practice & policy*. 2012. Baltimore: Johns Hopkins

References

1. Adamczyk A. Understanding the effects of personal and school religiosity on the decision to abort a premarital pregnancy. J Health Soc Behav. 2009;50:180–95.
2. Allen JD, Pérez JE, Tom L, Levya B, Diaz D, Idalí TM. A pilot test of a church-based intervention to promote multiple cancer-screening behaviors among Latinas. J Cancer Educ. 2014;29(1):136–43.
3. Belanger-Levesque M, Dumas M, Blouin S, Pasquier J. "That was intense!" Spirituality during childbirth: a mixed-method comparative study of mothers' and fathers' experiences in a public hospital. BMC Pregnancy Childbirth. 2016;16:294.
4. Best M, Butow P, Olver I. Doctors discussing religion and spirituality: a systematic literature review. Palliat Med. 2016;30(4):327–37.
5. Bockting WO, Cesaretti C. Spirituality, transgender identity, and coming out. J Sex Educ Ther. 2001;26(4):291–300.
6. Breen GV, Price S, Lake M. Spirituality and high-risk pregnancy: another aspect of patient care. AWHONN Lifelines. 2006;10(6):467–73.
7. Brewster ME, Velez BL, Foster A, Esposito J, Robinson MA. Minority stress and the moderating role of religious coping among religious and spiritual sexual minority individuals. J Couns Psychol. 2016;63(1):119–26.
8. Buser JK, Goodric KM, Luke M, Buser TJ. A narratology of lesbian, gay, bisexual and transgender clients' experiences addressing religious and spiritual issues in counseling. J LGBT Issues Couns. 2011;5(3–4):282–302.
9. Christman LK, Abernathy AD, Gorsuch RL, Brown A. Intrinsic religiousness as a mediator between fatalism and cancer-specific fear: clarifying the role of fear in prostate cancer screening. J Relig Health. 2014;53(3):760–72.
10. Copeland M, Rose D. Struggling in good faith: LGBTQI inclusion from 13 American religious perspectives. Woodstock: Skylight Paths Publishing; 2016.
11. Cotton S, Zebracki K, Rosenthal SL, Tsevat J, Drotar D. Religion/spirituality and adolescent health outcomes: a review. J Adolesc Health. 2006;38(4):472–80.
12. Cotton S, Berry D. Religiosity, spirituality, and adolescent sexuality. Adolesc Med. 2007;18(3):471–83.
13. Crowther S, Hall J. Spirituality and spiritual care in and around childbirth. Women Birth. 2015;28(2):173–8.
14. Dowshen ND, Forke CM, Johnson AK, Kuhns LM, Rubin D, Garofalo R. Religiosity as a protective factor against HIV risk among young transgender women. J Adolesc Health. 2011;48(4):410–4.
15. Drake BF, Shelton RC, Gilligan T, Allen JD. A church-based intervention to promote informed decision making for prostate cancer screening among African American men. J Natl Med Assoc. 2010;102(3):164–71.
16. Friedman DB, Thomas TL, Owens OL, Hébert JR. It takes two to talk about prostate cancer: a qualitative assessment of African American men's and women's cancer communication practices and recommendations. Am J Mens Health. 2012;6(6):472–84.
17. Gaydos LM, Page PZ. Religion and reproductive health. In: Idler E, editor. Religion as a social determinant of public health. Oxford; 2014. p. 179–202.

18. Golub SA, Walker JJ, Longmire-Avital B, Bimbi DS, Parsons JT. The role of religiosity, social support, and stress-related growth in protecting against HIV risk among transgender women. J Health Psychol. 2010;15(8):1135–44.
19. Grossoehme DH, Teeters A, Jelinek S, Dimitriou SM, Conrad LA. Screening for spiritual struggle in an adolescent transgender clinic: feasibility and acceptability. J Health Care Chaplain. 2016;22(2):54–66.
20. Hall J. Spiritual care: enhancing meaning in pregnancy and birth. Pract Midwife. 2013;16(11):26–7.
21. Hampton MC, Halkitis PN, Mattis JS. Coping, drug use, and religiosity/ spirituality in relation to HIV serostatus among gay and bisexual men. AIDS Educ Prev. 2010;22(5):417–29.
22. Handzo G, Koenig HG. Spiritual care: whose job is it anyway? South Med J. 2004;97(12): 1242–4.
23. Hogue L, Hogue C. Anthony Comstock: a religious fundamentalist's negative impact on reproductive health. In: Idler E, editor. Religion as a social determinant of public health. Oxford; 2014. p. 154–74.
24. Holt CL, Wynn TA, Darrington J. Religious involvement and prostate cancer screening behaviors among southeastern African American men. Am J Mens Health. 2009;3(3):214–23.
25. Holt CL, Wynn TA, Litaker MS, Southward P, Jeames S, Schulz E. A comparison of a spiritually based and non-spiritually based educational intervention for informed decision making for prostate cancer screening among church-attending African-American men. Urol Nurs. 2009;29(4):249–58.
26. Husaini GA, Reece MC, Emerson JS, Scales S, Hull PC, Levine RS. A church-based program on prostate cancer screening for African American men: reducing health disparities. Ethn Dis. 2008 Spring;18(2 Suppl 2):S2 – 179–84.
27. Idler EL. Religion as a social determinant of public health. Oxford; 2014.
28. Isaac K, Hay J, Lubetkin E. Incorporating spirituality in primary care. J Relig Health. 2016;55(3):1065–77.
29. Koenig HG. Religion, spirituality, and health: the research and clinical implications. Int Sch Res Netw Psychiatry. 2012:278730, 33 pages. https://doi.org/10.5402/2012/278730.
30. Lofters AK, Vahabi M, Fardad M, Raza A. Exploring the acceptability of human papillomavirus self-sampling among Muslim immigrant women. Cancer Manag Res. 2017;9:323–9.
31. Mann JR, Mannan J, Quiñones LA, Palmer AA, Torres M. Religion, spirituality, social support, and perceived stress in pregnant and postpartum Hispanic women. J Obstet Gynecol Neonatal Nurs. 2010;39(6):645–57.
32. Marin DB, Sharma S, Powers R, Fleenor D. Richard Powers, David Fleenor. Spiritual care and physicians: understanding spirituality in medical practice. 2017, HealthCare Chaplaincy Network and Spiritual Care Association.
33. Matthews AK, Berrios N, Darnell JS, Calhoun E. A qualitative evaluation of a faith-based breast and cervical cancer screening intervention for African American women. Health Educ Behav. 2006;33(5):643–63.
34. McCord G, Gilchrist VJ, Grossman SD, King BD, McCormick KF, Oprandi AM, Schrop SL, Selius BA, Smucker WD, Weldy DL, Amorn M, Carter MA, Deak AJ, Hefzy J, Srivastava M. Discussing spirituality with patients: a rational and ethical approach. Ann Fam Med. 2004;2(4):356–61.
35. National Center for Transgender Equality. The report of the 2015 U. S. transgender survey. Washington, DC. 2016.
36. Nguyen AB, Hood KB, Belgrave FZ. The relationship between religiosity and cancer screening among Vietnamese women in the United States: the moderating role of acculturation. Women Health. 2012;52(3):292–313.
37. Padela AI, Peek M, Johnson-Agbakwu CE, Hosseinian Z, Curlin F. Associations between religion-related factors and cervical cancer screening among Muslims in Greater Chicago. J Low Genit Tract Dis. 2014;18(4):326–32.

38. Pargament KI, Hoenig HG, Tarakeshwar N, Hahn J. Religious coping methods as predictors of psychological, physical and spiritual outcomes among medically ill elderly patients: a two-year longitudinal study. J Health Psychol. 2014;9(6):713–30.
39. Pew Research Center, May 12, 2015, "America's Changing Religious Landscape."
40. Puchalski CM. The FICA spiritual history tool #274. J Palliat Med. 2014;17(1):105–6.
41. Puchalski CM, Vitillo R, Hull SK, Reller N. Improving the spiritual dimension of whole person care: reaching national and international consensus. J Palliat Med. 2014;17(6):642–56.
42. Puchalski CM, Blatt B, Kogan M, Butler A. Spirituality and health: the development of a field. Acad Med. 2014;89(1):10–6.
43. Romeiro J, Caldeira S, Brady V, Timmins F, Hall J. Spiritual aspects of living with infertility: a synthesis of qualitative studies. J Clin Nurs. 2017;26(23–24):3917–35.
44. Rosenkrantz DE, Rostosky SS, Riggle ED, Cook JR. The positive aspects of intersecting religious/ spiritual and LGBTQ identities. Spiritual Clin Pract. 2016;3(2):127–38.
45. Ross L, Kohler CL, Grimley DM, Green BL, Anderson-Lewis C. Toward a model of prostate cancer information seeking: identifying behavioral and normative beliefs among African American men. Health Educ Behav. 2007;34(3):422–40.
46. Singh AS, McKleroy VS. "Just getting out of bed is a revolutionary act." The resilience of transgender people of color who have survived traumatic life events. Traumatology. 2011;17(2):34–44.
47. Tanyi R, McKenzie M, Chapek C. How family practice physicians, nurse practitioners, and physician assistants incorporate spiritual care in practice. J Am Acad Nurse Pract. 2009;21(12):690–7.
48. The Joint Commission. The source for joint commission compliance strategies. 2018;16(1):6–12. https://www.nationalcoalitionhpc.org/wp-content/uploads/2020/07/NCHPCNCPGuidelines_4thED_web_FINAL.pdf. Accessed March 18, 2022.
49. Tuthill Z. Negotiating religiosity and sexual identity among Hispanic lesbian mothers. J Homosex. 2016;63(9):1194–210.
50. Wang T, Geffen S, Cahill S. The current wave of anti-LGBT legislation: historical context and implications for LGBT health. Boston: Fenway Institute; 2016.
51. Williams TT, Pichon LC, Campbell B. Sexual health communication within religious African-American families. Health Commun. 2015;30(4):328–38.
52. Winslow GR, Wehtje-Winslow BJ. Ethical boundaries of spiritual care. Med J Aust. 2017;186(10 Suppl):563–6.
53. Yudell M, Roberts D, DeSalle R, Tishkoff S. Taking race out of human genetics. Science. 2016;351(6273):564–5.

Part III
Sexual and Reproductive Health for Transgender and Gender Non-binary Patients
- Section Reviewer Zil Goldstein, FNP-BC

Chapter 14
Gender-Affirming Medical Care for Transgender and Gender Nonbinary Patients

Linda Wesp, A. C. Demidont, Jelinek Scott, and Zil Goldstein

Contents

L. Wesp (✉)
Clinical Assistant Professor, University of Wisconsin Milwaukee – College of Nursing,
Milwaukee, WI, USA
e-mail: lmwesp@uwm.edu

A. C. Demidont
Principal Medical Scientist, HIV Prevention Medical Affairs, New England, (CT, RI, MA,
VT, NH, ME, Upstate NY), USA
e-mail: ac.demidont@gilead.com

J. Scott
Pediatric Resident Physician, Department of Pediatrics, Icahn School of Medicine at Mount
Sinai, New York, NY, USA
e-mail: scott.jelinek@icahn.mssm.edu

Z. Goldstein
Associate Medical Director, Callen-Lorde Community Health Center, New York City, NY,
USA
e-mail: Zgoldstein@callen-lorde.org

© Springer Nature Switzerland AG 2022
J. Truglio et al. (eds.), *Sexual and Reproductive Health*,
https://doi.org/10.1007/978-3-030-94632-6_14

Introduction

Transgender and gender nonbinary (TGNB) people often experience discrimination, homo−/transphobia, ineffective care from the healthcare system, and other broad structural determinations of health that place TGNB people at increased risk for poor health outcomes. This is particularly true for sexual and reproductive health. It is therefore important for all clinicians to be familiar with the basics of providing sexual and reproductive care to transgender and gender nonbinary (TGNB) people and to be comfortable taking an appropriate history and managing any medical issues that may arise. Historically, clinician education programs lack adequate training on the healthcare needs of TGNB people. As a result, TGNB patients have received poor care and often faced discrimination from the healthcare system. One-third (33%) of respondents to the US Trans Health Survey reported having at least one negative experience with a healthcare clinician in the past year related to being TGNB, such as being refused treatment, verbally harassed, physically or sexually assaulted, or having to teach the provider about TGNB people in order to get appropriate care [16]. TGNB patients have many of the same health needs as all patients, but clinicians need to have up-to-date knowledge about best practices in the medical management of the unique healthcare needs of TGNB patients. This includes a basic understanding of the approach to gender-affirming hormones as well as the impact of hormones on sexual and reproductive health. This chapter reviews the basics of taking a comprehensive sexual history, and provides an overview of gender-affirming hormone therapy and non-hormonal transitions practices, and discusses current management approaches to common sexual and reproductive health needs. While this chapter generally applies to patients of all ages, unique aspects of caring for TGNB adolescents and young adults are described in the final portion.

General Approach to TGNB Sexual and Reproductive Health

Talking about sexual practices will often be uncomfortable for individuals who have previously experienced discrimination, assumptions, or judgment about their sexual practices, especially if this occurred in the healthcare setting. For the transgender community, mistrust of medical providers due to past discrimination may lead to feeling unsafe when talking about sensitive topics. Therefore, the primary care clinician should take specific steps toward maintaining a gender-affirming and trauma-informed approach to these discussions.

More specifically, trauma-informed care means that the clinician validates patients' experiences and reactions while simultaneously minimizing any potential further trauma during the healthcare encounter [27]. Beginning the sexual history with an explanation that these questions are asked of all patients and some validation that answering certain questions may be uncomfortable can create an environment of mutual respect and understanding.

Taking a Sexual and Reproductive Health History

People may describe their sexual orientation in a wide variety of ways. Understanding and providing comprehensive sexual healthcare involves understanding how people are having sex so the clinician may ascertain the types of screening and prevention measures that would be appropriate to promote and maintain health. Instead of asking "do you have sex with men, women, or both," the clinician should approach questions from a more general perspective that validates the wide diversity of sex and gender. Asking a broad question such as "are you sexually active?," "what are the genders of your sexual partners?," and "how do you like to have sex?" can present a more open-ended question that allows for more accurate representation of the patient's history.

It is important to also ask about behavior, as identity does not determine how people have sex. When taking a sexual history, clinicians should ask which body parts their patient are using and coming in contact with when they have sex, such as "what types of sex are you having?," what parts of your body do you use for sex?," or simply asking, "when you have sex, what goes where?" This will provide necessary information to determine what types of STI screening to provide, which body parts to assess, and type of pregnancy prevention counseling to offer.

Clinicians should also conduct an "organ inventory" to establish which organs their patient currently has, organs present at birth or expected at birth to develop, organs surgically enhanced or constructed, and organs hormonally enhanced or developed. Options include the breasts, cervix, ovaries, uterus, vagina, penis, prostate, and testes. This is true for all patients regardless of their gender identity.

Reproductive Health Needs and Considerations

When discussing reproductive health, it is important to ask all patients, especially those who are TGNB, about their history of reproductive health as well as their current reproductive health needs. Clinicians should not assume TGNB patients do not have reproductive needs and desires; this is often overlooked and both patients and clinicians can have inaccurate beliefs that go unchallenged. Asking about desire for pregnancy and discussing options for future fertility preservation are important aspects of primary care, especially for people who are about to start or are currently on hormone therapy. Options for preserving gametes, such as egg or sperm preservation, are available via reproductive technology although not always financially viable or covered by insurance. This is a conversation clinician should have with all their patients before hormones are started.

Both clinicians and patients should also be aware that while testosterone can lead to suppression of menses, fertilization can still occur as testosterone is not a failsafe contraceptive and some transmasculine patients may continue to ovulate. As a result, clinicians should still counsel patients on contraceptive options since endogenous testosterone can be teratogenic. Box 14.1 provides some suggestions for how to approach taking a comprehensive, gender-affirming, and trauma-informed sexual and reproductive health history.

Box 14.1 Taking a Sexual and Reproductive Health History
Starting out:
"As your primary care clinician, I want to consider all aspects of your health, so I always ask my patients some questions about their sexual history and current practices."

"It is ok to not answer these questions today."

"I understand if some of these questions might feel uncomfortable. I am asking them so we can talk together about whether you might want to do any screenings or talk about ways to stay healthy."

"Do you have any specific concerns or questions we can start with, about your sexual health or sexual practices?"

Specific practices:
"How do you like to have sex?"

"What body parts go where when you are sexually active?"

"How many sexual partners do you have?"

"Do you/How often do you use condoms/barriers/dental dams/finger cots/etc.?"

"Do you currently exchange sex for money, housing, food, or something you needed?"

Specific reproductive health needs:
"Are you currently having a type of sex where pregnancy could occur?"

"Do you use anything for pregnancy prevention?"

"Are you interested in or planning for pregnancy now or in the future?"

"Would you like to discuss options for pregnancy prevention/contraception?"

Gender Inclusive Language

Combining information from the review of systems with the sexual history may reveal areas that require further inquiry. If a more detailed review is required to evaluate abnormal signs or symptoms, the clinician should follow the patient's lead when using language to describe body parts. For example, when discussing genital symptoms, people may refer to "pain in the lower region" or say that they are having "discharge down there." Following up by asking for a more specific description using generic terms will avoid labeling body parts in a way that the patient does not relate to, for example, "when you say you are having discharge down there, do you mean it is coming from the front or the back? What kind of discharge is it?" or "when you say you are having pain in your lower region, is it on the inside or the outside?" Transmasculine people may use the term "front hole" to describe the vagina, "outer folds" to describe the labia, "internal organs" to describe uterus or ovaries, or "chest" to describe breasts.

Inequities in Sexual Health and Outcomes

Multiple inequities in sexual and reproductive health are observed in TGNB patients. These include increased exposure to intimate partner violence and sex work and worse mental health outcomes in TGNB patients compared with cisgender patients. One in eight respondents to the US Trans Health Survey reported doing sex work at some point during their lifetime, of which 63% were trans women or nonbinary people with male assigned on their birth certificate and 36% were trans men or nonbinary people with female assigned on their birth certificate [16]. TGNB people who are doing sex work are more likely to be living in poverty, at greater risk for intimate partner violence, and at greater risk for HIV and other STIs and experience greater levels of stigma within the healthcare encounter [17, 32, 34]. Screening for past or current sex work in the primary care setting means asking nonjudgmental questions such as "how do you support yourself?" or "have you ever exchanged sex for money, food, or housing?" The primary care clinician will gain a greater understanding about the lives of their patients and also have an opportunity to provide harm reduction and sexual health-related resources. However, it is important to approach this topic in a nonjudgmental fashion and discuss occupational health and safety issue rather than immediately encouraging someone to stop all together.

Additionally, 50% of TGNB people responding to the US Trans Health Survey have experienced some form of intimate partner violence [16]. According to 2016 data from the National Coalition of Anti-Violence Programs, TGNB people of color were 3.3 times more likely to experience intimate partner violence than survivors who did not identify as people of color or TGNB (2017). Clinicians should be aware that TGNB people also experience high rates of police violence and discrimination, leading to mistrust of law enforcement for reporting purposes [19]. Significant gaps in the literature exist around the issue of intimate partner violence for people of transmasculine experience [41]. Asking routinely about experiences of intimate partner violence can allow for discussions about safety planning and other supportive services.

Physical Exam Considerations

Physical examination of genital/pelvic areas is often extremely sensitive and especially uncomfortable for TGNB people who experience dysphoria around their genitals or who have had prior traumatic experiences in healthcare. About 15% of transgender people reported being asked invasive and inappropriate questions, often about their genitals or transgender status, during a medical encounter [16]. Therefore, previous negative and discriminatory experiences often shape mistrust and hesitation, and a trauma-informed approach to the physical exam is paramount. Often, a comprehensive and accurate history and symptom review can reveal important information that allows the clinician to explain what exactly will be examined and why the exam will be informative can be helpful to establish trust.

Clinicians can also be creative in the development and maintenance of a safe and trusting relationship with their patients. People with skin issues may have already taken photos on their cell phones, which can provide helpful diagnostic information. Offering the option for self-collection of vaginal and anal swabs allows for diagnostic testing without invasive examination. Deferring portions of the exam until after the patient and provider have established trust and rapport allows the patient to proceed on their own timeline and can make the patient more comfortable. Maintaining open communication and transparency about what information the physical exam will provide and letting the patient choose to do none, some, or all of the exam can create an equitable power dynamic and establish trust. As with all patients a pelvic or genital exam should never be conducted against the patient's will, and they should always be offered the opportunity to stop the exam at any time.

Medical Considerations of Gender-Affirming Interventions

Transition is the time when a person begins living as the gender with which they identify, rather than the sex they were assigned at birth. "Transitioning" is a process and not a singular event, and the approach one takes to affirm their gender is unique to every individual person and can evolve over time. Current best practice supports gender affirmation as a determinant of health, meaning TGNB people must have the right to access all potential avenues for gender affirmation across social, psychological, medical, and legal domains [42]. Therefore, TGNB people may seek hormones and/or various other interventions such as social transition, binding or tucking with use of clothing or other materials, surgery, facial hair removal, or voice therapy. There are many ways in which healthcare providers can be part of affirming a patient's gender identity so the best way to start may be simply asking, "How can I be a part of affirming your gender identity?"

Social and Nonhormonal Transition

Many patients will begin with transitioning socially by changing their outward gender expression to affirm their gender identity. This may involve wearing clothing and hairstyles and perhaps acquiring a new name. Simple steps can help clinicians create a gender-affirming environment. It is essential for all clinicians to ask all patients their preferred name and gender pronouns, ideally at the beginning of the visit and/or on an intake questionnaire, and then to use the name and pronouns throughout the visit, in the medical record, and when referring to the patient with others.

Clinicians should also be familiar with typical methods of social and nonhormonal transitioning. Transmasculine people also often bind their chest, using compression garments to flatten and masculinize the appearance of their chest. It is important to assess for binding discomfort and discuss ways to minimize daily time binding the chest as that will help avoid pain due to binding. Using specialty garments designed to help bind may also reduce comfort compared to other methods such as tightly winding an elastic bandage around the chest.

Some transfeminine patients practice "tucking," which is a gender affirming practice of using tight clothing or undergarments to create a feminine genital contour by placing the testicles upward into the inguinal canal and the penis/scrotum posteriorly toward the anus. A clinician should ask if a patient is experiencing any testicular or scrotal pain associated with tucking, as acute pain may be associated with testicular torsion, infection, or trauma. Urinary tract infections are not uncommon due to proximity of urethral meatus to the anus. Some transwomen may use a special undergarment called a *gaff* or tight-fitting clothing or tape for tucking purposes, which may also lead to skin breakdown or tinea cruris.

Gender-Affirming Hormones

Gender-affirming hormones are one of many potential interventions that are medically necessary for transgender people [46]. The approach to gender affirmation interventions is individualized, and although most transgender people in the USA desire access to hormone therapy (James et al. 2015), some may not. A more detailed overview of the impact of hormones on sexual and reproductive health will be the focus of this section, with an overview of gender-affirming hormone medications in Table 14.1 and a summary of hormone impacts relevant to sexual and reproductive

Table 14.1 Gender- affirming hormone options

Feminizing	Masculinizing	Puberty suppression
Estrogens:	**Androgens:**	**GnRH analogues:**
Oral 17-B estradiol	Injectable testosterone	Injectable leuprolide
Transdermal estradiol patch	cypionate	acetate
Injectable estradiol valerate	Transdermal testosterone	Implanted histrelin
Anti-androgens:	gel or patch	
Spironolactone		
Alpha-reductase inhibitors		
(i.e., finasteride, dutasteride)		
Micronized progesterone		
Medroxyprogesterone acetate		

Table 14.2 Impact of hormones related to sexual and reproductive health

Feminizing hormones	Masculinizing hormones
Decreased libido	Increased libido
Reduced erectile function	Cessation of menses
Lessened or absent ejaculatory fluid	Change to ovulation (may or may not
Reduced testicular size	include anovulation)
Potential permanent loss of sperm motility and	Atrophic change to cervix/vaginal tissue
production (with estrogen)	Growth of clitoral tissue

> **Box 14.2 Resources for Management of Gender-Affirming Hormones**
> Center of Excellence for Transgender Health, University of California San Francisco. Guidelines for the Primary and Gender-Affirming Care of Transgender and Gender Nonbinary People; second edition. Available at www.transhealth.ucsf.edu/ guidelines
> Endocrine treatment of gender-dysphoric/gender-incongruent persons: An Endocrine Society clinical practice guideline. The Journal of Clinical Endocrinology & Metabolism. Hembree, W. C. et al. [14]. Available at https://academic.oup.com/jcem/article-lookup/doi/10.1210/jc.2017-01658

health found in Table 14.2. For more information about detailed evidence-based guidelines for hormone management, see Box 14.2 for a list of resources.

Common Approaches to Gender-Affirming Hormones

For adolescents and adults who have completed puberty, gender-affirming hormone therapy involves the administration of hormones that cause the development of secondary sex characteristics which align with the gender identity of the individual. In general, the goal for feminizing hormone therapy is development of female secondary sex characteristics and minimization of male secondary sex characteristics. Treatment regimens usually include estradiol (in the form of a pill, transdermal patch, or injection) and anti-androgens (spironolactone is most commonly prescribed in the USA). Through a combination of estrogen and anti-androgen therapy the following changes are expected to occur: breast development, body fat redistribution, decrease in muscle mass, slowing or thinning of body and facial hair (although not complete elimination), and a slowing or possible reversal of scalp hair balding.

The goal for masculinizing hormone therapy is development of male secondary sex characteristics and minimization of female secondary sex characteristics. The treatment regimen is administration of parenteral testosterone alone, either injectable or transdermal. With testosterone therapy, expected changes include growth of facial and body hair, cessation of menses, deepening of the voice, muscle development, body fat redistribution, and possible scalp hairline recession (male pattern baldness).

Impact of Gender-Affirming Hormones on Sexual and Reproductive Health

Feminizing hormone therapy impacts sexual and reproductive health in several ways. In feminizing hormone therapy, lower serum testosterone levels lead to changes in libido, a reduction in erectile function, lessened or absent ejaculatory fluid, and (over time) a reduction in testicular size. Adjustments in anti-androgen treatment and/or administration of erectile dysfunction medications may lessen any undesired impacts on sexual function. Some people may also experience hypoactive sexual desire disorder (HSDD), which in one small observational study was not associated with hormone regimen, duration of hormone treatment, or satisfaction with hormone therapy [44].

Additionally, feminizing hormone therapy leads to decreased sperm production as exogenous estrogen administration has been associated with a permanent reduction in sperm production [9, 38]. The timing of when sperm production decreases is not firmly established. Therefore, patients should also be counseled that it is still possible for pregnancy to occur if they are sexually active in a manner that could lead to pregnancy. Best practices involve counseling about the option of sperm banking through cryopreservation and other options for preservation of future fertility [9] as well as a thorough sexual health practices history and education about family planning before initiating feminizing hormone therapy (see section above for more details on taking a sexual health history). No literature to date has found a permanent impact of spironolactone or progestogens on future sperm count or motility. Of note, primary care clinicians should also be aware that TGNB adolescents and adults who received GnRh analogues during early puberty, followed by estrogen for feminizing hormone therapy, are unlikely to have had maturation of gametes and will not have any capacity for sperm production in adulthood [14].

Administration of testosterone causes sexual and reproductive health changes including an increase in libido, cessation of menses, changes to ovulation patterns that may or may not include anovulation, atrophic changes to cervix and vaginal mucosal tissue, and growth of clitoral tissue. Clitoral enlargement can be uncomfortable at times. Atrophic changes to the cervix and vaginal mucosal tissue may lead to dryness and friability. As discussed in more details in the below section on diagnostic testing people on masculinizing hormone therapy who have a cervix should be followed with routine cervical cancer screening according to national guidelines.

Expanded Differential Diagnosis for Common Sexual and Reproductive Health Concerns in TGNB Patients

A clinician's approach to the review of systems in the TGNB population should take into consideration the usual differential diagnosis for any given symptoms, but it should be modified based on the individual patient's medication and surgical history and organ inventory. Table 14.3 presents common sexual and reproductive health concerns followed by how the differential diagnosis would broaden in the TGNB population. Gender-affirming hormones can at times cause some of these symptoms that are related to a patient's complaint.

Pelvic Pain

TGNB people taking masculinizing hormone therapy often experience pelvic pain after initiating hormone therapy. Testosterone dosing being too high or too low can be related to cyclical cramping and return of menses (or lack of amenorrhea in people just starting on testosterone). Asking about testosterone dosing, self-administration techniques, and expiration dates of testosterone vials can be helpful information to determine if testosterone dose is contributing to symptoms. Pain may be associated with vaginal bleeding or discharge and may occur intermittently, cyclically, and/or with orgasm. Causes of pelvic pain in TGNB people may include atrophic or other types of vaginitis, sexually transmitted infections or pelvic

Table 14.3 Expanded differential diagnosis for common sexual and reproductive health concerns in TGNB patients

Symptom	Associated gender-affirming hormone	Associated gender-affirming practice
Scrotal pain	Estrogen	Tucking
Irregular vaginal bleeding	Testosterone	
Pelvic pain	Testosterone	Packing
Recurrent urinary tract infections		Tucking
Chest pain	Estrogen	Binding

inflammatory disease, gonadal or uterine pathology, bladder dysfunction, or musculoskeletal disorders. Evaluation for pregnancy or ectopic pregnancy should be considered if supported by sexual history and current anatomy.

Endometrial or ovarian cancer must always be considered as possible causes of pelvic pain and in the appropriate clinical context whenever these organs are present, regardless of the patient's gender identity or gender expression. Invasive diagnostic testing such as endometrial biopsy or pelvic ultrasound may be met with resistance and fear due to negative experiences with healthcare providers or significant dysphoria, and providers should ensure trauma-informed care is provided throughout this process.

Chest Pain

Transmasculine people who bind may experience musculoskeletal pain in the thoracic region due to the binder restricting movement of the rib cage and spine. It is important to assess for binding discomfort and discuss ways to minimize daily time binding the chest as that will help avoid pain due to binding. Clinicians may provide references to physical therapy or deep breathing exercises which can be done during times the binder is off, to reduce or prevent pain.

Transfeminine patients who start taking estrogen will begin to develop breast buds beneath their nipples that can be slightly painful and sensitive. Clinicians should advise patients this can happen intermittently, this is an entirely normal course of breast development, and that the pain should diminish over time.

Scrotal Pain

TGNB people on feminizing hormone therapy may often experience testicular or scrotal pain. Pain is sometimes associated with "tucking," as described above. Scrotal pain is also a common complaint related to the onset of estrogen therapy; however, the etiology of this symptom is unknown. This pain is generally benign and patients can be provided with reassurance that the pain should improve spontaneously.

Diagnostic Testing for Sexual Health

Determination of diagnostic testing for sexual health-related issues in TGNB populations is based on a thorough sexual history without assumption of sexual practices based on gender identity, review of symptoms, cultural competence regarding the sex lives of TGNC individuals, a sex-positive approach, and if necessary a physical exam. Keeping in mind the diverse gender affirmation experiences of TGNB people, establishing trust, overcoming one's own bias or lack of education regarding sexual practices of TGNB individuals, and accurate history taking are keys to understanding whether risk for various sexually transmitted infections is present. Data evaluating pre-exposure prophylaxis (PrEP) uptake in individuals across the gender spectrum reveal that Assigned Female at Birth Non-Binary (AFABNB), Assigned Male at Birth Non-Binary (AMABNB), TGW, and TGM chose cisgender men as their sex partner of choice >50% of the time, over >50% had engaged in exchange sex, and > 30% routinely engaged in receptive anal sex. This reminds us that STI/HIV screening should view each person's individual risk (Morris S et al. AIDS 2020. San Francisco). HIV testing is recommended at least once for all people of ages 13–64, and more frequent testing should be considered based on risk [45]. Various data sets reveal that, despite actively engaging healthcare settings for GAHT, TGNB often do not have HIV testing completed as recommended by the CDC. A retrospective chart review of TGM attending a large FQHC focusing on sexual and gender minority patients showed that only about 50% of the TGM had received HIV testing. The same study showed that for TGN identifying as Black who only are sexually active with cisgender men, HIV prevalence rates were > 11% (Radix et al. CROI 2020. Boston). Gonorrhea and chlamydia testing should always be site-specific depending on the type of sex the person is having and screening completed for all sites which are used for sexual behavior (three-site testing). For people who are having oral or anal sex without condoms or dental dams, pharyngeal and anal swab testing for gonorrhea and chlamydia are necessary. Urine testing will only accurately determine gonorrhea, chlamydia, and trichomonas for symptomatic patients or known urethral or vaginal exposures. In the case of patients who have undergone vaginoplasty, vaginal swabs are necessary to collect an adequate specimen.

Cancer Screening

Cervical cancer screening is an important diagnostic test for TGNB people with a cervix, and routine clinical guidelines for cervical cancer screening should be followed [2]. However, transmasculine people are less likely to be up to date on cervical cancer screening [25]. This is also complicated by the fact that atrophic changes are associated with a higher prevalence of unsatisfactory samples for cytology among TGNB people with a cervix who take testosterone [26]. Transmasculine people may also have a low uptake of conventional cervical cancer screening because the exam may cause discomfort/worsening of dysphoria and healthcare clinicians are often misinformed about the need for routine screening in this population [1, 28]. Self-collected swabs to screen for high-risk HPV DNA offer a more patient-centered approach for individuals who are unable or unwilling to have a speculum exam or who have previously had inadequate cytology results. In a study testing the acceptability and performance of self-collected high-risk HPV DNA swabs with transmasculine people, 90% of participants preferred the self-collected swab, which had a sensitivity of 71.4% and specificity of 98% [31]. This is comparable to studies of self-collected swabs testing for high-risk HPV DNA among cisgender women, which had a sensitivity of 74% and specificity of 88% [21]. Therefore, because transmasculine people may be less up to date on cervical cancer screening with increased rates of inadequate specimens due to atrophic changes from testosterone, self-collected HPV screening is an important alternative screening option that should be considered for this population [31].

While there is controversy and at times conflicting guidelines regarding screening for breast cancer and prostate cancer, clinicians should generally follow current USPSTF guidelines and base recommendations on the organs and tissue each patient has, as opposed to their individual gender identity, with each patient's individualized medical and surgical history as well as preferences taken into account. Masculinizing chest reconstructing surgery does not typically remove all breast tissue. Direct communication between the primary care clinician and the surgeon can help ensure appropriate screening methods are used for breast cancer. For transgender women, Fenway and the University of California San Francisco guidelines both recommend screening mammography starting at age 50 in the presence of additional risk factors, including estrogen and progesterone use for greater than 5 years, a family history of breast cancer, or a body mass index greater than 35 kg/m^2, whereas the European Endocrine Society recommends following current cisgender screening guidelines.

HIV Prevention

Primary care clinicians are in a unique position to reduce many of the health inequities seen in TGNB populations. One such inequity is HIV. Convenience samples and meta-analyses suggest transgender women bear a disproportionate burden of HIV infection, especially transgender women of color [3, 15, 16]. Additionally, transgender men who have sex with cisgender men may have similar risk pathways to HIV as cisgender men who have sex with men [33]. National surveillance about HIV prevalence among TGNB people has been lacking due to inadequate population level data collection for gender identity in the overall census population as well as epidemiologic data. The first publication of national surveillance data from 2009 to 2014 has shown that of the newly diagnosed HIV infections, 84% identified as transgender women and over half were among Black/African American identified individuals [5].

The primary care clinician is in an important position to evaluate for HIV risk and offer HIV prevention counseling, condoms, and medication if appropriate, particularly if the primary care clinician is also the practitioner who prescribes GAHT in the primary care setting. HIV prevention tools now include pre-exposure prophylaxis, or PrEP, a once daily medication that has been approved by the FDA for prevention of HIV among high-risk populations. Emtricitabine-tenofovir 200–300 mg (Truvada) and emtricitabine-tenofovir alafenamide 200–25 mg (Descovy) are combination antiretroviral medications that, if taken daily, prevent acquisition of HIV. Studies thus far show no interactions between current gender-affirming hormone treatment and either Truvada or Descovy. Data from HPTN 083, which evaluated the use of long-acting cabotegravir injections every 2 months, proved superior to Truvada for HIV prevention in TGW (Landovitz, R et al. AIDS 2020). Additional trials of long-acting injectible agents of PrEP and HIV treatment for all TGNB individuals are expected to happen in the near future. Guidelines for use of PrEP can be found at the CDC's website (https://www.cdc.gov/hiv/risk/prep/index.html). Although TGNB people were not adequately accounted for or include in the original PrEP trials and therefore not listed specifically in FDA approval as an "at-risk group" [13], a re-examination of data found that transgender women who took PrEP daily had similar efficacy to the other study participants [12]. PrEP is an important HIV prevention tool, yet one study of transgender men identified a major barrier to accessing PrEP was that clinicians avoided discussions about sexual health [36]. Additionally, a major barrier for PrEP access among studies with transgender women was found to be a lack of gender affirmation in healthcare settings [39]. In fact, a prospective, cohort evaluation of uptake and adherence to Truvada for PrEP in TGW who attended a primary care setting for GAHT showed that the when asked the predominant reason that women who meet CDC criteria to initiate PrEP (47% in FIRED-UP) were not already on PrEP was because their provider neither initiated the conversation (68%) nor provided information on option to pay for PrEP (68%) (Golub, S et al. CROI 2020). Ending the Epidemic (ETE) commissions of many citys and states have specifically focused portions of their plans on improving culturally competent care for TGNB as a crucial part of improving rates of HIV testing/screening, TasP, and PrEP, as well as to utilize phylogenetic transmission clustering data to identify pattern of HIV transmission to TGW (Ragonnet-Cronin, M et al.). Clinicians can use the gender-affirming skills presented in this chapter to ensure they are providing their TGNB patients with the appropriate sexual and reproductive preventative services and learn to help advocate for and encourage sexual health for TGNC patients.

Transgender and Gender Nonbinary Youth

While the vast majority of recommendations discussed above apply to TGNB patients of all ages, clinicians treating adolescents and young adults (AYAs) who identify as transgender or gender expansive should seek out additional knowledge and skills specific to this population. The American Academy of Pediatrics (AAP) calls for all pediatric providers to be familiar with this emerging area and "take steps toward use of a gender-affirming, developmentally appropriate framework that can improve early identification and positive health interventions for a historically vulnerable population" [29]. Providers should use a gender-affirming model of care in their practice (described further below), where patients can explore their gender identity and providers normalize the experience and model for caregivers ways of providing affirmation and support. Gender affirming care provides TGNB earlier access to mental health support and gender affirming medical/surgical care, as well as reduces the sense of shame and isolation many TGNB youth often experience.

TGNB youth report an awareness of difference in their gender experience at an average age of 8.5 years, but delay disclosing until an average age of 10 years later [23]. Increasing numbers of adolescents though have already started living in their affirmed gender role upon entering high school [6]. Research has shown that youth who have earlier access to gender-affirming care have better mental health outcomes, including lower rates of depression, self-harm, and suicide ideation and attempts, compared to youth 15 years and older [40]. Referral to a qualified gender-affirming mental health professional can be vital in assisting TGNB youth with their dysphoria and assessing their readiness to transition.

Gender-Affirming Model of Care

Similar to adults, healthcare clinicians for TGNB youth should personalize and individualize their support based on a patient's unique gender experience, questions, concerns, and goals. The goal of the gender-affirming model of care is to "listen to the child and decipher with the help of parents or caregivers what the child is communicating about both gender identity and gender expressions". Healthcare clinicians should strive to optimize a youth's gender health, which is defined as a child's opportunity to live in the gender that feels most real or comfortable and to express that gender with freedom from restriction, aspersion, or rejection. For gender-expansive youth, determining what is most comfortable is often a fluid process, and can change over time, especially as the child matures and develops. Clinicians should encourage ongoing communication, problem-solving, and acceptance between families and the child, particularly during this time that can often be confusing and socially challenging. This will provide the child the space and time for exploration and self-acceptance [30].

Research shows that children who are not allowed these freedoms by agents within their developmental systems (e.g., *family, peers, school, healthcare*) are at later risk for developing a downward cascade of psychosocial adversities including depressive symptoms, low life satisfaction, self-harm, isolation, homelessness, incarceration, posttraumatic stress, and suicide ideation and attempts. Subsequent studies found that TGNB youth who reported their families as being strongly supportive of their gender identity and expression in childhood endorsed more positive mental health, less depressive symptoms, high self-esteem, and life satisfaction in later adolescence compared with those whose families were nonsupportive.

All pediatric clinicians should have at least a basic understanding of how to facilitate a conversation about and treatment options for gender dysphoria, which is the emotional distress TGNB AYA may experience due to the disconnect between one's gender identity and their outward manifestation of gender, including their primary and/or secondary sex characteristics. Providers should acknowledge and validate patients' feelings of gender dysphoria and possible desires to transition.

A gender-affirming model of care takes into consideration what is developmentally appropriate for the patient (given their age, progression of puberty), focuses on an individual's unique gender experience, and uses a strengths-based and family-centered approach. A healthcare clinician can play an important role in a TGNB youth's life, especially as they try and navigate understanding their own identity and getting support from the systems and structures in their lives. A clinician can start by simply asking, "what role can I play in helping you affirm your gender identity?"

Social Transitioning

The process of gender affirmation is unique and different for all patients and the management considerations can vary widely. Some clinicians may not feel comfortable or knowledgeable enough to assist TGNB youth with their transition plans, but all clinicians should be familiar with basic concepts and be able to refer patients to another physician with experience or expertise around gender-affirming care. TGNB youth face many barriers accessing desired medical therapies, and their primary care clinician should serve as an advocate and not be one of the barriers.

Every patients' gender journey is different, but many youth will begin with transitioning socially by changing their outward gender expression to affirm their gender identity; this may involve wearing preferred clothing and hairstyles and perhaps acquiring a new name. The optimal timing for social transitioning differs among individuals as they each assess their social and psychological supports and level of safety and comfort. A provider should counsel and support patients and their families as they make decisions regarding the timing and process of any gender role changes and work through the options and implications. One study measured the positive mental health effects of prepubescent transgender children (ages 3–12) who transitioned socially, and the median age was 7.7 years old. The study found that socially transitioned transgender children who are supported in their gender identity have developmentally normative levels of depression, only minimal elevations in anxiety, and notably lower rates of internalizing psychopathology compared to reports of children who had not socially transitioned [24]. Another study found that TGNB who were able to use their chosen/preferred name at work, school, or at home experienced a reduction in depressive symptoms, suicidal ideation, and suicidal behavior [37].

Gender-Affirming Medical Treatment Options

Medical treatment options for gender transition can be separated into three phases: fully reversible, partially reversible, and irreversible phase. Outlining and explaining the different phases to AYAs is helpful to understanding goals of the AYA and setting expectations. Moving from one phase to the next should not happen until there has been adequate time for AYAs and their parents/caregivers to fully assimilate the effects of earlier interventions.

Fully Reversible

When adolescents with gender dysphoria approach puberty, many experience an increase in stress and anxiety as they anticipate the development of unwanted secondary sex characteristics. Pubertal suppression may be accomplished through the use of gonadotropin-releasing hormone (GnRH) analogs ("puberty blockers") to quell estrogen or testosterone production and consequently delay the onset of puberty and the development of secondary sex characteristics, thereby relieving the distress of pubertal development. The suppression is fully reversible, meaning if treatment were stopped, an adolescent would experience full pubertal development in their sex assigned at birth.

Pubertal suppression gives adolescents more time to explore options and live in the experienced gender before making the decision to proceed with gender-affirming sex hormones [43]. Treating adolescents with gender dysphoria who are entering puberty with puberty blockers has been shown to significantly improve psychological functioning and decrease depressive symptoms and behavioral and emotional problems [11]. Starting puberty blockers in early puberty also improves physical outcomes and reduces the need for future surgeries since adolescents never develop the undesired and irreversible secondary sex characteristics such as advanced breast development, lowering of the voice, and outgrowth of the jaw and brow [7]. Clinicians can also use puberty blockers with adolescents in later pubertal stages to stop menses in transmasculine youth and prevent facial hair growth in transfeminine youth.

The Endocrine Society Clinical Practice Guidelines recommend clinicians to begin pubertal hormone suppression when patients first exhibit physical changes of puberty (Tanner stage II for both genitals and breasts) and pubertal levels of estradiol and testosterone. The Endocrine Society believes that having adolescents experience the onset of puberty will allow them and their parents/caregivers to make an informed decision. For those individuals assigned female at birth, the first physical sign of puberty is the budding of the breasts followed by an increase in breast and fat tissue, and in individuals assigned male at birth it is testicular growth >4 mL. Puberty suppression may continue for a few years, at which time a decision is made to either discontinue all hormone therapy or transition to a feminizing/masculinizing hormone regimen. Providers should inform and counsel all adolescents considering gender-affirming medical treatment about options for fertility preservation prior to initiating puberty suppression and prior to treating with hormonal therapy [14].

An alternative reversible treatment is the use of progestins, commonly medroxyprogesterone, or other medications, like spironolactone, that decrease the masculinizing effects of androgens. Continuous oral contraceptives or depot medroxyprogesterone acetate (DMPA) may be used to suppress menses, but some transmasculine patients may opt not to use a "female" hormone because of concerns it would exacerbate dysphoria.

Partially Reversible

Gender transition may be achieved using gender-affirming hormones that induce the onset of the desired puberty and development of masculine or feminine secondary sex characteristics aligned with one's gender identity. If an adolescent requests gender-affirming hormones, the clinician should assess the readiness of the AYA and carefully review if there are any contraindications to their use. The World Professional Association for Transgender Health (WPATH) Standards of Care 7 and the Endocrine Society recommend that providers may add gender-affirming hormones after a multidisciplinary team has confirmed the persistence of gender dysphoria, any co-existing psychological, medical, or social problems that could interfere with treatment have been addressed, and the adolescent has sufficient mental capacity to give informed consent to this partially irreversible treatment [14, 46]. While most adolescents have this capacity by age 16 years old, some specialty clinics and experts now recommend that the decision to initiate gender-affirming hormones be decided based more on state of development of each individual patient rather than a specific chronological age, despite the fact that there are minimal published studies of hormone treatments administered before age 13.5 to 14 years [10] [35]. This informed consent model can be more empowering to the patient, gives them increased ownership of their own transition, and allows the adolescent to undergo their desired puberty closer to the age of their peers rather than waiting until age 16. Also, note that at the time of this writing, the WPATH Standards of Care are undergoing revisions, and clinicians should look for the new Standards of Care, Version 8, at www.wpath.org to stay the most up to date with current practice guidelines.

The Endocrine Society recommends initiating puberty using a gradually increasing dose schedule of testosterone for transmasculine youth and estrogen for transfeminine youth. Since the initial levels of hormones will not be high enough to suppress endogenous sex steroid secretion, continuation of treatment with "puberty blockers" is advised until gonadectomy. For transwomen, sometimes an androgen inhibitor, such as spironolactone, is used in addition to estrogen [22]. Transmasculine patients may still have some pregnancy risk since testosterone is not a fail-safe contraceptive and some may continue to ovulate. Providers should counsel these patients to consider contraceptive options such as an etonogestrel implant, a progesterone IUD, or DMPA [18]. A systematic review found that the physical changes induced by gender-affirming hormones are usually accompanied by an improvement in mental well-being [8]. Physical changes that are expected to occur were outlined above in Table 14.2.

Irreversible Intervention

Some AYAs may desire surgical options to further affirm their gender identity. AYAs should be given sufficient time and opportunity to experience and socially adjust in their desired gender role before undergoing irreversible surgery. WPATH guidelines state, at a minimum, patients should have lived continuously for at least 12 months in the gender role that is congruent with their gender identity and reached the legal age of majority in a given country [46]. Various irreversible interventions include breast augmentation, masculinizing chest reconstruction, fat grafting/transfer, facial feminization, tracheal shave, orchiectomy, vaginoplasty, hysterectomy, metoidioplasty, or phalloplasty.

Conclusion

This chapter has provided a comprehensive review of providing medical care to TGNB people, including a review of the effects of gender-affirming hormones, how to take an appropriate sexual and reproductive health history, considerations for sexual and reproductive health screenings, contraception options, and HIV prevention. Clinicians must be aware of the unique considerations due to the effects of hormones on reproductive and sexual functioning that have been discussed here. Additionally, establishing trust and maintaining a harm reduction and trauma-informed approach to clinical care will improve access to care and overall health of this population. All clinicians caring for TGNB people should maintain a thorough and up-to-date understanding of these topics so we can continue to meet the specific sexual and reproductive health needs of our patients.

References

1. Agenor M, Peitzmeier SM, Bernstein IM, McDowell M, Alizaga NM, Reisner SL, et al. Perceptions of cervical cancer risk and screening among transmasculine individuals: patient and provider perspectives. Cult Health Sex. 2016;18(10):1192–206. https://doi.org/10.108 0/13691058.2016.1177203.
2. American College of Obstetricians and Gynecologists. Committee Opinion no. 512: health care for transgender individuals. Obstet Gynecol. 2011;118(6):1454–8. https://doi.org/10.1097/ AOG.0b013e31823ed1c1.
3. Baral SD, Poteat T, Stromdahl S, Wirtz AL, Guadamuz TE, Beyrer C. Worldwide burden of HIV in transgender women: a systematic review and meta-analysis. Lancet Infect Dis. 2013;13(3):214–22. https://doi.org/10.1016/S1473-3099(12)70315-8.
4. Center of Excellence for Transgender Health, University of California San Francisco. Guidelines for the Primary and Gender-Affirming Care of Transgender and Gender Nonbinary People; second edition. Deutsch MB, ed. (2016). Available at http://www.transhealth.ucsf.edu/ guidelines.
5. Clark H, Babu AS, Wiewel EW, Opoku J, Crepaz N. Diagnosed HIV infection in transgender adults and adolescents: results from the national HIV surveillance system, 2009–2014. AIDS Behavior. 2017;21(9):2774–83. https://doi.org/10.1007/s10461-016-1656-7.
6. Cohen-Kettenis PT, Pfäfflin F. Transgenderism and intersexuality in childhood and adolescence: making choices. 2003. https://doi.org/10.4135/9781452233628.

7. Cohen-Kettenis PT, Van Goozen SHM. Sex reassignment of adolescent transsexuals: a follow-up study. J Am Acad Child Adoles Psychiatry. 1997;36(2):263–71. https://doi. org/10.1097/00004583-199702000-00017.

8. Colizzi M, Costa R. The effect of cross-sex hormonal treatment on gender dysphoria individuals' mental health: a systematic review. Neuropsychiatr Dis Treat. 2016;12:1953–66. https:// doi.org/10.2147/ndt.s95310.

9. De Roo C, Tilleman K, T'Sjoen G, De Sutter P. Fertility options in transgender people. Int Rev Psychiatry (Abingdon, England). 2016;28(1):112–9. https://doi.org/10.3109/09540261.201 5.1084275.

10. de Vries ALC, McGuire JK, Steensma TD, Wagenaar ECF, Doreleijers TAH, Cohen-Kettenis PT. Young adult psychological outcome after puberty suppression and gender reassignment. Pediatrics. 2014;134(4):696–704. https://doi.org/10.1542/peds.2013-2958.

11. de Vries ALC, Steensma TD, Doreleijers TAH, Cohen-Kettenis PT. Puberty suppression in adolescents with gender identity disorder: a prospective follow up study. J Sex Med. 2011;8(8):2276–83. https://doi.org/10.1111/j.1743-6109.2010.01943.x.

12. Deutsch MB, Glidden DV, Sevelius J, Keatley J, McMahan V, Guanira J, et al. HIV pre-exposure prophylaxis in transgender women: a subgroup analysis of the iPrEx trial. The Lancet HIV, available online 6 Nov 2015. 2015. https://doi.org/10.1016/S2352-3018(15)00206-4; M3: https://doi.org/10.1016/S2352-3018(15)00206-4; 07 https://doi.org/10.1016/ S2352-3018(15)00206-4

13. Grant RM, Sevelius JM, Guanira JV, Aguilar JV, Chariyalertsak S, Deutsch MB. Transgender women in clinical trials of pre-exposure prophylaxis. J Acquir Immune Defici Syndr (1999). 2016;72 Suppl 3, 226. https://doi.org/10.1097/QAI.0000000000001090.

14. Hembree WC, Cohen-Kettenis PT, Gooren L, Hannema SE, Meyer WJ, Murad MH, et al. Endocrine treatment of gender-dysphoric/gender-incongruent persons: an Endocrine Society clinical practice guideline. J Clin Endocrinol Metab. 2017;102(11):3869–903. https://doi. org/10.1210/jc.2017-01658.

15. Herbst JH, Jacobs ED, Finlayson TJ, McKleroy VS, Neumann MS, Crepaz N, Team, H. A. P. R. S. Estimating HIV prevalence and risk behaviors of transgender persons in the United States: a systematic review. AIDS Behav. 2008;12(1):1–17. https://doi.org/10.1007/ s10461-007-9299-3.

16. James SE, Herman JL, Rankin S, Kiesling M, Mottet L, Anafl M. The report of the 2015 U.S. transgender survey. Washington, D.C.: National Center for Transgender Equality; 2016.

17. Kaplan RL, McGowan J, Wagner GJ. HIV prevalence and demographic determinants of condomless receptive anal intercourse among trans feminine individuals in Beirut, Lebanon. J Int AIDS Soc. 2016;19(3 Suppl 2):20,787. https://doi.org/10.7448/IAS.19.3.20787.

18. Light AD, Obedin-Maliver J, Sevelius JM, Kerns JL. Transgender men who experienced pregnancy after female-to-male gender transitioning. Obstet Gynecol. 2014;124(6):1120–7.

19. Mallory C, Hasenbush A, Sears B. Discrimination and Harassment by Law Enforcement Officers in the LGBT Community. 2015. Retrieved from http://williamsinstitute.law.ucla. edu/wp-content/uploads/LGBT-Discrimination-and-Harassment-in-Law-Enforcement-March-2015.pdf.

20. National Coalition of Anti-Violence Programs. A crisis of hate: a mid year report on lesbian, gay, bisexual, transgender and queer hate violence homicides. 2017. Retrieved from http://avp. org/wp-content/uploads/2017/08/NCAVP-A-Crisis-of-Hate-Final.pdf.

21. Ogilvie GS, Patrick DM, Schulzer M, Sellors JW, Petric M, Chambers K, et al. Diagnostic accuracy of self collected vaginal specimens for human papillomavirus compared to clinician collected human papillomavirus specimens: a meta-analysis. Sex Transm Infect. 2005;81(3):207–12. https://doi.org/10.1136/sti.2004.011858.

22. Olson J, Forbes C, Belzer M. Management of the transgender adolescent. Arch Pediatr Adolesc Med. 2011;165(2):171–6. https://doi.org/10.1001/archpediatrics.2010.275.

23. Olson J, Schrager SM, Belzer M, Simons LK, Clark LF. Baseline physiologic and psychosocial characteristics of transgender youth seeking care for gender dysphoria. J Adoles Health. 2015;57(4):374–80. https://doi.org/10.1016/j.jadohealth.2015.04.027.

24. Olson KR, Durwood L, Demeules M, McLaughlin KA. Mental health of transgender children who are supported in their identities. Pediatrics. 2016;137(3):e20153223. https://doi.org/10.1542/peds.2015-3223.
25. Peitzmeier SM, Khullar K, Reisner SL, Potter J. Pap test use is lower among female-to-male patients than non-transgender women. Am J Preventive Med. 2014a;47(6):808–12. https://doi.org/10.1016/j.amepre.2014.07.031.
26. Peitzmeier SM, Reisner SL, Harigopal P, Potter J. Female-to-male patients have high prevalence of unsatisfactory Paps compared to non-transgender females: implications for cervical cancer screening. J General Intern Med. 2014b;29(5):778–84.
27. Poteat T, Singh A. Conceptualizing trauma in clinical settings: Iatrogenic harm and bias. In: Eckstrand KL, Potter J, editors. Trauma, resilience, and health promotion in LGBT patients: what every health care provider should know. Cham: Springer; 2017. p. 25–33.
28. Potter J, Peitzmeier SM, Bernstein I, Reisner SL, Alizaga NM, Agenor M, Pardee DJ. Cervical cancer screening for patients on the female-to-male spectrum: a narrative review and guide for clinicians. J Gen Intern Med. 2015;30(12):1857–64. https://doi.org/10.1007/s11606-015-3462-8.
29. Rafferty J. Committee on Adolescence; Section on Lesbian, Gay, Bisexual, and Transgender Health and Wellness. Ensuring comprehensive care and support for transgender and gender-diverse children and adolescents. Pediatrics. 2018;142(4):e20182162.
30. Rafferty JR, Donaldson AA, Forcier M. Primary care considerations for transgender and gender-diverse youth. Pediatr Rev. 2020;41(9):437–54. https://doi.org/10.1542/pir.2018-0194.
31. Reisner SL, Deutsch MB, Peitzmeier SM, White Hughto JM, Cavanaugh TP, Pardee DJ, et al. Test performance and acceptability of self- versus provider-collected swabs for high-risk HPV DNA testing in female-to-male trans masculine patients. PLoS One. 2018;13(3):e0190172. https://doi.org/10.1371/journal.pone.0190172.
32. Reisner SL, Poteat T, Keatley J, Cabral M, Mothopeng T, Dunham E, et al. Global health burden and needs of transgender populations: a review. Lancet. 2016;388(10042):412–36. https://doi.org/10.1016/S0140-6736(16)00684-X.
33. Reisner SL, White Hughto JM, Pardee D, Sevelius J. Syndemics and gender affirmation: HIV sexual risk in female-to-male trans masculine adults reporting sexual contact with cisgender males. Int J STD & AIDS. 2015; https://doi.org/10.1177/0956462415602418.
34. Roche K, Keith C. How stigma affects healthcare access for transgender sex workers. Br J Nurs (Mark Allen Publishing). 2014;23(21):1147–52. https://doi.org/10.12968/bjon.2014.23.21.1147.
35. Rosenthal SM. Approach to the patient: transgender youth: endocrine considerations. J Clin Endocrinol Metab. 2014;99(12):4379–89. https://doi.org/10.1210/jc.2014-1919.
36. Rowniak S, Ong-Flaherty C, Selix N, Kowell N. Attitudes, beliefs, and barriers to PrEP among trans men. AIDS Educ Prev. 2017;29(4):302–14. https://doi.org/10.1521/aeap.2017.29.4.302.
37. Russell ST, Pollitt AM, Li G, Grossman AH. Chosen name use is linked to reduced depressive symptoms, suicidal ideation, and suicidal behavior among transgender youth. J Adolesc Health. 2018;63(4):503–5. https://doi.org/10.1016/j.jadohealth.2018.02.003.
38. Schulster M, Bernie AM, Ramasamy R. The role of estradiol in male reproductive function. Asian J Androl. 2016;18(3):435–40. https://doi.org/10.4103/1008-682X.173932.
39. Sevelius JM, Deutsch MB, Grant R. The future of PrEP among transgender women: the critical role of gender affirmation in research and clinical practices. J Int AIDS Soc. 2016;19(7(Suppl 6)):21105. https://doi.org/10.7448/IAS.19.7.21105.
40. Sorbara JC, Chiniara LN, Thompson S, Palmert MR. Mental health and timing of gender-affirming care. Pediatrics. 2020;146(4):e20193600. https://doi.org/10.1542/peds.2019-3600.
41. Stephenson R, Riley E, Rogers E, Suarez N, Metheny N, Senda J, et al. The sexual health of transgender men: a scoping review. J Sex Res, 2017;54(4–5), 424–45. https://doi.org/10.1080/00224499.2016.1271863.
42. The Lancet. Transgender Health and Well-Being. 2016. Retrieved from http://www.thelancet.com/pb/assets/raw/Lancet/infographics/transgender-health/transgender-health.pdf.

43. Waal HD-VD, Cohen-Kettenis PT. Clinical management of gender identity disorder in adolescents: a protocol on psychological and paediatric endocrinology aspects. Eur J Endocrinol.
2006;155:S131–7. https://doi.org/10.1530/eje.1.02231.

44. Wierckx K, Elaut E, Van Hoorde B, Heylens G, De Cuypere G, Monstrey S, et al. Sexual desire
in trans persons: associations with sex reassignment treatment. J Sex Med. 2014;11(1):107–18.
https://doi.org/10.1111/jsm.12365.

45. Workowski KA, Bolan GA. Sexually transmitted diseases treatment guidelines, 2015.
MMWR Recommen Rep. 2015;64(3):134134p. Retrieved from https://ezproxy.lib.uwm.edu/
login?url=http://search.ebscohost.com/login.aspx?direct=true&AuthType=ip,uid&db=rzh&A
N=109799990&site=ehost-live&scope=site.

46. World Professional Association for Transgender Health. Standards of care for the health of
transsexual, transgender, and gender non-conforming people. 7th ed. WPATH. 2011.

Chapter 15
Gender-Affirming Surgery: Perioperative Care for the Primary Care Clinician

Asa Radix and Sangyoon Jason Shin

Contents

Introduction

A large national survey indicated that about 40% of transmasculine and 30% of transfeminine people have already undergone some type of gender-affirming surgery with many more planning on having surgeries in the future [23]. A recent publication has demonstrated a steady increase in gender-affirming surgeries being performed in the United States [5] related to improved insurance coverage as well as an increase in qualified surgeons nationally. TGNB people may seek out surgeons who are located at some distance from their homes, some even traveling overseas, increasing the probability that they will return home to their primary care clinicians with postoperative concerns. Medical clinicians should therefore be familiar with

A. Radix (✉)
Callen-Lorde Community Health Center, New York, NY, USA
e-mail: aradix@callen-lorde.org

S. J. Shin
Icahn School of Medicine at Mount Sinai, New York, NY, USA

Mount Sinai Downtown – Union Square, New York, NY, USA

© Springer Nature Switzerland AG 2022
J. Truglio et al. (eds.), *Sexual and Reproductive Health*,
https://doi.org/10.1007/978-3-030-94632-6_15

the various surgical options including necessary preoperative preparation and potential immediate and long-term postoperative healthcare concerns. Primary care clinicians should ensure that patients have a plan in place to deal with serious postoperative complications. This is even more important when the surgeons are not geographically close. This includes their surgeon's emergency contact details and names of alternative providers in their home area, who preferably have some expertise in transgender care. This chapter provides an overview of the preoperative care of patients seeking gender-affirming surgery, followed by overviews of common surgical approaches along with their respective postoperative care.

Preoperative Assessment and Care

A comprehensive pre-surgical evaluation addresses the perioperative management of active medical conditions, anticipates potential complications, offers interventions to reduce risk, and engages the patient and clinician in shared decision-making.

Optimizing TGNB (transgender and gender nonbinary) surgical patients can present unique challenges that require a tailored approach while using existing guidelines. In this section, we aim to explore an evidence-based approach which focuses not only on cardiac risk factors but other relevant risk factors that may impact the patient's perioperative risk and postoperative recovery.

Initial Evaluation

The initial evaluation should occur with the patient's primary care clinician about 3 months prior to surgery. This initial phase includes infectious disease management, hormone management, bariatric considerations, and reproductive planning.

Infectious Disease Management

We recommend risk assessment based on current anatomy and sexual behaviors, awareness of symptoms consistent with common sexually transmitted infections (STIs), and screening for asymptomatic STIs based on behavioral history and sexual practices.

Serologic screening recommendations for transgender patients do not differ from non-transgender patients and include HIV, hepatitis B and C, and syphilis and are described in more detail in Chap. 6.

Screening intervals should be based on risk, with screening every 3 months in individuals at high risk (multiple partners, condomless sex, transactional sex/sex work, sex while intoxicated) [43].

Hormone Management

The goal of hormonal therapy in transgender patients is to develop secondary sex characteristics of affirmed identity and to suppress secondary sex characteristics that are incongruent with identified sexual identity.

There is no consensus about hormone management in the preoperative period. Some clinicians do not stop hormones unless there is a history of thromboembolic or thrombophilic conditions, while others advise cessation 2 weeks prior to surgery.

Bariatric Considerations

Based on surgical technique and surgeon preference, body mass index (BMI) may be a limitation to gender-affirming surgery. Elevated BMI is associated with cardiac, pulmonary, and endocrine morbidity, increasing perioperative risk. If questions exist regarding optimizing the patient's BMI prior to surgery, the primary clinician should communicate directly with the primary surgeon [17].

Reproductive Planning

Reproductive planning should be discussed during preoperative planning. Patients are encouraged to explore all preserving options prior to the procedure. Family planning is discussed in more detail in Chap. 5 of this book.

Mental Health

Mental health is a critical aspect preparing for gender-affirming surgery. In some cases a patient may be referred to a primary care clinician by a mental health specialist to aid in the medical aspects of preparing for a gender-affirming surgery. Other times a primary care clinician may refer a patient to mental health specialist. In either event, the primacy care clinician should play an active role in assessing the mental health needs of the patient. Mental health in TGNB patients is discussed in more detail in Chap. 16 of this book.

Hospital-Based Pre-admission Testing and Evaluation

Hospital-based pre-admission testing and evaluation should occur about 2 weeks prior to the planned procedure. A comprehensive preoperative medical evaluation at the facility performing the procedure should focus on stratification of cardiac as well as noncardiac risks.

Based on the preoperative testing and risk stratification, interventions can be identified to help reduce the risk of perioperative complications.

Cardiac Risk Stratification

The approach to cardiac evaluation in patients undergoing transgender surgery is similar to those patients undergoing other types of noncardiac surgery. The America College of Cardiology and American Heart Association published the ACC/AHA 2014 Guidelines on Perioperative Cardiovascular Evaluation [47], which note that the goals of the preoperative cardiac evaluation are:

- Assessment of perioperative major adverse cardiac events
- Determination of the need for changes in management
- Identification of cardiovascular conditions or risk factors requiring longer-term management

Changes in management can include the decision to modify existing medical therapies, the decision to perform further cardiovascular interventions, or recommendations about postoperative monitoring. Further discussions may be needed with the perioperative team about the optimal location and timing of surgery or alternative strategies.

Strong cardiac contraindications to proceeding with gender affirmation surgery are the same as other surgeries and include recent myocardial infarction, decompensated heart failure, severe valvular disease (such as severe aortic stenosis or symptomatic mitral stenosis), high-grade heart block, and poorly controlled arrhythmias (e.g., atrial fibrillation with rate > 110).

In the absence of these so-called cardiac "red flags," the clinician must then estimate the risk of major adverse cardiac events (MACE). The Revised Cardiac Risk Index (RCRI) is perhaps the most widely used validated risk stratification tool, identifying six major predictors of postoperative MACE, including a history of ischemic heart disease, heart failure, stroke, diabetes requiring insulin, preoperative creatinine equal or greater than 2.0, and high-risk surgical procedures. Gender-affirming surgeries are generally considered to carry a low to intermediate procedure-specific risk.

Other risk stratification tools have been developed which allow more precise calculation of surgical risk (Fig. 15.1). Newer tools such as American College of

RCRI	MICA	ACS NSQIP Surgical Risk Calculator
• Simple scoring system using six independent predictors • Stratifies into low/elevated risk categories • Simple, easy to use • Non-gender based • Recommended for inpatients with at least two day stays	• Uses five independent predictors • Calculates perioperative risk of MI and cardiac arrest in % • Non-gender based	• Procedure CPT code and twenty one patient-specific variables incorporated into calculating % risk and relative risks for cardiac complications, as well as nine other significant outcomes • Gender based

Fig. 15.1 Comparison of the RCRI, the American College of Surgeons NSQIP MICA, and the American College of Surgeons NSQIP Surgical Risk Calculator [47]

Surgeons National Surgical Quality Improvement Program (NSQIP), Myocardial Infarction and Cardiac Arrest (MICA), and American College of Surgeons NSQIP Surgical Risk Calculator have shown better predictive performance than Revised Cardiac Risk Index (RCRI) calculator. ACS NSQIP calculator also offers the added benefit of assessing for other significant complications as well. RCRI and MICA cardiac risk calculators are non-gender based and can be more readily used for our transgender and gender nonbinary (TGNB) patients.

Low risk for major adverse cardiac events is defined as risk of MACE or MI below 1%. Patients whose calculated risk of MACE is ≥1% are considered elevated risk [47].

Noncardiac Risk Evaluation and Mitigation of Existing Risks

Other organ systems have proven to be relevant when evaluating overall fitness and safety of transgender patients for affirming procedures. In this section, we will briefly outline noncardiac risk screening tools and risk mitigation that is applicable to transgender surgical patients.

Pulmonary

The goal of a preoperative pulmonary assessment is to minimize postoperative pulmonary complications (PPC) in the recovery phase. Medical clinicians, through detailed history taking and examination, should identity modifiable risks and optimize underlying conditions. A pulmonary abnormality could result in clinically significant disease or dysfunction. Common PPCs include atelectasis, infection, respiratory failure, exacerbation of underlying chronic lung disease, bronchospasm, pulmonary edema, pulmonary embolism, and transfusion-related acute lung injury (TRALI).

Several risk assessment tools exist to determine the overall risk of PPCs and identify patients likely to benefit from risk reduction interventions. The Assess Respiratory Risk in Surgical Patients in Catalonia (ARISCAT) score identifies seven independent risk factors for postoperative pulmonary complications, including age, preoperative SpO2, respiratory infection in the past month, preoperative Hgb <10, type of surgical incision, duration of surgery, and emergency status of surgery [4].

The Gupta Postoperative Respiratory Failure Risk calculator can also provide a risk estimate of postoperative respiratory failure (PRF) for surgical patients.

Postoperative respiratory failure (PRF) is considered as failure to wean from mechanical ventilation within 48 hours of surgery or unplanned intubation/reintubation in the postoperative setting. Preoperative variables associated with increased risk of PRF include type of surgery, emergency case, dependent functional status, sepsis, and higher ASA class. The validated risk calculator provides a risk estimate of PRF and is anticipated to aid in surgical decision-making and informed patient consent [16].

Obstructive sleep apnea (OSA) screening can identify known or suspected cases for targeted recovery. Documenting CPAP/BiPAP settings, mask type, amount of oxygen, and compliance should be included in a detailed history. For patients of unknown status, providers should use the STOP-BANG questionnaire tool to screen for obstructive sleep apnea [7].

Pulmonary specialists should be consulted for uncontrolled dysfunction or for conditions such as pulmonary hypertension, restrictive lung disease, cystic fibrosis, history of lung transplant, and severe OSA.

Smoking cessation is recommended for improved postoperative pulmonary status as well as for acceleration of wound healing. All patients anticipating surgery are advised to quit smoking as soon as possible. Since there is no harm in discontinuing cigarette use for a short duration, all patients anticipating transgender surgery should quit smoking as soon as possible. When time allows, a longer duration of cessation is preferred [13, 31].

Hematology

TGNB patients undergoing gender-affirming procedures face unique hematological risks based on their profile. As the majority of patients choose to be on affirming hormonal therapy, careful risk assessment of its effects should be considered.

The Modified Caprini Risk Assessment Model is widely used to calculate estimated baseline risk (EBR) for venous thromboembolism (VTE) in patients undergoing surgical procedures. This model has been validated for and applied to patients undergoing general and abdominal/pelvic surgery, making it suitable for patients undergoing primary or "bottom" surgeries.

• Very low risk or Caprini score of 0 corresponds to an EBR <0.5 percent
• Low risk or Caprini score 1–2 corresponds to an EBR of about 1.5 percent
• Moderate risk or Caprini score 3–4 corresponds to an EBR of about 3 percent
• High risk or Caprini score of ≥5 corresponds to an EBR of at least 6 percent

Majority of TGNB patients undergoing affirming procedures would fall into the moderate risk category given that affirming hormonal therapy is ongoing with a history of negative thromboembolism. For low-risk patients, mechanical methods of VTE prophylaxis are adequate. For moderate-risk patients, pharmacologic prophylaxis is recommended along with mechanical measures. For patients at high risk of VTE, we suggest pharmacologic prophylaxis at minimum and consider extended therapy as indicated; however, it is not routinely recommended [15].

As highlighted in this section, understanding and stratifying the risk of different procedures is essential for assessing the overall fitness of a surgical patient. Below, we further explore the techniques used as well as the risks and benefits associated with existing procedures.

Gender-Affirming Surgeries

Transmasculine Chest Surgery

About 40% of transmasculine people have undergone top surgery [23], also termed chest wall recontouring/reconstruction or chest masculinization. Top surgery is probably the most common procedure sought out by transgender clients [25]. The surgery usually involves bilateral mastectomy with free nipple grafts or nipple transposition on a pedicle. Sometimes the patient may opt for mastectomy without retention of the nipples. For those with smaller chest sizes the periareolar (keyhole) technique can be used [38, 42]. The first postoperative visit is usually with the surgeon. If surgical drains (usually Jackson-Pratt drains) were placed, these will be removed between 5 and 10 days after surgery, when the drainage has stopped or becomes less than approximately 25 ml/day. Primary care clinicians should be acquainted with early postoperative care as well as drain removal techniques as patients may opt to travel home before the drains have been removed. Arrangements with a local surgeon should be made for early postoperative co-management should the primary clinician be unfamiliar with drain removal or should complications arise. Complications may occur in as many as 25% of individuals following top surgery [10]; however, these are usually minor and may include hematomas, hypertrophic scarring, seromas, depigmentation of the nipple areolar complex, or more serious concerns, e.g., nipple necrosis. During the first postoperative visit (usually within 7–10 days), the clinician will remove the dressings and assess the surgical site area for infection or other issues such as hematomas or seromas. A seroma is a collection of subcutaneous fluid that causes swelling. It often resorbs however may need to be aspirated, especially if it is large or compromising skin integrity. If the drains are to be removed, the provider should follow standard techniques [24]. Medical clinicians should refer patients to a surgeon for aspiration of large hematomas or seromas if they do not have expertise to do this. Patients may experience a temporary loss of sensation over the chest wall for several weeks after surgery. Clinicians should caution their clients to avoid inadvertent burns, e.g., to carefully test water temperature while showering, until sensation has returned. Cosmetic issues such as "dog ears" (residual tissue at the lateral chest wall) can be revised at a later date [29]. Hypertrophic scars, or keloids, may be treated with intralesional steroids, and patients can be referred to plastic surgeons or dermatologists for treatment. Patients frequently need minor revisions to remove excess tissue, repair nipple ptosis, or other concerns. Although these are not urgent, they can result in significant emotional distress. Clinicians should facilitate referrals so that revisions can occur in a timely manner.

There are insufficient data regarding cancer screening in transmasculine individuals who have undergone top surgery. Although much of the breast tissue is removed, there is still a possibility of cancer. Recent systematic reviews have reported cases of transgender men who have developed breast cancer after top surgery [9, 39] although the risk appears to be less than in cisgender women or transgender men who have not had surgery. Clinical recommendations for breast cancer screening have included annual clinical chest wall examinations, a discussion of the limitations of mammography in the postoperative chest, and consideration of ultrasound or MRI examination [6, 9, 39]. Primary care clinicians should discuss options for screening with the patient after assessing their known risk factors for cancer, including advanced age, family history, and genetic factors.

Transfeminine Breast Surgery

Transgender women may opt for breast surgery, regardless of hormone use. About one in ten transgender women have undergone breast augmentation procedures [23]. The surgeries are similar to those undertaken in cisgender women, with the use of implants (either silicone or saline filled) that are inserted usually through an incision in the inframammary fold, although circumareolar or axillary approaches may also be used. Due to the wider chest, a larger implant is often chosen and inserted using subglandular, subfascial, or subpectoral placement [38]. Patients are usually seen by their surgeons within 2 weeks after surgery. Primary care clinicians should be aware of potential complications after breast surgery. Early issues may involve skin and soft tissue infections, hematomas or seromas. Patients should be referred back to their surgeon for evaluation of serious issues if indicated. Longer-term complications can include implant rupture, leakage of silicone, capsular contracture, and even implant-related cancer. Symptoms of rupture can include sudden change in breast size, redness, swelling, or pain. Capsular contracture results in hardening or distortion of the breast. All of these complications will require referral to a breast surgeon for further evaluation and treatment.

Medical clinicians should discuss breast cancer screening with their patients. There have been no prospective studies or clinical trials evaluating mammography in transgender women receiving hormones, with or without breast surgery. There have been case reports however of transgender women on estrogen therapy developing breast cancer [9, 18] as well as case reports of breast implant-associated anaplastic large cell lymphoma [8, 32]. Medical clinicians should be aware that many transgender women have injected soft tissue fillers into the breasts, often resulting in granulomatous lesions that may not be easily removed during breast surgery [30]. The residual silicone may make it difficult to interpret mammograms or breast ultrasounds [34, 37]. Current guidelines recommend that transgender women on hormone therapy receive routine breast cancer screening using accepted guidelines as for cisgender women [21]. This is discussed in more detail in Chap. 14. For those with a history of silicone or soft tissue fillers injected into the breast, it may be advisable to have further imaging using MRI if mammography cannot be adequately interpreted.

Transmasculine Genital Surgery

The proportion of transgender men who have undergone either metoidioplasty or phalloplasty is low, about 2–3% for either procedure [23], even though many more, up to 45%, want one of these surgeries eventually [23]. Clinicians should first be aware that these surgeries are highly individualized in order to meet patient goals. For example, an individual can undergo a metoidioplasty (clitoral release procedure), with or without urethral lengthening, and may or may not have a hysterectomy, oophorectomy, or vaginectomy. Phalloplasty is generally a multistage procedure over many months or years and can involve using tissue flaps from the forearm, chest wall, or thigh. Although most individuals undergo total hysterectomy and vaginectomy before phalloplasty surgery, some may opt to retain their internal organs and vagina. This has consequences for long-term care and cancer screening. Primary care clinicians should be fully aware of all surgeries undertaken and what organs remain, in order to offer appropriate preventive care services.

Long-term preventive care is highly individualized and depends on the organs that have been retained. The cervix is not retained after vaginectomy; however, if the individual has not had a vaginectomy, and still has a cervix, cervical cancer screening will need to continue using established guidelines. In the United States, the US Preventive Services Task Force recommendations for cisgender women at average risk for cervical cancer are to screen for cervical cancer at age 21–65 years with cytology (Pap smear) every 3 years. For those 30–65 years the screening interval can be extended to every 5 years if cytology is done in combination with human papillomavirus (HPV) testing or HPV testing alone [40]. For transgender men receiving testosterone, initial studies indicate that they are more likely to have unsatisfactory cytology specimens, likely due to testosterone-induced cervical atrophy [33]. After metoidioplasty, cytology collection is further complicated by narrowing of the introitus, causing technical difficulties performing the Pap as well as discomfort in many individuals. Performing vaginal exams usually requires patience and a very small speculum. If this is not possible (technical issues or patient refusal), then screening can be performed using a self-collected swab for high-risk HPV. Although HPV testing alone has not been accepted into national screening guidelines for those under the age of 30, it was found to be a viable option for transgender men [36].

An age-based approach to the sexual history and screening, diagnosis, and treatment of sexually transmitted infections are discussed in detail in Part 1 and Chap. 6 of this book, respectively. As described in Part 1 of the book, taking a comprehensive sexual history is paramount and should include the genders of the patient's sexual partners, the body parts used for sexual activity, whether barrier protection is used, and whether the person is on (or wishes to start) HIV pre-exposure prophylaxis. The Centers for Disease Control and Prevention (CDC) states that STI screening in transgender individuals should be based on anatomy and sexual behaviors [43]. For transgender men who have undergone metoidioplasty with urethral lengthening and have retained their cervix and vagina, a urine specimen will be inadequate to detect gonorrhea or chlamydia cervicitis. In this clinical scenario a cervical swab will need to be obtained. For transgender men who have retained internal organs, there should also be a discussion about fertility, pregnancy potential, and contraception options, if indicated. A complete discussion on contraception is found in Chap. 5.

Common complications after both metoidioplasty and phalloplasty include urethral strictures and fistulae. On initial and subsequent visits medical clinicians should ask patients about difficulty voiding including poor stream, dysuria, incontinence, or leakage of urine from a non-meatal opening. The area should be examined for signs of infection, swelling, or redness or fistulae. Soft tissue infection or urinary retention should be evaluated urgently. Most complications will require evaluation by the primary surgeon or an alternative specialist, e.g., a urologist who is familiar with the procedures.

Transfeminine Genital Surgery

Transgender women may opt to undergo genital surgery. In one survey, 12% had undergone vaginoplasty and about half wanted it someday [23]. Most vaginoplasty surgeries involve a combination of penile and scrotal tissue to create the neovagina. A second surgical technique uses intestinal tissue (e.g., sigmoid colon graft). The differences in the tissue used for surgery have great importance for long-term follow-up.

After surgery the patient will usually spend the initial postoperative course in the hospital. A vaginal stent of packing is placed during surgery and removed at about 5–7 days. After this the patient will need to start using vaginal dilators. Usually this continues lifelong to prevent vaginal stenosis.

Primary care clinicians should be aware of early and long-term clinical issues associated with vaginoplasty surgeries. At initial visits medical clinicians should ask about difficulty urinating, including dysuria, frequency and inability to void, bleeding, odor, fecal matter on the dilator, or gas. They should also inquire about pain management, frequency of, and any difficulty with dilations. In the early postoperative period, within 4 weeks, issues such as skin and soft tissue infections and urinary tract infections may develop. It is common for the urinary stream to be irregular, which often resolves over time. Patients should be aware that after surgery tissue swelling persists for many months. Another common issue is persistent granulation tissue of the neovagina and/or neo-labia, which may be associated with bleeding or odor. Many of the minor postoperative medical concerns can be treated by primary care clinicians, including assessment and treatment of urinary tract infections and treatment of granulation tissue with silver nitrate. If there is any suspicion about more serious complications, e.g., rectovaginal fistula, the patient should be referred immediately to a colorectal surgeon.

Rare complications include urinary stenosis, urinary retention, and fistulae, including rectovaginal fistulae. If women report pain with dilations, they should be assessed for strictures or infection. They can be advised to try a smaller dilator or to apply a small amount of lidocaine gel to the dilator tip. After patients have adequately healed, on average 8–12 weeks, the surgeon will advise patients when they may safely have vaginal intercourse. Clinicians should ask about sensation, orgasm, and satisfaction with sex at subsequent visits. Several studies have indicated that overall satisfaction and sexual function is high for those undergoing vaginoplasty [27, 46].

Hormones are usually restarted the week following surgery when patients are fully ambulatory. During genital surgeries the testes are removed; therefore, androgen blockers can usually be stopped. There are some providers who reduce the estrogen doses following gonadectomy; however, this has not been fully evaluated and may result in untoward effects, such as osteopenia.

The prostate is not removed during the vaginoplasty procedure; therefore, transgender women are potentially at risk for prostate issues. Prostate cancer appears to be rare in transgender women who have received estrogens and androgen blockers and who have undergone orchiectomy; however, there are case reports in the literature [14]. Primary care clinicians should be aware that the prostate-specific antigen (PSA) test is unreliable in the setting of androgen blockers or gonadectomy. The prostate can be examined intravaginally, palpating the anterior wall.

Since vaginoplasty surgery does not result in a cervix, there is no recommendation to perform cervical cancer screening. It is still good practice to visually inspect the vagina each year to examine the tissue for lesions, ulcers, etc. There have been case reports of genital warts (condyloma acuminata) [3, 26, 28, 45], gonorrhea [1, 19, 41], herpes simplex [11], chlamydia trachomatis [35], and squamous cell carcinomas [2, 12] of the neovagina. Medical providers should have a low threshold for screening individuals at risk for STIs. The preferred method is to send a vaginal swab for testing. Genital warts can be treated using usual methods, but patients should be referred for biopsy if the lesions are atypical or do not respond to treatment.

If the vaginoplasty is performed using an intestinal graft, there are additional clinical concerns for long-term management. There have been case reports of adenocarcinoma [22, 44] as well as a host of other issues such as neovaginal inflammatory bowel disease, diversion colitis, and polyps [20]. Most of these conditions can be evaluated and treated by a gastroenterologist, using similar techniques as for native bowel tissue, including biopsy, polyp removal, and steroid douches.

After vaginoplasty, or gonadectomy, patients are at risk for osteopenia and osteoporosis if they discontinue their hormone therapy. Current osteoporosis screening recommendations are to screen using bone densitometry. When applying the FRAX® tool, the consensus is that assigned birth sex should be used to assess bone density [21].

Conclusion

As more and more transgender people access gender-affirming surgeries, there will be a heightened need for primary care clinicians to be more knowledgeable about immediate and long-term clinical issues and to play a greater role in preparation for surgery and short- and long-term postoperative management.

Primary care clinicians should be aware of the available gender-affirming surgery techniques, as well as the impact of hormonal and surgical interventions on preventive care guidelines. Providers should know what organs have been retained and appropriately apply screening recommendations, e.g., for cervical, breast, or prostate cancer screening if indicated. Many immediate complications can be assessed and treated by primary care clinicians, often with guidance from surgeons and other specialists.

References

1. Bodsworth NJ, Price R, Davies SC. Gonococcal infection of the neovagina in a male-to-female transsexual. Sex Transm Dis. 1994;21(4):211–2.
2. Bollo J, Balla A, Rodriguez Luppi C, Martinez C, Quaresima S, Targarona EM. HPV-related squamous cell carcinoma in a neovagina after male-to-female gender confirmation surgery. Int J STD AIDS. 2018;29(3):306–8. https://doi.org/10.1177/0956462417728856.
3. Buscema J, Rosenshein NB, Shah K. Condylomata acuminata arising in a neovagina. Obstet Gynecol. 1987;69(3 Pt 2):528–30.
4. Canet J, Gallart L, Gomar C, Paluzie G, Vallès J, Castillo J, et al. Prediction of postoperative pulmonary complications in a population-based surgical cohort. Anesthesiology. 2010;113(6):1338–50. https://doi.org/10.1097/ALN.0b013e3181fc6e0a.
5. Canner JK, Harfouch O, Kodadek LM, Pelaez D, Coon D, Offodile AC 2nd, et al. Temporal trends in gender-affirming surgery among transgender patients in the United States. JAMA Surg. 2018;153(7):609–16. https://doi.org/10.1001/jamasurg.2017.6231.
6. Center of Excellence for Transgender Health, D. o. F. a. C. M., University of California San Francisco. Guidelines for the primary and gender-affirming care of transgender and gender nonbinary people, M. Deutsch (Ed.). 2016. Retrieved from www.transhealth.ucsf.edu/
7. Chung F, Yegneswaran B, Liao P, Chung SA, Vairavanathan S, Islam S, et al. STOP questionnaire: a tool to screen patients for obstructive sleep apnea. Anesthesiology. 2008;108(5):812–21. https://doi.org/10.1097/ALN.0b013e31816d83e4.
8. de Boer M, van der Sluis WB, de Boer JP, Overbeek LIH, van Leeuwen FE, Rakhorst HA, et al. Breast implant-associated anaplastic large-cell lymphoma in a transgender woman. Aesthet Surg J. 2017;37(8):Np83–np87. https://doi.org/10.1093/asj/sjx098.
9. Deutsch MB, Radix A, Wesp L. Breast cancer screening, management, and a review of case study literature in transgender populations. Semin Reprod Med. 2017;35(5):434–41. https://doi.org/10.1055/s-0037-1606103.
10. Donato DP, Walzer NK, Rivera A, Wright L, Agarwal CA. Female-to-male chest reconstruction: a review of technique and outcomes. Ann Plast Surg. 2017;79(3):259–63. https://doi.org/10.1097/sap.0000000000001099.
11. Elfering L, van der Sluis WB, Mermans JF, Buncamper ME. Herpes neolabialis: herpes simplex virus type 1 infection of the neolabia in a transgender woman. Int J STD AIDS. 2017;28(8):841–3. https://doi.org/10.1177/0956462416685658.

12. Fernandes HM, Manolitsas TP, Jobling TW. Carcinoma of the neovagina after male-to-female reassignment. J Low Genit Tract Dis. 2014;18(2):E43–5. https://doi.org/10.1097/LGT.0b013e3182976219.
13. Goltsman D, Munabi NC, Ascherman JA. The association between smoking and plastic surgery outcomes in 40,465 patients: an analysis of the American College of Surgeons National Surgical Quality Improvement Program Data Sets. Plast Reconstr Surg. 2017;139(2):503–11. https://doi.org/10.1097/prs.0000000000002958.
14. Gooren L, Morgentaler A. Prostate cancer incidence in orchidectomised male-to-female transsexual persons treated with oestrogens. Andrologia. 2013; https://doi.org/10.1111/and.12208.
15. Gould MK, Garcia DA, Wren SM, Karanicolas PJ, Arcelus JI, Heit JA, Samama CM. Prevention of VTE in nonorthopedic surgical patients: antithrombotic therapy and prevention of thrombosis, 9th ed: American College of Chest Physicians Evidence-Based Clinical Practice Guidelines. Chest. 2012;141(2 Suppl):e227S–77S. https://doi.org/10.1378/chest.11-2297.
16. Gupta H, Gupta PK, Fang X, Miller WJ, Cemaj S, Forse RA, Morrow LE. Development and validation of a risk calculator predicting postoperative respiratory failure. Chest. 2011;140(5):1207–15. https://doi.org/10.1378/chest.11-0466.
17. Gurunathan U, Myles PS. Limitations of body mass index as an obesity measure of perioperative risk. Br J Anaesth. 2016;116(3):319–21. https://doi.org/10.1093/bja/aev541.
18. Hartley RL, Stone JP, Temple-Oberle C. Breast cancer in transgender patients: a systematic review. Part 1: male to female. Eur J Surg Oncol. 2018; https://doi.org/10.1016/j.ejso.2018.06.035.
19. Haustein UF. Pruritus of the artificial vagina of a transsexual patient caused by gonococcal infection. Hautarzt. 1995;46(12):858–9.
20. Heller DS. Lesions of the neovagina–a review. J Low Genit Tract Dis. 2015;19(3):267–70. https://doi.org/10.1097/lgt.0000000000000110.
21. Hembree WC, Cohen-Kettenis PT, Gooren L, Hannema SE, Meyer WJ, Murad MH, et al. Endocrine treatment of gender-dysphoric/gender-incongruent persons: an Endocrine Society* clinical practice guideline. J Clin Endocrinol Metabol. 2017;102(11):3869–903. https://doi.org/10.1210/jc.2017-01658.
22. Hiroi H, Yasugi T, Matsumoto K, Fujii T, Watanabe T, Yoshikawa H, Taketani Y. Mucinous adenocarcinoma arising in a neovagina using the sigmoid colon thirty years after operation: a case report. J Surg Oncol. 2001;77(1):61–4.
23. James SE, Herman JL, Rankin S, Keisling M, Mottet L, Anafi M. The report of the 2015 U.S.Transgender survey. Retrieved from Washington, D.C. 2016
24. Knowlton MC. Nurse's guide to surgical drain removal. Nursing. 2015;45(9):59–61. https://doi.org/10.1097/01.NURSE.0000470418.02063.ca.
25. Lane M, Ives GC, Sluiter EC, Waljee JF, Yao TH, Hu HM, Kuzon WM. Trends in gender-affirming surgery in insured patients in the United States. Plast Reconstr Surg Glob Open. 2018;6(4):e1738. https://doi.org/10.1097/gox.0000000000001738.
26. Liguori G, Trombetta C, Bucci S, De Seta F, De Santo D, Siracusano S, Belgrano E. Condylomata acuminata of the neovagina in a HIV-seropositive male-to-female transsexual. Urol Int. 2004;73(1):87–8. https://doi.org/10.1159/000078811.
27. Massie JP, Morrison SD, Van Maasdam J, Satterwhite T. Predictors of patient satisfaction and postoperative complications in penile inversion vaginoplasty. Plast Reconstr Surg. 2018;141(6):911e–21e. https://doi.org/10.1097/prs.0000000000004427.
28. Matsuki S, Kusatake K, Hein KZ, Anraku K, Morita E. Condylomata acuminata in the neovagina after male-to-female reassignment treated with CO2 laser and imiquimod. Int J STD AIDS. 2015;26(7):509–11. https://doi.org/10.1177/0956462414542476.
29. McEvenue G, Xu FZ, Cai R, McLean H. Female-to-male gender affirming top surgery: a single surgeon's 15-year retrospective review and treatment algorithm. Aesthet Surg J. 2017;38(1):49–57. https://doi.org/10.1093/asj/sjx116.

30. Murariu D, Holland MC, Gampper TJ, Campbell CA. Illegal silicone injections create unique reconstructive challenges in transgender patients. Plast Reconstr Surg. 2015;135(5):932e–3e. https://doi.org/10.1097/prs.0000000000001192.

31. Myers K, Hajek P, Hinds C, McRobbie H. Stopping smoking shortly before surgery and postoperative complications: a systematic review and meta-analysis. Arch Intern Med. 2011;171(11):983–9. https://doi.org/10.1001/archinternmed.2011.97.

32. Patzelt M, Zarubova L, Klener P, Barta J, Benkova K, Brandejsova A, et al. Anaplastic large-cell lymphoma associated with breast implants: a case report of a transgender female. Aesthet Plast Surg. 2018;42(2):451–5. https://doi.org/10.1007/s00266-017-1012-y.

33. Peitzmeier SM, Reisner SL, Harigopal P, Potter J. Female-to-male patients have high prevalence of unsatisfactory Paps compared to non-transgender females: implications for cervical cancer screening. J Gen Intern Med. 2014;29(5):778–84. https://doi.org/10.1007/s11606-013-2753-1.

34. Peters W, Fornasier V. Complications from injectable materials used for breast augmentation. Can J Plast Surg. 2009;17(3):89–96.

35. Radix AE, Harris AB, Belkind U, Ting J, Goldstein ZG. Chlamydia trachomatis infection of the Neovagina in transgender women. Open Forum Infect Dis. 2019;6(11). https://doi.org/10.1093/ofid/ofz470.

36. Reisner SL, Deutsch MB, Peitzmeier SM, White Hughto JM, Cavanaugh TP, Pardee DJ, et al. Test performance and acceptability of self- versus provider-collected swabs for high-risk HPV DNA testing in female-to-male trans masculine patients. PLoS One. 2018;13(3):e0190172. https://doi.org/10.1371/journal.pone.0190172.

37. Scaranelo AM, de Fatima Ribeiro Maia M. Sonographic and mammographic findings of breast liquid silicone injection. J Clin Ultrasound. 2006;34(6):273–7. https://doi.org/10.1002/jcu.20235.

38. Schechter LS. Gender confirmation surgery: an update for the primary care provider. Transgend Health. 2016;1(1):32–40. https://doi.org/10.1089/trgh.2015.0006.

39. Stone JP, Hartley RL, Temple-Oberle, C. Breast cancer in transgender patients: a systematic review. Part 2: female to male. Eur J Surg Oncol. 2018. https://doi.org/10.1016/j.ejso.2018.06.021.

40. U.S. Preventive Services Task Force. U.S. Preventive Services Task Force. Retrieved from https://www.uspreventiveservicestaskforce.org/Page/Name/home.

41. van der Sluis WB, Bouman MB, Gijs L, van Bodegraven AA. Gonorrhoea of the sigmoid neovagina in a male-to-female transgender. Int J STD AIDS. 2015;26(8):595–8. https://doi.org/10.1177/0956462414544725.

42. Whitehead DM, Weiss PR, Podolsky D. A single Surgeon's experience with transgender female-to-male chest surgery. Ann Plast Surg. 2018;81(3):353–9. https://doi.org/10.1097/sap.0000000000001536.

43. Workowski KA, Bolan GA. Sexually transmitted diseases treatment guidelines, 2015. MMWR Recomm Rep. 2015;64(RR-03):1–137.

44. Yamada K, Shida D, Kato T, Yoshida H, Yoshinaga S, Kanemitsu Y. Adenocarcinoma arising in sigmoid colon neovagina 53 years after construction. World J Surg Oncol. 2018;16(1):88. https://doi.org/10.1186/s12957-018-1372-z.

45. Yang C, Liu S, Xu K, Xiang Q, Yang S, Zhang X. Condylomata gigantea in a male transsexual. Int J STD AIDS. 2009;20(3):211–2. https://doi.org/10.1258/ijsa.2008.008213.

46. Zavlin D, Schaff J, Lelle JD, Jubbal KT, Herschbach P, Henrich G, et al. Male-to-female sex reassignment surgery using the combined vaginoplasty technique: satisfaction of transgender patients with aesthetic, functional, and sexual outcomes. Aesthet Plast Surg. 2018;42(1):178–87. https://doi.org/10.1007/s00266-017-1003-z.

47. Fleisher L A et al. J Am Coll Cardiol. 2014;64(22):e77–e137.

Chapter 16
Mental Health for Transgender and Gender Nonbinary Patients

Eric Yarbrough

Contents

Introduction

There is an intimate relationship between sexual and reproductive health and mental health. This relationship is at times amplified in gender-diverse patients. Given the contemporary and historic oppression of transgender and gender nonbinary (TGNB) patients and the resulting inequities in mental health, there are particular areas that a primary care clinician should be familiar with when addressing the mental health needs of this population. Gender-diverse people have typically experienced a lifetime of being invalidated and even having their mental stability questioned because of their gender identity. Nearly half of TGNB patients have attempted suicide at least once in their life, compared with 20% of patients who identify as lesbian, gay, or bisexual, and under 5% of the general population [5]. While research continues to be lacking in the area of transgender mental health, it is clear that gender-diverse people do not experience such inequities in mental health inherently because they are transgender but as a result of lived experiences within an unaccepting and potentially hostile world. In a society intent on maintaining a gender dichotomy of male

E. Yarbrough (✉)
Department of Psychiatry, NYU School of Medicine, New York, NY, USA

© Springer Nature Switzerland AG 2022
J. Truglio et al. (eds.), *Sexual and Reproductive Health*,
https://doi.org/10.1007/978-3-030-94632-6_16

and female, breaking such rules unjustly invites scrutiny and isolation. Growing up TGNB in a larger cisgender world creates an internal mental struggle in that TGNB people are taught – through media, family, or friends – that being gender diverse is abnormal or "crazy." Over time such minority stress experienced by TGNB patients can result in internalized transphobia – the internalization of negative thoughts, feelings, and attitudes about transgender people. It is a mostly unconscious process that can have lasting psychological effects leading to the previously mentioned symptoms of depression, anxiety, trauma, and even suicidal ideation [11].

Such social and structural drivers of mental health inequities have been amplified by a strained relationship between mental health professionals and gender-diverse people. Historically gender diversity was seen as something to diagnose and treat. The most recent edition of the *Diagnostic and Statistical Manual of Mental Disorders* (DSM), the DSM-5, continues to struggle to find gender-diverse people an avenue to care while, at the same time, not stigmatizing their identity as a mental illness. The term "Gender Dysphoria" is currently used to describe and diagnose those who experience dysphoric symptoms from a sex assigned at birth that does not align with their gender identity [1].

Despite progress away from treating gender-diverse patients as having an illness to be cured, mental health professionals will often have to prove themselves to be understanding of the gender spectrum and overall gender-diverse culture in order to connect with TGNB patients. While there are many mental health professionals who are competent to work with gender-diverse people, the supply of knowledgeable clinicians does not in any way meet the need [3]. Primary care clinicians therefore need to have basic knowledge and skills to provide effective primary mental healthcare to TGNB patient.

The approach to primary mental healthcare presented in this chapter will offer clinicians the opportunity to think outside the usual gender box and will tell them how to approach patients on an individualized level. This chapter will cover the following basic mental health areas for clinicians providing primary sexual and reproductive healthcare for TGNB patients:

1. Application of basic primary care mental health skills within a gender-affirming and trauma-informed framework
2. Considerations of mental health in TGNB patients with sexual dysfunction
3. Assessment of mental health symptoms in patients receiving gender-affirming hormone therapy
4. Supporting patients going through gender-affirming procedures

Application of Basic Primary Care Mental Health Skills Within a Gender-Affirming, Trauma-Informed Framework

Transgender and gender nonbinary patients experience complex mental and physical health concerns. A 2016 US survey of over 27,0000 transgender-identified people revealed marked increase rates depression, anxiety, PTSD, and suicide attempts

[5]. Despite this increased risk for mental health issues, TGNB people may be hesitant to convey their psychiatric symptoms for a wide variety of reasons, related and unrelated to their gender identity. These include prior negative experiences with the healthcare system and fear that disclosure might cause their primary care clinician to withhold access to hormones or gender-affirming treatments. TGNB people are also subject to high rates of repeated trauma and violence, including intimate partner violence, physical assault, hate crimes, police violence, and even murder. Whether the trauma be physical, verbal, or sexual in nature, acute and chronic trauma may lead to symptoms of depression, anxiety, and post-traumatic stress disorder (PTSD). As such the approach to mental health in TGNB patient must be both gender affirming and trauma informed.

Gender-affirming mental health clinicians are competent in the language of gender diversity, are open to the individualistic nature of the gender spectrum, and are knowledgeable of gender-affirming treatments such as hormone therapy and gender-affirming surgeries. Trauma-informed care is grounded in and directed by a thorough understanding of the neurological, biological, psychological, and social effects of trauma in persons who seek and receive health services. It takes into account knowledge about trauma – its impact, interpersonal dynamics, health and mental health effects, and paths to recovery – and incorporates this knowledge into all aspects of service delivery. Trauma-informed care recognizes that certain approaches may re-traumatize patients and family members. Gender-affirming, trauma-informed care is thus a person-centered response focused on improving an individuals' all-around wellness rather than simply treating symptoms of illness.

Trauma-informed care supports safety; emphasizes trust, transparency, and collaboration; and recognizes cultural and historical contexts [6]. The four R's of trauma-informed primary care are effective guidance for clinicians treating TGNB patients [7]:

1. *Realization* about trauma and understanding how trauma can affect TGNB individuals and their families and relationships.
2. *Recognizing* the signs of trauma which can include excessive anxiety and depression, difficulty concentrating, trouble sleeping, nightmares, feeling chronically tired, chest pain, difficulty breathing, substance misuse, stomachaches, headaches, and general physical pain with no apparent cause.
3. *Responding* by sensitively assessing if the patient has experienced any acute trauma, has past experiences they have found to be traumatic, or is experiencing minority stress in anticipating rejection, mistreatment, or the threat of violence. In these cases, making a referral for appropriate treatment will be critical to insuring health and mental health recovery.
4. *Resist re-traumatization* is also essential in insuring that the TGNB patient feels safe and supported by their primary care provider. This may include understanding sensitivities to touch, to body parts that may not reflect a patient's current gender identity, to using the correct name and gender pronouns, and to making sure that the practice environment is also safe and supportive for those patients.

Box 16.1 provides some examples of an integrated gender-affirming, trauma-informed approach to primary mental healthcare in TGNB patients.

For more information and best practices at assessing and addressing trauma and minority stress for TGNB patients in healthcare settings, an excellent resource is the Fenway Institute's training module in LGBT trauma-informed care which can be found at http://www.lgbthealtheducation.org/wp-content/uploads/Trauma-Informed-Care.pdf

Box 16.1 Suggested Approaches for Gender-Affirming, Trauma-Informed Primary Mental Healthcare

Goal	Suggested language
Ask about prior experiences with clinicians, especially mental health clinicians, and explore how these experiences inform the patient's current care-seeking behaviors	"I recognize many of my patients have had negative experiences with doctors and other healthcare clinicians, which can sometimes make it hard to seek care when they need it. What have been your prior experiences with healthcare?"
Reinforce confidentiality	"I want to reassure you about confidentiality in our relationship you, which means that everything we discuss stays between you, me, and your healthcare team, unless I feel we need to get extra help to keep you safe."
Reinforce that having a mental health diagnosis rarely if ever results in being unable to continue with gender-affirming medical or surgical treatments	"Many of my patients on gender-affirming hormone treatment worry that if they express feelings of depression or anxiety we will 'blame the hormones' and stop treatment. I want you to know this rarely, if ever, needs to be done, and we always approach these types of decisions together as a team." "It's important that you feel comfortable sharing any changes in how you are feeling with me so that we can find the best way to address them together."
Offer to be an advocate for the patient – helping to educate other clinicians and mental health specialists on the patient's needs, including their gender identity	"It can be hard to start with a new specialist who does not know you or your past. I am more than happy to help communicate your needs and preferences to other doctors before you see them – it will be up to you how much I tell them."
Acknowledge trauma and/or stress in normalizing suicidal ideation screening	"Some people who have a lot of stress in their life sometimes feel like they don't want to live anymore or that they would like to end their life. Have you ever felt this way? Have there been times recently that you have felt this way?"

For patients in need of more support or a referral to a mental health specialist, primary care clinicians should familiarize themselves with local TGNB-affirming mental health resources. National resources include the Trevor Project helpline for adolescents and young adults (https://www.thetrevorproject.org/get-help-now/) and the National LGBT Hotline (https://www.glbthotline.org/hotline.html). TGNB patients and their friends and family members in need of referrals and support can also contact National PFLAG at https://pflag.org/needsupport. For patients expressing suicidal ideation, there are a variety of safety plans offered to clinicians which can be utilized [8] in addition to local protocols. Should a patient need an urgent referral or hospitalization, the primary clinician can contact the receiving clinical team and inform them of basic information such as the name and pronouns the patient uses. Small actions like these can lead to big differences in patient experience.

Considerations of Mental Health in Transgender and Gender Nonbinary Patients with Sexual Dysfunction

There are several unique factors that influence sexual functioning in TGNB patients. Gender-affirming hormone therapy can lead to differences in sexual desire, arousal, and functioning, many of which relate to overall mental health; transgender men and women who have undergone genital confirmation surgeries may have anxiety about using and potentially damaging new organs; transgender women may find postoperative vaginal dilation painful potentially leading to muscle tension and consequent pain during sex [4]. An inclusive approach to sexual dysfunction is described in Chap. 7 of this book. A comprehensive approach to any form of sexual dysfunction includes an assessment for any mental health symptoms that may cause, contribute to, or arise from the patient's sexual dysfunction. This approach is no different when caring for TGNB patients. The same gender-affirming trauma-informed framework described above should be used in exploring potential mental health concerns related to sexual dysfunction. Some questions and ways to approach sexual dysfunction include the following:

- "Many of my patients have concerns about sex and sexuality, do you have any concerns you'd like to bring up today?"
- "In order to better understand how to help, I'll need to ask more specific questions which may involve sensitive questions about your body. If you feel uncomfortable or would like to me use different words please let me know."

Most people are anxious when describing sexual concerns to clinicians. Everybody has different ways in which they describe their body and bodily functions. Don't assume just because you are someone familiar with a colloquial term, you know exactly what a person means. Approach each person with sensitivity with willingness to understand.

Assessment of Mental Health Symptoms in Patients Receiving Gender-Affirming Hormone Therapy

Gender-affirming hormone therapy symbolizes the metaphorical red herring of diagnosing psychiatric symptoms in TGNB patients. Many clinicians will blame hormone treatment for observed depression, anxiety, mania, or psychosis in their patients. This may be because iatrogenic causes are some of the first diagnoses to be ruled out. Testosterone and estrogen, the main two hormones prescribed in gender-affirming care, can contribute to some mild to moderate changes to mood and anxiety [2]. They do not, however, cause the levels of mania or psychosis which many clinicians are quick to conclude. Each and every person has some levels of estrogen and testosterone within their system, yet they are rarely looked to as causes of psychiatric symptoms in cisgender people.

Should new or worsening mental health symptoms coincide with initiation or titration of hormone therapy the hormones may be causative. In such cases stopping the hormone therapy is rarely the best course of action. Hormones have been shown to have a significant positive impact on the lives of gender-diverse people [9]. The risks of the new symptoms would need to be very severe to outweigh the benefits of treatment. A specialized psychiatrist should be consulted to help in this decision. If one is not available for consultation, the primary clinician in conjunction with the patient can consider adjusting the dose of hormone therapy, monitoring hormone levels, and trending both mental health and physical symptoms.

Supporting Patients Going Through Gender-Affirming Procedures

One area that primary care clinicians and mental health professionals will, at least for the present time, need to collaborate closely is providing letters of support for gender-affirming procedures. Depending on state regulations, insurance policies, and specific surgeon stipulations (see Chap. 18), gender-diverse patients will require some level of mental health input in order to get access to gender-affirming surgical treatments. The World Professional Association of Transgender Health (WPATH) is a group of experts in transgender medicine who provide guidelines for the requirements necessary depending in the type of surgery that is being sought out.

Psychiatrists, psychologists, and other mental health professionals are required to perform an assessment of capacity regarding the risks and benefits of surgical treatment and the recovery that is involved. Psychotherapy and hormones were previous requirements for procedures but have since been considered optional treatments. Some insurance providers may still require a patient to see a psychotherapist weekly for at least a year before they will pay for a procedure. A clinician can advocate for patients in these moments when they think that such requirements are putting up an unnecessary barrier to care. A legal consenting adult who understands the risks and benefits of treatment has the autonomy to make decisions about their care. When a person is a minor, this evaluation can get more complicated and will involve parents or guardians. Discussions around requirements continue to evolve as WPATH meets regularly to update their Standards of Care ("WPATH," [10]).

Conclusion

TGNB people fall into a specialized branch of physical and mental health treatment. While any clinician can be competent in working with gender-diverse people, the first step is to understand that gender identity and sexuality need to be looked at from an individual standpoint and generalizations made during a patient visit will likely lead to mistakes. Assumptions should not be made about gender identity, pronouns, or body parts. Clinicians will need to provide time and space to create a comfortable environment for gender-diverse people to express their identity and their concerns. Disclosure of mental health concerns or psychiatric symptoms in a primary care visit could happen if the patient is comfortable with the clinician. Only by doing this can clinicians be rest assured they have provided gender-affirming treatment as well as quality healthcare.

References

1. Diagnostic and statistical manual of mental disorders. 5th ed. Arlington: American Psychiatric Publishing; 2013.
2. Ettner R, Monstrey S, Coleman E. Principles of transgender medicine and surgery. 1st ed. Routledge; 1996;101–6.
3. Frazer MS, Howe EE. LGBT health and human services needs in New York state: a report from the 2015 LGBT health and human services needs assessment. The Lesbian, Gay, Bisexual & Transgender Community Center: New York; 2016.
4. Holmberg M, Arver S, Dhejne C. Supporting sexuality and improving sexual function in transgender persons. Nat Rev Urol. 2019;16:121–39. https://doi.org/10.1038/s41585-018-0108-8.
5. James SE, Herman JL, Rankin S, Keisling M, Mottet L, Ana M. The report of the 2015 U.S. transgender survey. Washington, D.C.: National Center for Transgender Equality; 2016.
6. Alex Keuroghlian, Behavioral Health Care for Transgender Adults. Webinar, the National LGBT Health Education Center, Fenway Institute, Boston. 2018. https://www.lgbthealtheducation.org/wp-content/uploads/2018/11/Behavioral-Health-Care-for-Transgender-Adults_November-2018_final.pdf. Accessed 11 Nov 2019.
7. Substance Abuse and Mental Health Services Administration. SAMHSA's concept of trauma and guidance for a trauma-informed approach. HHS publication no. (SMA) 14-4884. Rockville: Substance Abuse and Mental Health Services Administration; 2014.
8. Stanley B, Brown GK. The safety plan treatment manual to reduce suicide risk: veteran version. Washington, D.C.: United States Department of Veterans Affairs; 2008.
9. White Hughto J, Reisner S. A systematic review of the effects of hormone therapy on psychological functioning and quality of life in transgender individuals. Transgender Health. 2016;1(1):21–31.
10. WPATH. (2017). Wpath.org. Retrieved 6 May 2017, from http://www.wpath.org/site_page.cfm?pk_association_webpage_menu=1351&pk_association_webpage=4655
11. Yarbrough E. Transgender mental health. Arlington: American Psychiatric Association Publishing; 2018. p. 44.

Chapter 17
Transgender and Gender Nonbinary Medicolegal Issues in the United States

Jill Weiss

Contents

Introduction

There are a number of legal issues associated with medical treatment for transgender and gender nonbinary (TGNB) patients. This chapter will discuss the right to access to care, informed consent, patient identification and medical records, and insurance issues. It should be noted that the following is not legal advice, which can only be provided by an attorney licensed in your state.

The World Professional Association for Transgender Health (WPATH) is considered the premier medical association for transgender medicine. Further information about the medicolegal issues involved in trans-related care can be found at their website.

J. Weiss (✉)
Law Office of Jillian T. Weiss, Brooklyn, NY, USA
e-mail: jweiss@jtweisslaw.com

© Springer Nature Switzerland AG 2022
J. Truglio et al. (eds.), *Sexual and Reproductive Health*,
https://doi.org/10.1007/978-3-030-94632-6_17

Right to Access to Care

There is increasing acceptance of the principle that one cannot be excluded from healthcare due to gender identity. At the time of this writing, more than half of the states have statutes and policies explicitly prohibiting gender identity discrimination in healthcare.[1] The federal government has also interpreted the Affordable Care Act,[2] prohibiting sex discrimination, to include discrimination based on gender identity. Thus, refusing care because of transgender status may create legal risk for medical providers.

Some providers have concerns about their level of medical knowledge regarding transgender medicine that may lead them to prefer not to treat TGNB patients. Refusal to treat TGNB patients due to perceived lack of expertise may be in violation of nondiscrimination law and poses a potential liability risk. It can also be problematic for TGNB health. It would be preferable for providers to access information on transgender care. Information on hormone replacement therapy, one of the most common trans-related treatments, is generally available to providers. This is particularly important in areas where there is not a large choice of providers.

In regard to complex surgical procedures, or gender-transition-related psychotherapy, expertise is an important consideration, and it is not inappropriate to refer patients to others in such situations. Where the provider provides the same treatment to non-transgender patients, however, such as breast enhancement, gynecological exams, or treatment for illness or infection, refusal to treat based on lack of expertise in transgender medicine may be considered discriminatory.

More TGNB youth are seeking trans-related care. WPATH has recognized the right of TGNB youth to receive trans-related care. Oregon was one of the first to allow TGNB youth to receive Medicaid coverage for hormone therapy and hormone blocking treatments.[3] Others states, like New York and Washington, have begun to follow suit.

Many people within the transgender umbrella do not consider themselves to be "transitioning" nor to be moving from one binary gender to another. This includes patients who would identify as a nonbinary identity, gender nonconforming, and gender fluid, among many others. When gender-affirming medical treatment began in the United States, the protocols were specifically designed for "transsexual" people who were transitioning from one binary gender to another, as these were the first people who presented themselves for treatment to the few doctors available. During the past half-century, both society and the medical profession have seen an increase in gender nonconforming gender expression and nonbinary identities. While it has

---

[1] See Transgender People, National Center for Transgender Equality, NATIONAL CENTER FOR TRANSGENDER EQUALITY, Know Your Rights-Health Care (October 2021) https://perma.cc/GZ6Z-QFBY https://transequality.org/know-your-rights/health-care

[2] 42 U.S.C. § 18116

[3] https://www.nytimes.com/2016/10/06/nyregion/new-york-moves-to-allow-medicaid-to-cover-hormone-therapy-for-transgender-youth.html

taken some adjustment, most medical professionals in the field of transgender medicine recognize that treatment is appropriate for these groups as well. They may experience and receive treatment for gender dysphoria. WPATH has recognized the right of nonbinary and gender nonconforming people who are not transitioning to receive treatment. While there is little law on the subject, some states have begun to recognize this principle. For example, the New York State Department of Health has found that nonbinary people are entitled to appropriate healthcare, in that case a reduction mammoplasty, as a medically necessary treatment for gender dysphoria. The decision stated that it is not a requirement of the law that one be transitioning from female to male or vice versa.[4]

On the other end of the spectrum from gender-affirming treatment is "reparative" or "conversion" therapy. These "treatments" purport to have the effect of changing one's gender identity or sexual orientation and include methods such as shaming, hypnosis, inducing vomiting, and electric shocks. They have been found to create great risk of negative mental health effects by many medical associations, particularly for gender and sexual minority youth. Medical associations condemning these treatments include the American Medical Association, the American Psychiatric Association, and the American Academy of Child and Adolescent Psychiatry, among others. Currently, over a dozen states and about two dozen cities have laws prohibiting such therapies.

Consent: Informed Consent, Parental Consent, and Sterilization Consent

Consent is a legally required part of all medical treatment, with rare exceptions for emergency situations. That consent must be one that is granted based on the information necessary to know the risks and benefits that may be obtained from a treatment. Information regarding risks and benefits may be provided by the clinician orally or in writing. Medical providers and facilities often require patient signatures on written risk/benefit information for certain higher-risk treatments to insure that there is proof that the necessary information was provided in case of a later legal claim. Failure to obtain informed consent prior to providing medical treatment creates risk of liability both civil and criminal. At the same time, this must be balanced against the principle that failure to provide treatment where there is both need and consent can fall short of medical protocols. There are accepted medical protocols setting out the types of risk/benefit information that are important.

The accepted medical protocol for transition-related treatment of transgender patients is that first established by the WPATH in 1979. The WPATH Standards of Care (SOC) is now in its seventh edition at the time of this writing. The early standards had fairly rigid requirements, preventing many trans patients from accessing

---

[4] http://otda.ny.gov/fair%20hearing%20images/2018-5/Redacted_7510067L.pdf

care. One requirement that has attracted controversy is the necessity of having letters from both a treating mental health professional and an evaluating mental health professional, attesting to the patient's fitness for gender-affirming surgeries. The current edition of the SOC, however, explicitly labels its protocols as "clinical guidelines." Similarly, the 2017 Gender Dysphoria/Gender Incongruence Guideline Resources of the Endocrine Society also recommends two letters prior to gender-affirming surgeries, one from a mental health provider and one from the clinician responsible for endocrine transition therapy. WPATH also has guidelines for evaluation by mental health professionals in order to access hormone replacement therapy and other medical treatments. There is explicit recognition that these may be modified by practitioners based on individual circumstances. Nonetheless, some practitioners consider the WPATH standards to be too restrictive and instead use a model known as "informed consent." This model allows transgender patients to access hormone treatments and surgical interventions, without mental health evaluation, after appropriate education and advisement about the benefits and risks of treatment. This model has been adopted at many centers that provide hormone replacement therapy. It should be noted that all medical treatment requires informed consent, so the "informed consent" model does not imply that other models skip informed consent. Rather, it means "informed consent only," in that evaluation by mental health professionals is not a prerequisite to treatment.

Treatment of youth always raises issues of parental consent, except where the youth has been legally emancipated. That means the parents of an underage person who seeks trans-related care must provide informed consent. It is important to determine that the presenting parent has the right to make medical decisions alone, particularly in situations of divorce and separation, or whether it is necessary to receive consent from both parents. For older adolescents, some states may permit treatment without parental consent under the "mature minor" doctrine pursuant to statute or court decisions. At the time of this writing, these states include Alaska, Illinois, Kansas, Maine, Massachusetts, Montana, South Carolina, Tennessee, and West Virginia.[5] Under this doctrine, minors who are able to understand the nature and consequences of the medical treatment offered are considered mature enough to consent to or refuse the treatment. However, a number of states are considering laws and policies restricting or criminalizing treatment of trans youth, and Texas, Alabama and Florida have enacted such laws and policies.[6] However, the U.S. Department of Health and Human Services issued a bulletin on March 2, 2022

---

[5] Ikuta, Emily, Overcoming The Parental Veto: How Transgender Adolescents Can Access Puberty-Suppressing Hormone Treatment In The Absence Of Parental Consent Under The Mature Minor Doctrine, 25 Southern California Interdisciplinary Law Review 179 (2015)

[6] Florida issues Texas-like guidance seeking to bar transition care for minors, NBC News, April 20, 2022, https://www.nbcnews.com/nbc-out/out-politics-and-policy/florida-issues-texas-guidance-seeking-bar-transition-care-minorsrcna25273, https://perma.cc/6KJE-5SAZ. The ACLU persuaded a Texas court to block the Texas guidance. https://www.aclu.org/press-releases/texas-court-blocks-state-investigating-families-transgender-youth, https://perma.cc/XN7YSRCG

stating that such laws are in violation of the Affordable Care Act, Section 1557.[7] The legal situation in those states is unclear at the time of this writing.

Informed consent for patients who will be undergoing genital surgery includes the issues of sterilization and the options regarding assisted reproductive technologies. Since many (though not all) genital surgeries will involve sterilization, explicit written consent should be received for that. While the risk-benefit information necessary for informed consent may generally be provided orally or in writing, at the discretion of the provider or facility, many states require specific forms to be signed for sterilization consent. In addition, many patients may not have considered that they have options to have children using their biological material. Patients should be informed well in advance about the options for future reproduction, including how to find providers that can assist them in harvesting and storing biological material appropriately.

Essential ID for Accessing Care, Documentation on Medical Records, Legal Name and Gender Marker Changes, and Use of Gender-Appropriate Facilities

Accessing care generally requires identification of the patient and inclusion of patient identity on medical records. US identification documents are governed by a patchwork of federal, state, and local jurisdictions and agencies. Some of these do not permit change of name or sex. Others permit full or partial changes (such as keeping old information with a note of the change). Some require documentation of various medical treatments. These legal requirements are also subject to change with some regularity. (See the Documents Center of the National Center For Transgender Equality, found online at https://transequality.org/documents, for more information.) As a result, patients may have incongruent identification of various kinds.

Incongruent identification causes problems for transgender people in that medical documentation may in some instances be required to use a "legal name," or "legal sex," though those terms are ambiguous. Every US state has law permitting persons to use any name that they wish, except for purposes of monetary fraud. A court-ordered name change is useful but not required. It can be shockingly expensive and time-consuming to obtain, if at all.

It is important for medical providers to obtain advice about their state laws and regulations and to make identification requirements as least restrictive for their trans patients as possible. Although a medical record may, in some states, require a name validated by formal identity documents, it is not necessary for non-mandated records to use such a name or for providers to address patients by that name. While

---

[7] https://www.hhs.gov/sites/default/files/hhsocr-notice-and-guidance-gender-affirming-care.pdf, https://perma.cc/3T5Q-NU5B

this introduces an element of administrative inconvenience, providers should understand that validation of transgender and gender nonbinary patient identity is important to medical outcome, particularly if trans patients stop medical care because of inappropriate identification by staff. Staff training is required to ensure that competent and inclusive care is provided.

Hospitals and healthcare institutions should have policies addressing the appropriate treatment of TGNB patients. State and local public accommodation non-discrimination laws may apply to hospitals and healthcare providers. Policies should include use of appropriate names and pronouns, particularly on hospital bracelets and other medical records. Failure to do so can sometimes lead to inappropriate treatment by staff that may create a legal risk of litigation. Policies should also address gender identity appropriate facilities, including use of restrooms, beds, screening centers, and other accommodations. For example, a trans woman should be allowed to use the women's restroom in her provider's office. She should be allowed to wear clothing that matches her gender identity. She should be referred to by appropriate titles (Ms. or Mr.), names (preferred name rather than a gender-incongruent name on a state driver's license), and pronouns (he, she, they, etc). Staff training is required to ensure that such policies are understood and followed.

Third-Party Payers, Insurance, and Billing Issues

It is generally understood that non-discrimination laws applicable to insurers include hormone replacement therapy and psychotherapy. It is sometimes unclear whether these also extend to transition-related surgery.[8] While some insurers still have exclusions for any transgender-related medical care, there is an increasing trend toward voluntary renunciation of such exclusions. The American Medical Association has called for an end to such exclusions.[9] A pre-authorization request to the insurer may be useful in determining whether the treatment will be covered by insurance.

With regard to Medicare, the US Department of Health and Human Services has issued a ruling stating that its previous blanket exclusion of transgender-related health care is no longer reasonable under the Agency's standards.[10] Such care may include provision of hormones (such as estrogen or testosterone), mastectomy, or genital surgery. By 2016, a number of states had also changed their Medicaid rules

---

[8] At the time of this writing, HHS has proposed a rule that would require insurers to provide appropriate gender confirming surgeries, but it has not yet been made final.

[9] See American Medical Association (AMA), Policy H-180.980 (opposing the denial of coverage based on sexual orientation or gender identity); see also AMA Policy H-185.950 (supporting public and private health insurance coverage for treatment of gender identity disorder as recommended by patient's physician).

[10] See Department of Health and Human Services Departmental Appeals Board Appellate Division NCD 140.3, Transsexual Surgery, Docket No. A-13-87, NCD Ruling No. 2576 (May 30, 2014).

to permit transgender adults to receive hormone treatments and other medical treatments.

Even insurers with transgender exclusions will sometimes override their exclusions after internal appeals by the patient. This will require documentation from a medical professional stating the treatment is medically necessary and reasonable. Sample language for such letters may be obtained from nonprofit advocacy organizations, such as the Transgender Law Center and Transcend Legal.

Providers generally recognize that more than one diagnosis code can sometimes be assigned. Different insurers interpret these diagnosis codes differently. Thus, a diagnosis code that may trigger one insurer's transgender exclusion may not trigger that of another insurer. Pre-authorization requests can be helpful in determining coverage, where practicable. Providers should use reasonable discretion in assigning diagnosis codes, and deliberately using a clearly incorrect diagnosis code may constitute healthcare fraud. Nonetheless, gender-affirming providers generally try to act as an advocate for their transgender patients so that medical outcomes are optimized.

Conclusion

The clinician must be prepared to address legal issues associated with medical treatment for gender dysphoria. This chapter provided general guidance on a number of issues of importance. Generally, TGNB patients have a right to access to care, and aside from treatments requiring specialty knowledge, it is not sufficient to decline care because one does not have experience treating TGNB people. Appropriate informed consent is required, with an explanation of risks, particularly for treatments involving sterilization. Information on reproductive options should be provided. Patient identification and medical records should be gender-affirming. Institutional policies should be in place to assure these outcomes. Staff training should be provided to ensure culturally competent care. Providers should educate themselves regarding insurance coverage issues faced by transgender patients and be prepared to assist with internal appeals to reverse coverage denials to ensure that medical outcomes are optimized.

Resource Table

Issue	Resource	URL
Institutional policies	Guidelines for the Primary and Gender-Affirming Care of Transgender and Gender Nonbinary People	http://transhealth.ucsf.edu/trans?page=guidelines-home
Institutional policies	Transgender-Affirming Hospital Policies	https://www.hrc.org/resources/transgender-affirming-hospital-policies
Insurance coverage	Finding Insurance for Transgender-Related Healthcare	https://www.hrc.org/resources/finding-insurance-for-transgender-related-healthcare

Issue	Resource	URL
Insurance coverage	Medicare Benefits and Transgender People	transequality.org/PDFs/MedicareAndTransPeople.pdf
Legal issues	Healthcare Rights and Transgender People	transequality.org/Resources/HealthCareRight_UpdatedMar2014_FINAL.pdf
Legal issues	Transgender Health and the Law: Identifying and Fighting Healthcare Discrimination	thecentersd.org/pdf/health-advocacy/identifying-transgender.pdf
Medical records	Preferred Names, Preferred Pronouns, and Gender Identity in the Electronic Medical Record and Laboratory Information System: Is Pathology Ready?	https://www.ncbi.nlm.nih.gov/pmc/articles/PMC5653959/
Reproductive health	Fertility and You	http://transhealth.ucsf.edu/pdf/2013-0514_Web_Trans-Persons-and-Fertility_ENG.pdf
Reproductive health	New York State Sterilization Consent Form	https://www.health.ny.gov/health_care/medicaid/publications/docs/ldss/ldss-3134.pdf
Staff training and cultural competence	10 Tips for Working With Transgender Patients	https://transgenderlawcenter.org/resources/health/10tips
Staff training and cultural competence	Acknowledging Gender and Sex	http://transhealth.ucsf.edu/video/story_html5.html?lms=1
Standards of care	Guidelines for the Primary and Gender-Affirming Care of Transgender and Non-Binary People	http://transhealth.ucsf.edu/trans?page=protocol-00-00
Standards of care	Informed Consent in the Medical Care of Transgender and Gender-Nonconforming Patients	https://journalofethics.ama-assn.org/article/informed-consent-medical-care-transgender-and-gender-nonconforming-patients/2016-11
Standards of care	WPATH Standards of Care Version 7	https://www.wpath.org/publications/soc
Youth and adolescents	Interactive Map: Clinical Care Programs for Gender-Expansive Children and Adolescents	https://www.hrc.org/resources/interactive-map-clinical-care-programs-for-gender-nonconforming-childr

Index

© Springer Nature Switzerland AG 2022
J. Truglio et al. (eds.), *Sexual and Reproductive Health*,
https://doi.org/10.1007/978-3-030-94632-6